Disease in Babylonia

Cuneiform Monographs

VOLUME 36

BRILL

Disease in Babylonia

Edited by
I. L. Finkel and M. J. Geller

BRILL

LEIDEN • BOSTON
2007

This book is printed on acid-free paper.

Library of Congress Cataloging-in-Publication Data

Disease in Babylonia / edited by Irving L. Finkel and Markham J. Geller.
p. ; cm. — (Cuneiform monographs ; 36)
Includes bibliographical references and index.
ISBN-13: 978-90-04-12401-1 (hardback)
ISBN-10: 90-04-12401-2 (hardback)
1. Medicine, Assyro-Babylonian. I. Finkel, Irving L. II. Geller, Markham J. III. Series. [DNLM—Ancient Lands. 3. History of Medicine—Ancient Lands. 4. Medicine, Traditional—history—Ancient Lands. 5. Superstitions—history—Ancient Lands. WZ 51 D611 2006]

R135.3.D57 2006
610.9—dc22

2006049182

ISSN 0929-0052
ISBN-10 90 04 12401 2
ISBN-13 978 90 04 12401 1

PRINTED IN THE NETHERLANDS

CONTENTS

Foreword vii

Fevers in Babylonia
Marten Stol 1

Between Magic and Medicine—Apropos of an Old Babylonian Therapeutic Text against the Kurārum Disease
Nathan Wassermann 40

Infantile and Childhood Convulsions and SA.GIG XXIX
J. V. Kinnier Wilson 62

On Stroke and Facial Palsy in Babylonian Texts
J. V. Kinnier Wilson & E. H. Reynolds 67

Hittite Rituals against Threats and Other Diseases and Their Relationship to the Mesopotamian Traditions
Volkert Haas 100

The Hands of the Gods: Disease Names, and Divine Anger
Nils P. Heessel 120

Epilepsy in Mesopotamia Reconsidered
Hector Avalos 131

Lamaštu—Agent of a Specific Disease or a Generic Destroyer of Health?
Walter Farber 137

Witchcraft, Impotence, and Indigestion
Tzvi Abusch 146

The Demon of the Roof
Theodore Kwasman 160

Phlegm and Breath—Babylonian Contributions to Hippocratic Medicine
Markham J. Geller 187

Women's Medicines in Ancient Jewish Sources: Fertility Enhancers and Inhibiters
John M. Riddle 200

Ancient and Contemporary Management in a Disease of Unknown Aetiology
Ellis Douek 215

FOREWORD

The present volume of papers originated as a conference held at the Wellcome Institute in London on 'Concepts of Disease in Ancient Babylonia', organised by Larry Conrad of the Wellcome Institute, Irving Finkel of the British Museum, Mark Geller of University College London, and Marten Stol of the Free University, Amsterdam. The conference, held 9–10 December, 1996, was jointly sponsored by the Wellcome Institute, the Department of the Ancient Near East in the British Museum, and the Institute of Jewish Studies of University College London.

A number of presentations were made at the conference which do not appear in the present volume, including papers read by Barbara Böck, Timothy Collins, Martha Hausperger, Erica Reiner, and Frans Wiggermann. The conference raised many important issues regarding the identification of diseases, particularly such general categories as 'epilepsy', 'fever' and 'infection'. The conference explored the role of demons (such as Lamaštu) and witchcraft as causes of disease, as well as astral influences on the course of illnesses. Other papers discussed diagnosis of disease, among which the diseases of women and neurological disorders. Attention was also paid to modern analogies to problems of diagnosis facing the ancient physician. The conference programme also included a general discussion of '*asûtu* vs. *āšipūtu*' in Babylonian diagnosis and treatment of disease.

In the years since our original conference, there has been a marked increase in the number of scholars who have turned to research on diagnostic and therapeutic resources, which has even engendered a journal devoted to this field, *Le Journal des Médicines Cunéiformes* published in Paris.

The unfortunate long delay in publishing the proceedings has meant that bibliographies and references are often not up-to-date. Nevertheless, this collection of articles makes many significant contributions to the study of ancient Babylonian medicine.

The consensus of this conference was that more meetings of this kind need to be held, with closer co-operation between historians of medicine and philologists working on ancient medical texts, both from the Near East and Classical world.

The editors and contributors are most grateful to the publishers, Brill, and to Michiel Klein Swormink, for finally bringing this volume to press, since the volume had been submitted to STYX Publications in 2001. Despite the long delay, the individual articles make importantly and timely contributions to the study of Babylonian medicine.

I. L. Finkel
M. J. Geller

FEVERS IN BABYLONIA

Marten Stol
Vrije Universiteit, Amsterdam

Very little has been written on fever in Babylonian texts. We only have the short article "Fieber" in the *Reallexikon der Assyriologie* (by R. Labat); nothing more. This dearth of information is due to two causes (a) few people have written on Babylonian medicine; (b) according to modern opinion, fever is not a disease; it is a reaction of the body to disease. In this contribution a first attempt will be made to describe fever in Babylonia. It primarily is a collection of many references, and often no medical interpretation can be given. It has all the characteristics of a first step on unexplored soil. I will first present all the information on fever and will proceed by discussing some diseases with fever as an important symptom.

I. *Fevers*

1. *"Fire" as Fever*

Feverish conditions are described by words indicating various degrees of being hot. They are attested in medical texts where they must have had a precise meaning (*ummu, ḫimiṭ ṣēti*). One such word for "fever" does not occur in such a "technical" context, namely the word "fire" (*išātu*). This "fire" is seen in incantations as a metaphor for feverish heat. A group of them has been published under the name "Fire Incantations", and the symptoms given there are not precise.[1] In Greek literature the word *pûr* "fire" in the meaning "fever" has a similar marginal position; the normal word is *puretós*.[2]

---

[1] W. G. Lambert, "Fire Incantations", *AfO* 23 (1970) 39–45. Two were translated again by B. R. Foster, *Before the Muses* (1996) 841f., "Against fever".
[2] Reinhold Strömberg, *Griechische Wortstudien* (1944) 70–88, "Zum Begriff des Fiebers".

The Babylonian incantations describe this "fire" as coming from forests, burning down reed thickets, eating (*akālu*) and gnawing (*kasāsu*) the human body, reducing humanity. The last qualification may point to an epidemic. Medical texts prescribe amulets for a "gnawing fire" (IZI *kāsistu*); again, this is not technical language. In Aramaic, "fire" is the normal word for fever.[3]

The word "fire" as a symptom of disease is perhaps attested in a group of Middle Babylonian letters from Nippur, which use the word "fires" (*išātātu*) and "fever" (*ummu*), even in the same context (BE 17 33); "fever" has been the interpretation of the word "fire" in these letters although recently, "abscess" has been suggested as a better translation. The letters have been translated more than once; lastly by S. Parpola.[4] They discuss the physical problems of girls, including fever (*ummu*). "The daughter of M., fever has seized her in the evening (*šimiti*), I made her drink a drug in the morning (*namāru*). Her fever is *mitḫar*, her feet are cold. She, who had a dry cough (*ganāḫu*) before, now [coughs no more]" (BE 17 32). Another letter says: "The abscesses (*išātātu*) of the daughter of M. are healed (*balṭā*), (and) although she was coughing before, she does not cough anymore" (BE 17 31:11–14). Abscess, or another word for fever? The letter continues: "The other abscess of the daughter of I., which persisted (*2 išātu ša uḫḫurātu*) (Labat: "das zweite Fieber"), has produced a . . . spot (*ši-i-pa ittadi*) (. . .). Half of the abscesses of the Aramean girl (still) persist. Of the abscesses of the daughter of B., those on her rib(s) persist, and she is coughing".

R. Labat saw fever in this "fire". He recognized in one passage, with the *2 i-ša-tu* in it, even the tertian fever: "das 'zweite' Fieber". He distinguished: "1. *ummu* = die Periode des Fieberausbruches oder eines andauerndes Fiebers, besonders wenn es näher als *mitḫar* 'gleichmässig, konstant' bezeichnet wird; 2. *išātātu* = 'die Fieberhitze', d.h. die aufeinanderfolgenden Fieberanfälle, die ein Wechsel- oder Rückfallfieber charakterisieren; 3. *šanû* = das 'zweite' Fieber, vielleicht zweimal am Tag auftretend, oder ein dreitägiges Wechselfieber (Anfall an einem Tag mit zwei Tagen Zwischenraum)".[5] However, E. Ritter

[3] The latest reference is found on an amulet; *'št'* in *Atiqot* 28 (1996) 162. See M. Jastrow, *Dictionary*.

[4] S. Parpola, *Letters from Assyrian scholars to the kings Esarhaddon and Assurbanipal*. Part II: *Commentary and appendices* (1983) 492–496.

[5] R. Labat, "Fieber", *RlA* III (1957) 61a.

and S. Parpola have translated "fire" here as "abscess," which would free us from a problem.[6] An important line may be, "The abscesses on the chest of PN have secreted sweat (*zu'tu*)" (PBS 1/2 71:10–11), for which Parpola suggests "(pus?)" instead of "sweat".

2. ummu *"Fever"*

The word *ummu* "fever" is normal in the medical texts, frequently used in a verbal form with the "iterative" (infix *-tan-*). We can render it either by "repeatedly", or by "all the time, continuously". "Repeatedly" would be an important indication of a remittent fever but grammatically one is never sure and there are many cases where it is impossible to decide. The word *ummu* literally means "heat" and derives from the verb *emēmu* "to be hot". The same root exists in Hebrew and Arabic as *ḥmm*; in Arabic *ḥumma* means "fever". The verb *emēmu* "to be hot" in medical texts is often contrasted with "to be cold" (*kaṣû*); in those cases the patient "is (now) hot, (then) cold" (*immim ikaṣṣi*). One cannot say that the verb means "to have a fever". The consequence of this observation would be that the substantive *ummu*, too, simply means "heat" in the body, and not "fever". This is not so. In everyday language the word *ummu* "heat" must have had the specific meaning "fever". On the other hand, the underlying verb *emēmu* never acquired a meaning "to have a fever".[7] The medical texts follow this usage. It is a problem that only one specific part of the body can have this "fever" while others do not; there, the fever is localised. Professor Walter Farber observed [oral communication] that this can be explained if we assume that *ummu* can mean "hot (local) spot": a part of the body that has an abnormally high temperature. The Editors of this book suggest that *ummu* means "high temperature", sometimes fever but not always.

It is important to remark that the medical texts never give *ummu* as a diagnosis because the word is too general,[8] and it is often one

[6] E. Ritter, *Studies Benno Landsberger* (1965) 317.

[7] Note, however, BAM 5 480 III 22, "If the head of a man is *hot* (*qaqqassu ēm*), and the hair of his head thins out: in order to [tear out] the *fever* of [his] head (*ummi qaqqadišu*) and to make stand up the hair that is going out". Duplicate: "[If the he]ad of a man is inflamed by sun-heat, and the hair of his skull thins out [..]" (BAM 1 9:23). Duplicate has sun-heat (*ṣētu*) instead of "hot".

[8] In medical texts, the Sumerogram NE is used for *ummu*. There is another NE, in the diagnosis NE MU.NI. This NE probably stands for *pendû*, see M. Stol, *JEOL* 32 (1991–92) 64.

of many symptoms: "the skull / the trunk holds fever" (*umma ukal*). In many parts of the body fever can be felt: the skull, the head, the face (TDP 74:34), the nose (BWL 52:20), the belly (*libbu*), the feet (BAM 2 121 III 1; CTN IV 117). A child-bearing woman has "fever of the entrails" (NE *irrī*) (BAM 3 240 rev. 39). It is often mentioned in one breath with sweat (*zu'tu*), in "he has / gets fever and sweat", or "after fever and sweat have left" (*paṭāru*) (TDP 156:4).

The nature of fever can be indicated by more or less impressionistic verbs. A body part "holds" fever (*kullu*), fever "seizes" (*ṣabātu*), comes to rest (*nâḫu*) (BAM 416 rev. 10). One of the letters says, "The princess whom fever repeatedly had seized, has now come to rest through the bandage and potion" (PBS 1/2 72:27–29). One text speaks of feet "holding" fever and "constantly getting" fever (BAM 120 III 1, 8). Note the following expressions: the stomach area is "loaded" with it (*ṣênu*) (AMT 39,1:27),[9] fever repeatedly "falls" upon him (TDP 66:68). More technical is "the fever has released him" (*muššuru*), perhaps temporarily, for one or more days; one may distinguish this verb from "to leave", i.e., to go away for good (*ezēbu*). It can be "torn out" (*nasāḫu*) (STT 2 300:22, NE-*ma ana* ZI-*ḫi*), "completely", "all of it" (*kališ*) (BAM 171:49). Head fever that "holds" a person is "torn out" or, according to a duplicating text, to "made to stand up (= go away)" (*tebû*) (BAM 5 480 II 64 with 3 II 36). A few times we read that fever is "stripped away" (*šaḫātu*, CAD Š/1 94a), once belly fever is "made to go up" (*elû* Š, BAM 6 597 I 11), or "made to go out" (*aṣû* Š, I 59).

Fever in a mild (?) illness (*sil'itu*) can "expand" (*epēšu*) into the ears making hearing/the ears (*nešmû/uznē*) "heavy" (BAM 503 II 58, 61), or to the head making the head "heavy" and a therapy makes it leave (*elû* Gt) (BAM 3 III 42, 45). It can expand towards the eyes, ears, abdomen (*emšu*), hips, feet (III 47, 50, IV 7, 9, 11). Fever indeed is more often associated with this mild (?) illness (STT 2 138 rev. 23, LKA 154 rev. 13).

2.a. *Texts on Fever* (ummu)

BAM 6 579

In some large medical texts we can follow the place of *ummu* among other feverish conditions.

---

[9] AMT 39,1:27 = BAM 6 579 I 27, cf. AHw 1081b, below.

BAM 6 579 was described by its editor as a text on "Krankheiten, die im Bereich des Oberbauches, des Leibs und des Unterleibs auftreten und häufig mit Fieber einhergehen" (F. Köcher). The sequence is: fever in the belly, fever in the upper belly (epigastric region), "belly fever".

I 1 "His *belly* is seized by fever (NE = *ummu*)"
I 4 "His upper [sic] belly is hot (NE = *ēm*), his belly is 'blown' (*napāḫu*)"
I 6 "His belly is hot"
I 8 "His belly holds fever, he does not accept bread or water"
I 11 "In order to make the fever of the belly go up"
I 13 "His belly is hot repeatedly"
I 15 "His belly is hot, he does not [..]"
I 20 "His *upper belly* [is seized by (?)] fever (*um-ma*)"
I 22 "His upper belly gets fever; in order to strip his upper belly from the fever"
I 25 "His upper belly holds fever, and [he does not accept (?)] bread or [water]"
I 27 "His upper belly is 'loaded with' fever; in order to [. . .] the fe[ver]"
I 30 "He gets *fever of the belly* repeatedly, he has been overcome by sun-heat (*ṣēta kašid*)"
I 34 "In order to tear out the flaring-up (*ṣiriḫtu*) of the fever of the belly"
I 39 "All these are medications (*bulṭu*) . . ."
A new section begins,
I 40 "He gets flaring-up of the belly, and his belly holds (?) fever" (and more symptoms); the remaining problems of column I are "fever of the belly".

Col. II is largely lost.

BAM 5 480

I 1 "His *brains* (*muḫḫu*; can also mean: upper part of the skull) hold fever" (and more symptoms)
II 10 "His brains are repeatedly hot"
II 12 "He gets [. . .] . . . fever, and his eyes are dim, hold blood"
II 19 "His brains are inflamed by sun-heat, [and his eyes are dim]"
II 21 "His brains are inflamed by sun-heat, and [his eyes are di]m and full of blood"
II 26 [. . . .] gives him pain, the hair of his head stands up"
II 61 "His *head* is hot repeatedly"
II 64 ["In order to make the fever] of the head go away"

2.b. *Forms of* ummu

Doctors distinguished some forms of *ummu*. In one sequence of fevers in a therapeutic text exclusively dealing with fever, the order seems to be from mild to severe forms. In the severer cases one resorts to magic (BAM 2 147, dupl. 148):

(1–12) "strong fever has seized him" (= "strong fever" / "strong fever *li'bu*", 5, 12)
(13–24) "in order to tear out strong fever"
(25–33) "fever has seized him continuously (*kajjāmān*)". The treatment is magical.
(34) (dupl. 148:34, K. 2581 obv. 7) "(. . .) has seized him the one day, has released him the other day". Magical treatment.

(Rev. 20) (dupl. 148 rev. 22) "Incantation for tearing out a never-ending fever"

Catchline: "Fever of confusion (*tēšû*) . . ."[10]

One text indeed speaks of a plurality of fevers: "fevers holds (singular !) him all day" (NE.MEŠ *ina kal ūme ú-gil-šu*, var. *ú-kal-šú*, BAM 575 III 32, var. 55:6–7).

Let us now have a look at these and more forms of fever.

1. "*Strong fever*" (*ummu dannu*) is associated with the feverish condition named *li'bu* (for which see below), as in a prayer: "Me, your servant, whom a strong fever (NE *dan-nu*), *li'bu*, has seized me" (E. Ebeling, AGH 8:4). Already in the earlier Middle Babylonian period we come across this combination, slightly differently: "flaring-up fever (*ummu ṣarḫu*), strong *li'bu*" (G. Meier, *ZA* 45 [1939] 208 V 17). These seem to be bad forms of fever. Note the sequence of both, with *mungu* inserted (*ummu mungu li'bu*, BAM 231:4; cf. *ummu mungu zu'tu sil'itu*, LKA 154 rev. 13). The therapeutic text just summarized strongly suggests that "strong fever" is identical with *li'bu* because its introduction speaks of "a strong fever that has seized him," and its therapy promises that "the *li'bu* that has seized him will be torn out" (BAM 147:1, 5). The next section offers "the strong fever, *li'bu* which has seized him, will be torn out" (12). The recipes following have the introduction "for tearing out the strong fever" (13, 22).

[10] NE *tēšû* NE *qablu*, BAM 147 rev. 26, 148 rev. 28; cf. W. G. Lambert, *AfO* 23 (1970) 44, "Fire of confusion, fire of battle".

2. "*Flaring-up fever*" (verb *ṣarāḫu*, substantives *ṣirḫu*, *ṣiriḫti ummi*). "Flaring-up" said of body parts must have been a visible symptom in view of this observation of the entrails of an animal: "if the innards flare up".[11] The number of references for the verb *ṣarāḫu* in medical texts increases if we accept the identification of the Sumerogram NE with this verb.[12] Examples of flaring-up fever:

"If an ill man is flaring-up with fever (UD GIG *um-ma-šu ṣa-ru-uḫ*), he bathes in sweat as (in) water: hand of Šamaš, hand of his vows" (R. Labat, MDP 57 242 no. III 4). Having "flaring-up fever, *liʾbu* (?) (KA-*ʾ-ba*)" means drinking and sweating a lot (BAM 66:21, 24). "If a man has a flaring-up fever and his innards are 'blown' [lit. inflated] (*napāḫu*), he is constantly hot (*emēmu*)" (BAM 3 201:23). A man has a constant "flaring-up of belly fever" (*ṣiriḫti* NE ŠÀ, BAM 2 145:16; Köcher: brennende Hitze im Inneren ["Brennfieber"]). One text differentiates simple "flaring-up" (*ṣiriḫtu*) (no fever) from normal fever (*ummu*): "If a man has flaring-up of the belly and his belly holds fever" (BAM 52:39). Symptoms can refer to being inflamed by sun-heat (BAM 6 579 I 40–41): his "head is flaring-up with fever" (KAR 211:4); a "fever of flaring-up fever" (NE *ṣiriḫtu*) settled in the eyes should be "cooled" by water (BAM 510 III 3).[13] "If a man's penis and stomach area hold a flaring-up fever" is preceded by, "If his stomach area is inflamed and he is hot" (*iḫammaṭsu u ēm*) (TDP 178:14, cf. 12). Is this milder? "If a baby is flaring-up with fever: hand of Gula" (TDP 228:90).

---

[11] J. Nougayrol, *RA* 65 (1971) 73:41: "the innards (*qer-bu*) flare up (*i-ṣa-ar-ra-ḫu*)". An omen describes the house and cattle yard as being *ṣariḫ*, literally, with the consequence that its owner metaphorically will be "repeatedly suffering form attacks of *ṣarāḫu*" (quoted CAD Ṣ 98f.).

[12] Thus N. J. C. Kouwenberg, *Gemination in the Akkadian Verb* (= Studia Semitica Neerlandica, Vol. [32]) (Assen, 1997) p. 405 note 26. Kouwenberg shows that the reading of NE-*úḫ* in TDP as *nuppuḫ* is not likely. Kouwenberg conjectures: *ṣurruḫ*. The lexical tradition has NE = *ṣarāḫu*. I tend to agree because the translation "feverish" for NE-*úḫ* fits a number of contexts but *napāḫu* has another meaning, "to be inflated". We can indeed use a form of *ṣarāḫu*. I have this small correction to Kouwenberg: since the D stem is very rare, read the G stem NE-*úḫ* as *ṣaruḫ*. The stative is *ṣariḫ* but in Middle Babylonian we find *ṣaruḫ*, in *um-ma-šu ṣa-ru-uḫ*, R. Labat, MDP 57 242 III 4. Contrast later NE *ṣa-ri-iḫ* in *SBTU* I 34:24 (TDP, Chapter XI). Compare older *maruṣ* and later *mariṣ*. The older form must have been *ṣaruḫ* and it seems that the traditional "archaic"sign -*úḫ* reflects Old Babylonian usage. Nils P. Heeßel wrote me that he prefers NE ÚḪ = *umma ṣariḫ* (in a letter dated 21 October 1997). Now Heeßel, *Babylonisch-assyrische Diagnostik* (2000) 162.

[13] See W. Farber, *JNES* 49 (1990) 312.

Interesting is this complex of symptoms:

> If an "oath" has seized a man and he constantly has fever and sweating, a lot (*magal*); the one day it seizes him, the other day it releases him, he has a fit of of fever repeatedly (*ḫajjātti ummi*): a fever *la ḫaḫḫāš* has seized him and [. . .] (BAM 2 174 rev. 29–30).

Medical historians will probably point out that tertian fever is described here. The following therapy is intended "to stop the fever and the flaring-up" (*ana ummi u ṣirḫa parāsi*). "Flaring-up" (*ṣirḫu*) seems to reflect the fever *la ḫaḫḫāš* (see below, under 5). This text is about the treatment of "oath" and we know that inflammation by sun-heat can turn into "oath" (BAM 174 rev. 25).

Compare now this passage with another one:

> If, ditto (= sun-heat has inflamed him) (*ṣētu uḫammassuma*), and it attacks him every day at a certain time (*ūmišamma ana ittišu*) [. . .], whenever it overwhelms (*ḫâṭu*) him, [he has] (?) a flaring-up fever (NE *ṣa*[*r*]!-*ḫ*[*a*] [TUKU] ?), [his muscles hurt him], sweat falls upon him and he comes to rest: That man [will be ill during] 21 days [. . .]" (BAM 4 416 rev. 8–10). (For a full treatment of this text, see below.)

This is a quotidian fever. What seems to make it "flaring-up" or *la ḫaḫḫāš* is that it is a high fever, remittent. "Remittent" as a meaning of "flaring-up" seems to be confirmed by a passage in the Diagnostic Handbook: "If he is ill two, three days, and flaring-up fever has left him (*paṭāru*), after it has left him, in / on [. . .] (SBTU I 37:30; Chapter XVI). "Flaring-up" is a generalized symptom, not that of one specific body part: "His entrails are raised, he is flaring-up with fever" (SBTU I 34:24; Chapter XI).[14]

3. "*Even fever*", always in the phrase "the fever is (not) even", *ummu (la) mitḫar*. Already attested in the letters from Nippur, "Fever has seized PN in the evening and at sunrise I made her drink a potion, her fever is even, her feet are cold" (BE 17 32:7). Two ancient commentaries seem to try to eludicate this expression. The one says "His

[14] S. Parpola wrote that the words *ṣarāḫu* and *ṣurḫu* in Neo-Assyrian letters do not speak of fever, but of heat; S. Parpola, *Letters from Assyrian scholars to the kings Esarhaddon and Assurbanipal.* Part II: *Commentary and appendices* (1983) 170. This means that one telling letter on so-called "fever" has lost its relevance (LAS 181 = SAA X 241); see how E. Ritter translated this text; *Studies Benno Landsberger* (1965) 319 b (2. a).

fever is equal = all of his body is seized", the other is fragmentary and obscure.[15]

The expression is rather frequent in the diagnostic texts. Light may be shed upon it by studying the passages where we find the related word *mitḫariš*, an adverb roughly meaning "equally". Most important is this line: "If a baby is *mitḫariš* hot" (TDP 220:31). For "is hot" one expects *ēm* but the form is in the dual, *em-ma*, which could mean that the baby is hot on both sides. "All of his body is seized", said the commentary. The following description presupposes exactly this by adding the exceptions: "The fever is even; the right of his buttocks and of his ears are cold" (TDP 244 D 10). The passage in the Nippur letter can be explained in a similar way: "Her fever is even, her feet are cold". We have seen above that "fever" can be limited to specific body parts; the "hot (local) spots", according to W. Farber.[16]

4. "*Never-ending fever*" (NE *lazzu*) can be stopped (*parāsu*) by incantations (AMT 63, 2:4; BAM 2 147 rev. 20); also mentioned in connection with "tearing out" Lamaštu.[17] The demon "Provider of Evil" is the reason why "fever is never ending in his body, but he rumbles (*leḫēbu*) a lot and has sweat" (BAM 6 520 II 9).

5. *Fever ḫaḫḫāš*. The Diagnostic Handbook says several times "the fever is not *ḫaḫḫāš*"; sometimes that a body part "is not *ḫaḫḫāš* by fever", example: "His belly has fever, the fever is not *ḫaḫḫāš*, he throws up black spittle" (TDP 180:31). "If a baby's head holds fever, his trunk is not *ḫaḫḫāš* by fever, he has no sweat" (TDP 218:10, cf. 230:115). This means that this fever is here not generalized but limited to one body part. Only once is the formula positive: "If his head is *ḫaḫḫāš* by fever, it leaves him one day, it is heavy upon him the other day" (TDP 22:46, 48, cf. 50).[18] According to J. V. Kinnier

[15] "His fever is equal = all of his body is seized": NE-*šú mit-ḫar* = DÙ SU-*šu ṣa-bit*, STT 2 403:55. The other commentary seems to comment NE *mitḫar* by these words: "[. . .] . . . head, third fever, . . ., new break", SBTU I 38:20, comm. on TDP 244 D 9–11.

[16] One more word on *mitḫariš*. We now have the variants *ištēniš* and *mitḫariš* (written TÉŠ.BI) said of fever: "a fever 'together' (1-*niš*) (dupl. TÉŠ.BI) 'rides' (*rakābu*) him/pours down (*reḫû*) upon him"; SBTU I 37:26, dupl. II 180 no. 44:23. We will study the entire passage below, under "*li'bu* of the mountain", e–f. ("tertian fever").

[17] D. Myhrman, *ZA* 16 (1902) 156 I 21.

[18] P. Adamson, *JRAS* 1979, 3 with note 22: "intermittent fever of tertian type";

Wilson [oral communication], B. Landsberger in his class with E. Ritter had explained *la ḫaḫḫāš* as "low fever". This is in line with the Chicago Assyrian Dictionary and F. Köcher's translation "(mit) niedrigen Temperaturen" for *ummu la ḫaḫḫāš*.[19] Let me suggest: a fever without a crisis. However, above, under 2, "Flaring-up fever", we have suggested that the "flaring-up" fever (*ṣirḫu*) seems to reflect the fever *la ḫaḫḫāš* (based on BAM 174 rev. 29–32). This is quite the reverse and seems to be confirmed by the lexical tradition, which links "to flare up" and this *la ḫaḫḫāš*. We see the equations a.NE.zal = *ṣarḫūtum*, a.NE.a.zal = *la ḫaḫḫāšūtum* (MSL 13 (1971) 78 Proto-Kagal 410–411).

The word *ḫaḫḫāš* is of unknown etymology. In therapeutic texts NE *la ḫaḫḫāš* seems to have become a noun indicating a specific kind of fever; it occurs only twice: "a fever *la ḫaḫḫāš* has seized him" (BAM 2 174 rev. 30); "he repeatedly gets fever *la ḫaḫḫāš*" (BAM 2 146:31; var. 145:5 omits the verb). It seems that the redactor of the Diagnostic Handbook *TDP* accepted this term as a technical term for a kind of fever.[20] At first sight, it looks as if he replaced this word for earlier *ṣarāḫu* (and *ṣirḫu*, *ṣiriḫtu*) but this is not true: the latter words are attested in *TDP*.

6. "*Not much fever*" (NE NU *ma-dam-ma*), M. Stol, *Epilepsy in Babylonia* (1993) 66:46.

Addendum: fever symptoms in new-born babies:

"If the trunk of a baby has fever *la ḫaḫḫāš*, his head has fever, he 'eats' the breast, and he . . . a lot, his teeth come through (. . .), TDP 230:115. He is teething?

"If a baby has no fever, his head is hot, his teeth come through (. . .)", 230:116.

"If a baby . . ., fever seizes him repeatedly, he is deficient at the breast: Oath has seized him", 230:119.

"malarial attacks?" Adamson used no more than CAD Ḫ and TDP as quoted there when studying this word: Adamson, *JRAS* 1979, 4: "In conclusion, it is proposed to consider *ḫaḫḫašu* as a technical medical term denoting a marked degree of fever. In certain cases the medical texts strongly support the diagnosis of malaria". The identification with malaria is not provable.

[19] In R.M. Boehmer, *Uruk. Die Gräber* (= *AUWE* 10) (1995) 213 (line 5).

[20] BAM 174 rev. 29–31, with NE *la ḫaḫḫāš* in it, sounds like a quotation from TDP!

"If a baby has no fever, his eyes stare, his hands and feet tremble", 230:120, cf. 121–122.

Remedies:

1.) Plants: Fox grape (*karān šēlebi*) and milk plant (*šizbānu*) "in order to tear out belly fever" (see CAD Š/3/148, s.v.). 2) Fumigation, salves, bandages, poultices, "If fever has seized a man", BAM 3 315 I 28–42. "The princess whom fever repeatedly had seized, has now come to rest through the bandage and potion (*ina naṣmatti u mašqīti ittuaḫ*)" (PBS 1/2 72:27–29). 3) A composite salve (EŠ *šá* NE; R. Labat, *RA* 54 [1960] 175 AO 17617:7). 4) Atypical is the salve in BAM 2 143.

3. li'bu

According to CAD L, the verb *la'ābu* behind this word means "to infect, said of *li'bu*-disease".[21] The noun *li'bu* is not translated: "(a disease)". Neither is the noun *la'bu*: "(a skin disease)". There is some confusion and we prefer to distinguish:

1. A skin disease *la'bu*.[22]
2. Odious matter; cf. Arabic *luʿābun* "Speichel, Spucke, Geifer".[23] "If the lungs of a man are hot for him, he is full of *la-'-ba* and [. . .] spittle: that man is ill of the lungs; sorcery has seized him" (AMT 55,2:4–5).[24] A medical text speaks of "stopping *la'bu*", and one is reminded of the well known "to stop (*parāsu*) bleeding". Again, some fluid matter may be meant.[25]

[21] An important passage for the verb *la'ābu* is BMS 12:51, with W. von Soden, *Iraq* 31 (1969) 87, and R. Borger, *BiOr* 32 (1975) 72a, on CAD L 35a: diseases *la-'a-bu-in-ni*.

[22] T. Abusch, *Babylonian Witchcraft Literature* (1987) 68–71: "disease disfiguring the skin". But also *li'bu*, as in GAN = *ga-ra-bu*, GAN.bu = *li-'-bu*, in F. Rochberg-Halton, *Aspects of Babylonian celestial divination: The lunar eclipse tablets of Enūma Anu Enlil* (1988) 272, EAE 22 Text c, II 8.

[23] See M. Ullmann, *Aufs Wasser schreiben* (1989) 26; Ullmann, *WKAS* II/14 (1986) 809–816.

[24] With Abusch, *Babylonian Witchcraft Literature*, 69 note 105: "a pus-like secretion". Sorcery is often associated with dirty matter, *lu'(a)tu* (M. Stol, *JEOL* 32 [1991–92] 47), and we now understand why a commentary equates *lu-'-a-ti* = *la-'-ba*(!) (text -*šu*), STT 2 403:44–46. These three lines elaborate upon TDP 24:51, "*li'bu* of the mountain (DIḪ KUR) has seized him; alternative: sorcery has seized him". Note that sorcery is also the cause of *li'bu* in TDP 176:1.

[25] Attested as [..] *la-'-ba* TAR-*si*, *Studies Abraham Sachs* (1988) 12 no. 9b rev. 11. AHw, s.v. *parāsu*, does not give the well known meaning "to stop (bleeding)"; note

3. A fever. Often mentioned after the word *ummu* "fever", possibly qualifying it, example: NE *li-ʾ-bu la-ba-ṣi*, LKA 20:5 (prayer to Gula; cf. BAM 4 338:21); "He has fever, *li-ʾ-ba*" (Stol, *Epilepsy in Babylonia* (1993) 67f., rev. 4, 7). Faulty (?) writings of the first syllable in: "If sun-heat has inflamed a man, and he gets a flaring-up fever, KA-*ʾ-ba*" (BAM 1 66:21); shorter: "If he is inflamed by sun-heat, and he gets *l*[*a*]-*ʾ-ba*" (BAM 2 146:46); cf. *la-ʾ-bi*, Stol, *Epilepsy* 66:50. The most important reference is found in BAM 2 147 indicating that "strong fever" (*ummu dannu*) is identical with *liʾbu*.[26]

Symptoms (hot vs. cold):

> "If a man's fles[h (?) is (now) h[ot] (?), (now) cold, he eats bread, he drinks beer, and (*-ma*) he vomits ([*i*]-*ár-rù*), he becomes nauseated (*i-t*[*a*?-*n*]*a-áš*), above his flesh is cold, his bone beneath (*šaplānu*) is flaring-up: That man, he has been overcome by sun-heat, and (*-ma*) he has the *liʾbu*-disease" (BAM 2 146:43–46).
>
> "If a baby holds fever *li-ʾ-ba* and repeatedly becomes cold" (TDP 224:51).
>
> "If the flesh of a baby has green/yellow spots, his innards are swollen (*ebēṭu*), his hands and feet are 'blown', he has *li-ʾ-ba* a lot: he is ill in the lungs. Hand of the god, he will live" (TDP 220:29).—Is this "lot of" *liʾbu* of the lungs the odious matter discussed under (2.)?
>
> A child bearing mother "constantly has (?) fever, *liʾbu*, and dark spots on her flesh and veins" (BAM 3 240:59).

3.a. liʾbu *"of the Mountain"*

A few times the texts specify this disease as: the *liʾbu* "of the mountain". This expression goes back to the Middle Babylonian period where we find the most telling text. Its first line says, "in order to tear out the *liʾbu* of the mountain (*li-ʾ-*[*bi* KU]R-*i*)", and a lengthy magical ritual follows.[27] The next case is fully described: "If *liʾbu*, seizure of the mountain (*ṣi-bit* KUR-*i*), has seized a man, and [it

---

also (*ana*) *su-a-lim* TAR-*si*, CAD S 340b. This "to stop" can also refer to stopping a disease, including fever. Above we have seen "to stop the fever and the flaring-up" (*ana ummi u ṣirḫa parāsi*), BAM 174 rev. 31.

[26] See above, p. (112). The identity of "strong fever" and *liʾbu* in this text was already seen by R. Labat, *BiOr* 24 (1967) 179b.

[27] G. Meier, *ZA* 45 (1939) 200–208, I 1–V 14, with the end of I 1 in KUB 37 84; dupl. KBo 36 35.

releases] him, and on the third day it seizes him, [. . . .] continually chases him,[28] he repeatedly gets flaring-up fever (*umma ṣarḫa*), strong (*dannu*) *li'bu*, and much sweat, his mild (?) illness becomes protracted and . . . . throws him: when its 'work' seizes him, you shall hold his head (. . . you shall mix in oil); where its 'work' begins, you shall recite the incantation (. . .). When his seizure has released him, you shall not change the oil or the incantation. Do this again and its 'work' will come to completion".[29] This looks like a remittent fever, or perhaps malaria.

Later references for this mountain fever are:

a) K. 2581 with Labat, *BiOr* 18 (1961) 151; copy by K. van der Toorn, *Sin and Sanction* (1985) Plate I "obv." 20–21, "If a man shakes (*i-tar-rak*) from his feet to his shoulders, *li'bu* of the mountain (*li-i-bu šá-di-i*) has seized that man". Dupl. AMT 43,7:1 (*li-ib* KUR-[. . . .]).
b) TDP 24:51, "If his head is hot, the tip of his nose, his hands and his feet are cold: *li'bu* of the mountain (DIḪ KUR) has seized him; ditto: sorcery has seized him; [he will . . . .]".[30] Note here the symptoms of hot vs. cold.
c) ABRT 1 81:14, cf. CAD A/2 326b (*tamītu*), "Saved from the evil of shivering fever and cold shivers, *li'bu* of the mountain, which weaken everything" (*ina* ḪUL *šuruppû u ḫurbašu* LIM-*bu šá* KUR-*i munaššir mimma šumšu* KAR-*ir*). Does "*li'bu* of the mountain" qualify the two diseases shivering fever and cold shivers? Rather, all three together are malaria. Later on, we will suggest that "shivering fever and cold shivers" are the *stadium frigoris* in malaria. The addition "weakening everything" points to an epidemic.
d) Maqlû II 56, cited in CAD L 182a.

3.b. *"Seizure of the Mountain"*

The Middle Babylonian texts also spoke of "*li'bu*, seizure of the mountain (*ṣi-bit* KUR-*i*)". We add the references for "seizure of the mountain" in more texts:

---

[28] Text: *ir-te-dá-aš-šu*; Labat, "Fieber", *RlA* III (1957) 61b: "die Temperatur steigt".

[29] Meier, 208f., V 15–29; note the translation in CAD S 263b. The next case, "ditto", VI 1, has a prescription duplicating BAM 2 159 VI 45–47: "If a ghost has seized a man". And indeed, the long incantation in our text, II 1ff., ascribes *li'bu* to a ghost.

[30] Comparable are some symptoms in the syndromes noted in M. Stol, *Epilepsy* 67f. rev. 4–5, 7–8: the patient shouts 'My belly', he opens and closes the eyes, he has fever, *li'bu*, he touches (*lapātu* D) tip of nose, the tips of fingers and toes are cold.

e) SBTU I 37:24–26, dupl. SBTU II 180 no. 44:21–23: "If it leaves (emend in both texts ŠUB into TAG_4!) him two days, and seizes him on the third day: whenever it seizes him, he becomes stiff (*magāgu*) all the time, after he has been stiff all the time [ditto], he gets trembling (*ra'ibu*), his limbs (UB.MEŠ) hurt him, his hands and feet are cold ($ŠED_7$-*a*!), afterwards a fever 'together' (1-*niš*) (dupl. TÉŠ.BI = *mitḫariš*, on both sides?) 'rides' him / pours down (*reḫû*) upon him and (*u*) sweat falls upon him, and he comes to rest (*nâḫu*): seizure of the mountain has seized him".
f) The following line, 28 (dupl., 24): "If it seizes him two days, on the third day it pours upon him: seizure of the mountain / (dupl. omits) he will die".[31]
Both e–f strongly remind us of the Middle Babylonian text, with the critical third day.
g) DIB KUR = *ṣi-bit*! [. . . .], *ṣa-ba-a-tum*, Th. Meek, RA 17 (1920) 141 K. 4229 rev. 9, cited CAD Ṣ 163b. This is the catchline at the end of a *ṣātu* commentary on Šumma Alu Tablet 76.

A plant used against *li'bu*, Ú NI.NE (cf. CAD *šūšu*), occurs in BAM 1 1 I 43; between the diseases UD.DA and *ḫa-am*-ME (see at the end of this contribution). The myth "Nergal and Ereshkigal" gives the names of the 14 gates of the Netherworld and differentiates between gate 13, god *Umma* ("Fever"), and gate 14, god *Li'ba*. In a list both words follow each other; cf. *Ugaritica* V 31 no. 17:23. The word *li'bu* occurs in lists among other diseases.[32]

Everything in *li'bu* points to an infectious disease, as suggested by the dictionary translation for the verb *la'ābu*. Taking up the three meanings suggested above, we have here an infectious skin disease (1), infecting sputum (2), and fever with infection (3). Astrological

[31] Note that the next omen has as diagnosis GIG *ki-is-sa-tú* GIG (I 37:28, after dupl. II 44:25).

[32] A new reference is found in the incantation against *šimmatu* K. 10770 (Geers N 90), a duplicate not used by W. von Soden in his edition in *JNES* 33 (1974) 341. After four lines beginning with *tu-* follows (10) *ra-'-i-bu* [. . .], (11) *li-'-bu* [. . .]. Line 11 is von Soden's line 14, *li-i*[*p*]-*ti*; based on the copy STT 2 136 I 14. Furthermore: I. L. Finkel, *Aula Or.* 9 (1991) 93 with 97 (f): ÉN *murṣu mišittu* (var. *miqtu*) *le-e-bi di-'u* (var. STT 2 138 rev. 21; BAM 4 338 rev. 6). Uncertain: SBTU III 166 no. 94:41: a sow PAP SAG.KI KA.BI KIŠIB.BI DUB (= diḫ = *li'bu*?) DIB-*bat*. R. D. Biggs, *Aula Or.* 9 (1991) 20: a mycotoxicose?

omens indeed show that *li'bu* reigned in "the country". A letter from Ugarit speaks of *mar-ṣú li-'-[bi]* and mentions an epidemic (*mūtānu*).[33] The *li'bu* of the mountain "weakens everything" (ABRT 1 81:14–15).

In Sumerian the word for *li'bu* is diḫ, the sign DUB which can be a feature on the skin, mainly in physiognomic texts. A man suffers from it; see the Sumerian "Letter of Sin-šamuḫ to Enki", 18.[34] Allow me to make a daring suggestion: that the well known Akkadian word *di'u* (*diḫu*) is a loan from this Sumerian diḫ.[35]

4. di'u *"malaria"*

Let us follow the suggestion that Sumerian diḫ = *li'bu* has become a loanword in Akkadian: the famous word *di'u*. This is a "literary" word and very rare in therapeutic or diagnostic texts, hence appearing in another context than *li'bu*; we admit, however, that *di'u* and *li'bu* are a few times mentioned together.[36] One can show that *di'u* is an epidemic disease, is seasonal, and that it may include malaria.

As an epidemic, it is often mentioned together with the other pestilences *šibṭu* and *mūtānu*.[37] It is also seasonal, "annual", literally "of the year (mu.an.na = *šattu*)",[38] as in a bilingual fragment: mu.an.na tu.ra = *di-' šat-ti*, "*di'u* of the year".[39] In CTN IV 63 IV 47–49 we come across this sequence: (47) *ina di-'-i* [. . .] (48) MU.AN.NA [. . .] (49) *šu-ru-u[p-pu-ú . . .]*. This is the *tamītu* IM 67629 and Professor W. G. Lambert kindly made available to me his transliteration, based on collations and a duplicate. He saw more. A short list of annual

---

33 F. Malbran-Labat, in P. Bordreuil, *Une bibliothèque au sud de la ville* (1991) 58 no. 25:13.

34 With B. Böck, *AOF* 23 (1996) 13 Anm. 17a, déḫe = *la'bu*, "eine schwere Hautkrankheit".

35 Note that S. Lieberman in his book on loanwords saw Sumerian diḫi "(a skin disease)" behind the Akkadian word *ziḫḫu*. See his *The Sumerian loanwords in Old-Babylonian Akkadian* I (1977) 203f.

36 STT 2 138 rev. 21; I. L. Finkel, *Aula Or.* 9 (1991) 93:12, Tablet IVf.; cf. p. 97 (f).

37 S. Maul, *Zukunftsbewältigung* (1994) 186 rev. 4'; BAM 4 322:77 (incant.); BAM 2 183:34 (9 amulets); D. A. Kennedy, *RA* 63 (1969) 81f. no. 10 (a salve); R. Caplice, *Or NS* 39 (1970) 118:1 (cited in AHw as "Catal. 1814:1"). Note also CT 39 9:2, cited CAD D 166a: "Ningišzida will inflict the *d.*-disease on the country".

38 CAD Š/2 206a gives one reference, "it is a seasonal disease" (now SAA X 236:11). Also SAA VIII 1:8 (RMA 257).

39 KAR 24 rev. 23, with E. Ebeling, *AfO* 16 (1952–53) 297.

diseases appears to be given here: (245) *ina di-ʾi* MU.AN.[NA (. . .)] *šu-ru-up-pe-e* [(. . .)] (246) MU.AN.NA [. . .] *ù na-ga-aḫ* MU.AN.NA (247) *šu-ru-u*[*p-pu-ú u ḫur-ba-a-šu* (?)] ŠI-*bi* (248) *šá* KUR-*i mu-na-šir* [*mim-ma šum-šú*]. CAD N/1 106a translated: "from *diʾu* disease of the year, chill of the year, and *nagāḫu* of the year". This evil disease goes into hiding when Sirius appears, and the critically ill recovers; *ina ta-*[*mar*]*-ti-šu* GIG *di-ʾ-i lemnu iḫḫazu tubqāti* GIG *nakdu iturru ašruššu*.[40]

We have seen that there is a condition called *liʾbu* "of the mountain", "seizure of the mountain". The *diʾu* also is said to come from the mountains, but the evidence is meagre. The diseases *sa-ma-nu* (NIM.NIM) and *de-e* (SAG.GIG.GE_4), for example, descended from the mountains.[41]

For Malaria, we quote from the Diagnostic Handbook:

> "If at the onset of a disease, after it has 'touched' him until it stops (*kalû*), in one respect (?) (1-*is-su*) he gets fever, in one respect (?) (1-*is-su*) he gets cold, in equal measure; after the fever and the sweat have been loosened (*paṭāru*), his limbs bring fever to him, and he gets fever as much as the former fever, and it is loosened; afterwards he gets cold and sweat: (it is) the in- and outgoing *di-ḫu*; he is inflamed by sun-heat. Seven days he will be mildly (?) ill, and he will live" (TDP 156:4–7).

This most interesting passage has been translated more than once.

(1) R. Labat, TDP (1951) 157. Labat, *RlA* III [1957] 61b: "Sumpffieber; in der ersten Phase TDP 168:100–103 als lästige fiebrische Magenstörung auftretend und in TDP 156:4–7 die zweite Stufe des Fiebers mit heftigen Anfällen, charakterisiert durch die drei Phasen: Kälte, Hitze, Schweiss". For TDP 168:100–103, see below, (4). (2) E. Ritter, *Studies Benno Landsberger* (1965) 305–6. (3) J. Bottéro, *Annuaire EPHE IVe Section*, 1969/1970 97 ("les principaux symptômes du paludisme secondaire"; following R. Labat, "Sumpffieber"). We do not understand the unique 1–*is-su* (AHw 1417b: *ištessu* "etwas von ihm"). We still do not understand the word *salāʾu* translated here as "to be mildly (?) ill", by E. Ritter as, "suffer severe pain", and by

---

[40] E. Burrows, *JRAS, Centenary Supplement* (1924) Plate 2:4, with M.-J. Seux, *Hymnes et prières aux dieux de Babylonie et d'Assyrie* (1976) 480. Now *or* NS 74 (2005) 52.

[41] STT 2 178:21–22; Dupl. AMT 61,7 rev. 8 (here *di-ḫu-um* / SAG.GIG.GA) etc.; I.L. Finkel in *Festschrift R. Borger* (1998), 87f.

CAD S 96 as, "to enter a critical stage of an illness". The writing of the words *di-ḫu e-ri-bu wa-ṣú-ú* "in- and outgoing *di-ḫu*" betray an Old Babylonian original, and it refers to "remittent" fever.[42] Elsewhere in this same chapter of the Diagnostic Handbook, "disease goes in and goes out" (TDP 160:34–40). As to the seven days, followed by recovery, see Hippocrates, *Epidemics* I 24: "The seven-day fever is long-lasting but not fatal".[43]

The next two passages in this chapter do not diagnose the ailment as *di'u* but are the continuation and deserve to be given here:

> "If at the onset of his disease his temples bring fever to him, and afterwards they take the fever and sweat away: mild (?) illness of/by sunheat; 2, 3 days he will have a mild (?) illness, and he will live" (TDP 156:8–9).
>
> "If at the onset of his disease he is flaring-up (NE-*úḫ* = *ṣaruḫ*; see footnote 12), he consumes much bread, beer, fruits, (but) it will not stay in his belly, he pours it out; he stretches out his fingers, he has his eyes open all the time, he pays attention to a noise, he (now) makes himself well (*damāqu*), he (then) is worried (ZI.IR = *ašāšu*) all the time, and his face becomes yellow/green all the time: a "lurking spirit" has hit him; after it has touched him it becomes tied to him; from the bread that he eats, he eats, from the water that he drinks, he drinks. That man will live 5, 7 days" (TDP 156ff.: 10–13).
>
> All this is difficult to understand.

One more remark on malaria. A *tamītu* text offers this sequence: *murṣu di'u ummu zu'tu ni-su-tum miḫiṣ ilūti*.[44] Can one think of phases in malaria: fever (*ummu*)—sweat (*zu'tu*)—going away (*nesû*)?[45]

We conclude this section on *di'u* by giving its symptoms according to medical texts. We have already studied the most important passage that pointed to malaria.

> (1) "His . . . are 'blown', his entrails . . . vertigo . . . middle (. . .) his knees hurt him, [. . . whatever] he eats and drinks, does not please him: that man is ill of the *di'u* illness (GIG *di-'* GIG). If that man wishes to

[42] Was Old Babylonian *diḫu* replaced by *li'bu* in the later medical terminology?

[43] Cited after *Hippocratic Writings* (Penguin Classics) (1978) 100. Note G. Sticker, *Archiv für Geschichte der Medizin* 22 (1929) 331: "die kurzen Fieber im engeren Sinne, febres acutae, entscheiden sich binnen 2 Wochen, meistens am 7. Tage".

[44] IM 67692:333, cited CAD N/2 276a, with the translation "illness, *di'u* disease, fever, sweat, *nisūtu*, attack of a demon". Dupl. AMT 17,9:5.

[45] "Going away" is a verb used once more for *di'u*. KAR 321 rev. 4, with CAD N/1 151a, (c), <*ša*> (?) *di-'-ú šak-nu-uš na-'-i-ri tuš-te-es-si*.

live (. . .)".[46] Rectal treatment. The formula "If that man wishes to live" (*šumma* TI.LA *ḫašiḫ*) is unique. Does this mean that curing is optional and that the illness is not life-threatening? The symptoms look like the prodome to malaria. Is *di'u* here incipient malaria?
(2) "If he is ill, and in his illness he speaks with his wife, son, daughter well (*damqiš*), as if he were healthy (?), he does not eat bread: *di-ḫu*: he will li[ve]", TDP 160:41–42 (end preserved in AMT 50,4:16).
(3) "[. . . .] . . . he is stiff all the time, he has been touched by *di'u* (*di-ʾ lapit*)", TDP 184:17.
(4) "If, from the morning until the evening, *di-ḫu* begins in his body, and he gets a mild (?) illness (*sil'itu*) of the belly, his intestine stand(s) up (*ir-ra-šú i-te-bu*) he belches (= throws up?), through the mouth, he vacates through the anus: a touch by sun-heat (TAG-*ti* UD.DA) which is not joined to his limbs. His disease (is) a mild (?) illness of 1 day" (TDP 168:100–103). R. Labat, already quoted above: "Sumpffieber; in der ersten Phase TDP 168:100–103 als lästige fiebrische Magenstörung auftretend, und in TDP 156:4–7 die zweite Stufe des Fiebers mit heftigen Anfällen, charakterisiert durch die drei Phasen: Kälte, Hitze, Schweiss".

At the end of this discussion of malaria it is good to point out that the prospects of *di'u* are not bad. "He will live", is the prognosis. If we really can see "malaria" in this disease, the data about malaria in the Classical texts become interesting. Scholars assume that a malignant variant of malaria reached the Greek world in about 400 B.C. Malaria may have existed before but was much milder because it is never mentioned, not even by Hesiod.[47] Is *di'u* that earlier mild malaria? And is "*li'bu* of the mountain" a severe variety?

---

[46] BAM 1 106:1–4, dupl. 108 rev. 1–7; dupl. AMT 39, 4 rev. 3–5 (not seen by F. Köcher).

[47] Mirko D. Grmek, *Les maladies à l'aube de la civilisation occidentale* (1983) 355–407, Chapitre X, "L'hyperostose poreuse du crâne, les anémies héréditaires et l'évolution du paludisme" (esp. p. 399ff.); P. F. Burke, "Malaria in the Greco-Roman world. A historical and epidemiological survey", *Aufstieg und Niedergang der römischen Welt (ANRW)* II, 37/3 (1996) 2252–2281 (hardly a word on Grmek!). Bibliography: M. D. Grmek, "Bibliographie chronologique des études sur la malaria dans la Méditerranée orientale préhistorique et antique (depuis la découverte des agents pathogènes et des vecteurs)", in: *Université Jean Monnet, Saint Etienne. Centre Jean-Palerne, Lettre d'informations* no. 24 (mai 1994).

5. šuruppû *"shivering fever"*

This word means "chills, shivers", according to the Chicago Assyrian Dictionary, following an earlier and commonly accepted opinion.[48] One connects the word with *šurīpu* "ice, frost".[49] Once we find it together with what seems to be its contrast: a plant is used both for this and for inflammation by sun-heat (*ḫimiṭ ṣēti*).[50] We suggest that in malaria this is the *stadium frigoris*. The passages in the *tamītu* texts support this interpretation: "Saved from the evil of shivering fever (*šuruppû*) and cold shivers (*ḫurbašu*), *li'bu* of the mountain, which weaken everything". We may see in *šuruppû* and *ḫurbašu* two forms of *stadium frigoris* preceding the *stadium caloris*. Greek texts distinguish a mild form of "frost" (*phríke*) and a severe form (*rhîgos*).[51] Elsewhere we find the sequence *di-i šuruppû* (SBTU III 44 no. 65 rev. 12).

6. ḫamāṭu *"to be Inflamed"*

We have seen above that the verb *emēmu* "to be hot" from which *ummu* "fever" is derived, is not a symptom of disease. It refers to high temperature, not necessarily fever. Unnatural heat is indicated by the verb *ḫamāṭu*, according to the dictionaries meaning "to burn, to be inflamed", "brennen, verbrennen", and we translate it here as "to be inflamed". It is sometimes used with the comparison "like fire" and in medical contexts it then refers to skin problems.[52] "Fire" and other diseases "fall" from heaven and "inflame the cattle" (*eli*

---

[48] "Kälteschauer, als Krankheit bzw. Seuche" (AHw); "Schüttelfrost"; "unter 'Schüttelfrost' abklingendes Fieber", Th. Kämmerer, U.-F. 27 (1995) 165; "feverish shivering", M. Stol, *Epilepsy in Babylonia* (1993) 38 ("prodrome of an epileptic attack"?).

[49] Technically, a derivation from *šarāpu* "to burn" is possible. This word seems to indicate a feverish condition in only one instance and the reading (*šarup*) has been doubted (*tarup*?); S. Dalley, OBTR no. 124:5, with W. von Soden, *NABU* 1991/54, and J. Eidem, *NABU* 1991/87.

[50] [*a-na š*]*u-ru-ub-bi-e* TAB UD.DA *u* [. . .], BAM 4 379 I 43, dupl. SBTU III 202 no. 106:18.

[51] R. Strömberg, *Griechische Wortstudien* (1944) 80f.; "die *phríke* scheint sich nur auf die Haut zu beziehen, das *rhîgos* betrifft hingegen den ganzen Körper".

[52] "Like fire": M. J. Geller, *Iraq* 42 (1980) 31:167–8. In broken medical context: [DIŠ NA x] IZI TAB-*ma*, BAM 2 170:8; GIM IZI TAB-*šu*, AMT 77,6:1. Difficult is "and the skull is inflamed like the nature (?) of fever (?) (GIM *ši-kin* NE-*im-ma ḫa-mi-iṭ*), his skin is full of boils (*bubu'tu*)", CT 46 45 IV 19–20, with W. G. Lambert, *Iraq* 27 (1965) 6–7; cf. P.-A. Beaulieu, *NABU* 1992/77; W. Heimpel, *RA* 90 (1996) 9, 16 in non-medical context ARM 27 142:27 (*išātam ḫummuṭ* "brulé par le feu").

kali būlim úḫ-ta-am-mi-iṭ).[53] The Sumerogram is TAB.[54] The following are references to "to be inflamed" in medical texts.

"His upper belly is inflamed for him (*iḫammatsu*)".[55]

"His upper belly is inflamed for him (*iḫammatsu*), gives him piercing pains (*dakāšu*)" (AMT 45,6:6; diagnosis sun-heat). The preceding case says "His upper belly burns him (*uṣarrapšu*)" (5), cf. "gnaws him" (*kaṣāṣu*) (12).

"His upper belly is inflamed for him, is burning him, is giving him a stinging pain" (*uḫammatsu uṣarrapšu uzaqqatsu*)" (STT 1 96:20). Note the same sequence in BAM 1 75:7–8.

"The region between his shoulder blades makes him inflamed (*uḫammatsu*) (D)" (AMT 45,6:9).

"If a man's mouth is inflamed" (YOS 11 28:1).

"If the hips of a man, either in his walking, or in his lying, 'touch' him, [his pen]is gives him a stinging pain (*zaqātu*), makes him inflamed (*uḫammatsu*), shakes (?) him (*i-tar-rak-šú*), after he has urinated [. . .]" (AMT 60,1:22–24).[56]

Once "to be inflamed" is followed by "to be hot" (*emēmu*): "If the upper belly of a man is inflamed for him (*iḫammatsu*) and (*u*) (he) is hot (NE-*im*), he eats bread, and it does not please (*alāku*) him, he drinks water, and it is not pleasant (*ṭābu*) for him, and (*u*) his skin is green/yellow: that man is ill of an illness of sexual intercourse (*nâku*)" (TDP 178:12–13; also 110:9–10). The next line, with the same diagnosis, says that his penis and upper belly have a flaring-up fever (NE *ṣarḫu*).

The plant *egengerû* is used for "inflamed anus" (Ú DÚR TAB) (BAM 4 380:47). Another plant is Ú DÚR *ḫa-am-ṭi* (text ME), BAM 1 1 III 17, with CAD M/2 102b.

---

53 YOS 11 7:5; later dupl. STT 2 136 III 35–6.

54 In a medical commentary: TAB = *ḫa-ma-ṭu*, E. Leichty, *AfO* 24 (1973) 83:17; also: MSL 9 (1967) 133:461–2: TAB ta-ab = *ṣa-ra-pu*, *ḫa-ma-ṭu*. MSL 3 (1955) 135:8: TAB ta-ab = *ḫa-ma-ṭu*, var. *ḫu-um-ṭu*. Rarely TAB is used in a finite verbal form (*a-šar* TAB.BA *ši-i Ea liq-* [. . .], BAM 5 503 I 15; *ina* ŠUB-*ti* TAB.TAB-*šú*, M. Stol, *Epilepsy in Babylonia* (1993) 58, Tablet XXVI:5). "To begin" (TAB = *šurrû*)?

55 UET 6/2 410 rev. 9 with O.R. Gurney, *Iraq* 22 (1960) 224; dupl. "His upper belly hurts him (KÚ-*šú*)", BAM 2 193 I 9–10.

56 Broken: [. . .] *ḫamiṭ*: BAM 2 146:19–23, also KUB 37 2:18–23. Probably [*ṣētam*] *ḫamiṭ* (sun-heat).

7. ḫimṭu *"Burn"*

The word *ḫimṭu* "unnatural heat" is derived from the verb *ḫamāṭu*. It is mainly attested in the expression *ḫimiṭ ṣētim* "inflammation by sun-heat" (see below). The references to simple *ḫimṭu* are few. *Ḫinṭu* (= *ḫimṭu)* is an independent ailment in the series *ḫimiṭ ṣēti kibbu ḫinṭu*.[57] More often it is mentioned in one breath with the word *kibbu* which is derived from *kabābu* "to burn, to char". Is *ḫimṭu* a burn? Remember that the verb (*ḫamāṭu*) is sometimes used with the comparison "like fire" and that in medical context it then refers to skin problems.

At first sight there seems to be an example of "inflammation by fever" (TAB NE = *ḫimiṭ ummi*) in a pharmacological handbook. It occurs among skin problems and it is more likely that we have to think of burns. In that case we read the signs differently, NE IZI = *ḫimiṭ išāti*, "a burn by fire". We give the passage; on the left side is the plant, on the right side the medical problem that it is used for (STT 1 92 III 13–15):

[Ú KA] A.AB.BA	=	Ú TAB IZI
[Ú SAḪ]AR (?) AN.ZÁḪ	=	Ú TAB IZI
Ú KUR.RA	=	Ú *ḫi-im-ṭi*

In a diagnostic text: "If the nature of an illness (is this): it is hot like an inflammation (*kīma ḫimṭi ēm*), and (. . .)".[58]

8. ḫunṭu *"Fever" (in Assyrian)*

There is one more word derived from *ḫamāṭu* that will interest us: *ḫunṭu*.[59] The word is Assyrian (not Babylonian), attested outside medical texts, and denotes fever. It is attested in letters.[60] We can read here interesting descriptions written by the ancient Assyrian experts of the seventh century B.C. We follow the latest translations by Simo Parpola.

---

[57] CT 4 3:15 with MSL 9 (1967) 106. Cf. *lu kibbu lu ḫinṭu*, F.A.M. Wiggermann, *Mesopotamian Protective Spirits. The ritual texts* (1992) 6:8, or *ḫintu kibbu*, BAM 4 338 rev. 12.

[58] GIM TAB NE-*ma*, SBTU IV 152:12–16.

[59] Cf. Sumerogram LUL.TU = *ḫu-un-ṭu*, STT 2 402 II 9 (after *ruṭibtu*).

[60] S. Parpola, *Letters from Assyrian scholars to the kings Esarhaddon and Assurbanipal. Part II: Commentary and appendices* (1983) 170 (he notes that *ṣurḫu* is "heat", not "fever").

Fever "held" in the bones (*eṣemtu*) leads to these complaints: "My arms and feet (= legs) are without strength. I cannot open my eyes; I am scratched (*marāṭu*) and lie prostrate (*karāru*)". The prognosis is this: "There is no fault (*laššu ḫīṭu*); his illness will go out" (SAA X 242).

"Let the king apply this clysma (*marḫaṣu*), and perhaps this fever will be loosened (*paṭāru*) from the king, my lord". "Perhaps the king will sweat". "I am also sending a salve. The king should anoint himself on the day of [his] (acute) period (of illness) (UD-*mu ša e-da-ni-š*[*ú*])" (SAA X 315, rev. 1–3, 14, 20).

"The king should not be afraid of this fever which has seized him (*ṣabātu*) two or three times; his pulse is normal and sound (*sakikkušu* DI *tariṣ*), he is well" (SAA X 320:9–12).

"His fever has come to rest (*pašāḫu*); there is no fault" (SAA X 213:7–8).

Fever "seizes" a person (239:2), it "leaves" him (*ramû* D; restored in 193:8).

There is "fever (?) in the eyes" (328:17–18; 243:5–6).[61]

II. *Sun-heat*

Sun-heat (*ṣētu*) is disease caused by the heat of the sun; it is a frequent diagnosis in medical texts. Sometimes it is caused by "the heat of the night".[62] We have seen that *ummu* "fever' is never a diagnosis; it is just a concomitant symptom. The word *ṣētu* actually serves as diagnosis. It often goes with the verb *ḫamāṭu*, translated by us as "to be inflamed". Note that *ummu* goes with the verb *ṣarāḫu*, translated by us as "to flare up". In a study of Babylonian fever, we have

[61] Parpola translated in 243:5 "inflammation of eyes"; thus also in S. Parpola, *Letters from Assyrian scholars to the kings Esarhaddon and Assurbanipal.* Part II: *Commentary and appendices* (1983) 174, on no. 183.

[62] Here belongs "If he is healthy all day, and at night he is ill: sun-heat (is) his disease; 27 days; hand of Ninurta" (TDP 164:75). So "sun-heat" can also strike at night. For the bad rays of the moon see Stol, *Epilepsy* 126f. Note "the heat of night", in: *i-na ṣe-et li-li-im tubbal*, UET 6/2 414:22; translated as "You should dry it in the cool of the evening", by B. R. Foster, *Before the Muses* I (1996) 92.—Astrological texts contrast "its UD.DA is burning like fire" and "its UD.DA is cold"; W. H. van Soldt, *Solar omens of Enuma Anu Enlil* (1995) 86 Tablet 27 II 11; 99 Tablet 28:43, and 87 Tablet 27 II 8; 100 Tablet 28:46. Cf. D. Arnaud, *Semitica* 45 (1996) 10:33', with p. 16; M. Dietrich, *WZKM* 86 (1996) 100f., § XII–XVII.

to investigate the meaning of "sun-heat", which appears to be a complicated matter.[63] The basic meaning "(bad) sun-heat" is clear from a Mari letter. Referring to a princess, walking outside in the afternoon (*muṣlalum*), it is said: "In the courtyard the sun-heat (*ṣé-tum*) touched (*lapātum*) her and since then she has been ill (*marṣa*[*t*])" (AEM 1/2 26 no. 298:47). Sun-heat can "reach" or "overcome" a person, used with verb *kašādu*, Sumerograms KUR and SÁ.DI (DI.DI). In medical texts, the diagnosis "sun-heat" can be based on a bewildering variety of symptoms, often found in the belly. It is more severe than fever, as the following case shows, in a text offering important information on the position of sun-heat in the scale of fevers. When treating gall disease, a test is made by provoking boils artificially. The colours of the boils give information on the prospects, and in this the text runs from mild to bad: "If the boil is white, his belly will come to rest (*pašāḫu*). If the boil is red, his belly will hold fever (*umma ukal*). If the boil is green/yellow, he has been overcome by sun-heat (UD.DA KUR-*id*); it will repeatedly return to him (GUR.GUR-*šu*). If the boil is black, it will make him ill and he will not live" (BAM 6 578 I 8–10). So sun-heat is worse than fever and it can return repeatedly (*târu* Gtn). It can be a long, protracted disease and a few important texts discuss its varying length computed in days. They have a parallel in the Diagnostic Handbook (Chapter XXXI).

We will present below everything known to us about "sun-heat", which will give the outsider an idea about Babylonian taxonomy of symptoms and diseases. We cannot attempt to discover the scientific guidelines or principles behind their categorisations.

We begin by making a few philological remarks on the Babylonian word for sun-heat, *ṣētu*. It literally means "what is coming out" and refers to the rising and shining sun; this way it got its meaning "heat of the sun".[64] It is mostly written with the Sumerogram UD.DA.[65]

---

[63] Greek *kaûsos*, frequent in contexts of fever, is not a specific fever but a complex; M. D. Grmek, *Les maladies à l'aube de la civilisation occidentale* (1983) 416ff. It would be interesting to compare the details with those of our "sun-heat".

[64] Sunshine vs. shadow in SAḪAR GIŠ.MI *u* UD.DA, STT 1 57:4; CTN IV 115:6; K. 2581:8, in K. van der Toorn, *Sin and sanction* (1985) Pl. I, dupl. BAM 2 147 rev. 5; "heat" vs. "cold" (*ṣētu* and *kuṣṣu*) in MSL SS 1 (1986) 84:249–250 (MBGT II).

[65] Not to be confused with UD.DA in *ana* UD.DA ḪUL *parāsi* "Folgen des Unheils", S. Maul, *Zukunftsbewältigung* (1994) 347:18'. Cf. UD.DA DU_8 UD.DA TIL, SBTU IV 153 III 11; contra E. von Weiher.

Sometimes in the medical corpus we come across *ṣētu* in its literal meaning when *materia medica* are said to be dried in "the heat of the sun".[66] Additionally, "coming out" in medical texts can be an excrescence on the skin, which should not be confused with sun-heat. The CAD rightly distinguishes between both, positing the second word as *ṣītu*.[67]

We will name this feverish condition "sun-heat".

Earlier opinions defining *ṣētu* are:

1. R. C. Thompson, *RA* 26 (1929) 49f., note 4: "the heat of the day", "the day".
2. B. Landsberger, *ZA* 42 (1934) 161f.: "Trockenheit", "Dürre" (with an unusual etymology); *ḫimiṭ ṣēti* "trockenes Fieber", corrected in *JNES* 8 (1949) 252 note 30: *ṣētu* als Krankheit etwa "Erkältung"; *ḫimiṭ ṣēti* "fiebrige Erkältung".
3. I. M. Diakonoff, *Rocznik Orientalistyczny* 41/2 (1980) 23: acute uraemia. Based on a very limited number of texts.
4. P. Herrero, *Thérapeutique mésopotamienne* (1984) 38: enfiévré par "la sécheresse (le grand soleil)"; "fièvre (?)".
5. P. B. Adamson, *JRAS* 1984, 11–12: heat exhaustion, rather than heat stroke; malignant malaria? In addition, trauma caused by the rays of the sun.
6. K. van der Toorn, *Sin and sanction in Israel and Mesopotamia* (1985) 69, with note 188 (p. 188): "exposure to the sun could lead to *muruṣ ṣēti*, a sunstroke".
7. J. C. Pangas, *Aula Orientalis* 7 (1989) 227 note 76: "Se trataría, en aparencia, de una afección debida a la *sobreexposición* solar, caterizada por dermatosis, vómitos, diarrea liquida y expulsión de sangre per la boca", citing *TDP* and secondary literature.

---

[66] *Ina* UD.DA UD.A (= *ina ṣēti tubbal*), BAM 5 436 VI 7; 482 I 22). See D. Goltz, *Studien zur altorientalischen und griechischen Heilkunde* (1974) 29–30. I do not understand UD.DA *di-kat*, examples: Clay (*qadūtu*): [IM.G]Ú UD.DA DI.DI GAZ, dupl. IM.GÚ *ša ina* UD.DA *di-kat* GAZ (BAM 5 480 II 62, dupl. BAM 1 12:28; cf. AMT 72,2:13 = BAM 6 571 II 25; BAM 6 584 II 28); also: Clod Ú LAG A.ŠÀ IM.GÚ *šá* UD.DA *di-kat*, BAM 6 578 I 11; not in CAD D *dâku* G, 4, nor in AHw 152.

[67] F. Köcher, in *Uruk. Die Gräber* (= AUWE 10) (1995) 211b, ad 15' (= BAM 4 409:12): *ṣītu* "Hautausschlag (Exanthem)", ist allem Anschein nach ein Allgemeinbegriff für entzündliche Hautveränderungen, die sich auf verschiedene Körperpartien ausbreiten. *ṣītū* [plural!] "ausbrechende, zum Vorschein kommende Ausschläge". Examples are CT 44 36:1 (*ṣi-i-ta* GIG), SBTU IV 152:104 (*ṣi-i-tum*, Hand of Gula. Between *samānu* and *ṣarrišu*). We suggest that UD.DU = è = *ṣí-nu-um* in a short lexical text listing skin diseases has the same etymology and meaning; UET 6/2 361:4; AHw 1091a under *ṣênum*, with a question mark. Also in A. Goetze, *JCS* 9 (1955) 10 HTS 2:6, with Th. Kämmerer, *U.-F.* 27 (1995) 163.

8. Th. Kämmerer, *U.-F.* 27 (1995) 164: "Austrocknung" des ganzen Körpers.
9. F. Köcher, *Festschrift für Heinz Goerke* (1978) 24: Hitzefieber (Sonnenstich).
10. F. Köcher, *Uruk. Die Gräber* (= AUWE 10) (1995) 214: "P. B. Adamson (*JRAS* 1984), S. 11f., spricht sich für "Hitzschlag" bzw. für "Hitzeermüdung" aus. Möglicherweise umspannt die Krankheitsbezeichnung eine Vielzahl von schweren Erkrankungen, die mit starkem Fieber, Gliederschmerzen sowie Magen- und Darmbeschwerden einhergehen". Köcher translates the sub-category "inflammation by sun-heat" (*ḫimiṭ ṣētim*) as "schwere fiebrige Erkrankungen, die durch widriges Sommerwetter (wie Gluthitze, Dürre oder Sand- und Gewitterstürme, einsetzende Kälte) verursacht werden" (p. 210, line 23)
11. J. V. Kinnier Wilson, *Journal of the Royal Society of Medicine* 89 (1996) 136: *ḫimiṭ ṣētim* = pulmonary tuberculosis.

1. *Texts about Sun-heat*

We will now give descriptions of sun-heat in the medical texts, beginning with those which look like systematic treatises solely devoted to ailments diagnosed as "sun-heat".

BAM 1 52

"If a man has flaring-up of the belly (*ṣirihti libbi*), and (*-ma*) his belly holds fever (*ummu*), his limbs [are] pou[red down], his chest 'gnaws' (*kasāsu*) him: That man is inflamed with sun-heat (UD.DA *ḫa-miṭ*)" (BAM 1 52:39–40).[68] The therapy is this: the patient has to drink fourteen plants and will vomit; this is "a potion for loosening Oath", so the text concludes. "Oath" indeed resides in the belly and vomiting drives it out. A following recipe "tears out" Oath by a clysma, applying it "two, three times"; it also works against fever [of the . . .], inflammation by sun-heat (*ḫimiṭ ṣēti*), blast by wind (*šibit šāri*) (52:58–59). "If the belly of a man is ill, and (*-ma*) the inside of his bone is coloured with green/yellow spot(s), his belly [is full of 'wounds']: That man has been overcome by sun-heat" (52:63–4; dupl. BAM 6 575 I 21–22). He has to swallow fourteen pills. Here, the symptoms of sun-heat are visible on the skin.

"If the innards (*qerbū*) of a man are 'blown', his entrails (*irrū*) make noise like that of (caused by) a 'big worm' (ascaris?): that man is ill of accumulation of wind (*nikimtu šāri*), sun-heat. Its 'work' will last long

[68] Dupl. 579 I 40–41. The transliteration by Herrero omits "[are] pou[red down]", DU[B.DUB]; P. Herrero, *Thérapeutique mésopotamienne* (1984) 38.

and (then) "hand of a ghost" (52:66–67, with dupls.).[69] The last remark means that ultimately the disease will "turn into" "hand of ghost".[70] A cocktail of eleven plants is inserted into his anus.

"If the innards of a man are full of accumulation of wind and sun-heat" (72); a rectal application of 23 plants follows.

The remainder of this text speaks of wind and gall diseases; the treatments are largely rectal.

AMT 45,6+ (= K. 6779+)
Several fragments that were part of one tablet.[71]

AMT 45,6

"If the upper belly of a man is inflamed for him, it gives him a piercing pain (*dakāšu*), his (?) saliva [. . .]: he has been overcome by sun-heat" (6–7)

"If the middle of the shoulders of a man is inflamed for him, he throws blood together with his saliva: [he has been overcome by sun]-heat (!)" (9)

"If a man eats bread (or) drinks beer, and his innards (!) 'gnaw' (*kaṣāṣu*) him, his belly is 'blown' [. . .]: he has been overcome by [sun-h]eat" (12–13)

AMT 48,3 + 23,5

"If a man is worried all the time, his worry falls upon him all the time, piercing pain (*dikšu*) touches him all the time, his saliva is much, he drinks [water a lot]: He has been overcome by sun-heat" (6–7 + 5–6)

"[If a man . . .] drinks beer, and his belly becomes swollen, they (= ?) are 'blown', he drinks water a lot: He has been overcome by sun-heat" (8–9 + 7–8)

AMT 48,1 + 78,3

"[If a man] eats bread (or) drinks beer, and his innards (!) become swollen, are 'blown' (?): he has been overcome by sun-heat" (7 + 4)
"[If] a man eats bread (or) drinks beer, and his innards become swollen, he retains (?) his urine: he has been overcome by sun-heat" (10 + 7)
"[If a man] eats bread (or) drinks beer, and his innards (!) become swollen, get cramps, he gets movement of the bowels: he has been overcome by sun-heat" (12 + 9)

[69] P. Herrero, *Thérapeutique mésopotamienne* (1984) 38; cf. AMT 52,4.
[70] M. Stol, *BiOr* 54 (1997) 408 (2).
[71] See R. C. Thompson, *RA* 26 (1929) 77ff. This tablet is in Köcher's terminology K. 6779+ (BAM 2 p. XX).

To this tablet may belong the fragment AMT 44,6 because it also has the unusual ŠÀ-*šú* instead of ŠÀ.MEŠ-*šú* ('innards') (as in AMT 48,1:7, 10, 12):

> "If a man eats bread (or) drinks beer, and his innards (!) become swollen, get cr[amps . . .]: he has been overcome by sun-heat" (AMT 44,6 II 1–2).

BAM 2 174

> "If a man is overcome by sun-heat, he has fever" (BAM 2 174:21). Therapy follows.[72]
>
> "If a man is overcome by sun-heat, he does not accept bread or beer" (174:23); vomiting.
>
> "If a man is worried all the time, his worry falls upon him all the time, he bites (?) his lips all the time, he drinks w[ater] a lot: he has been overcome by sun-heat" (174:25–26). Therapy is rectal. F. Köcher gives a comparable passage: "If a man is worried (*ašāšu*) all the time, his worry (*ašuštu*) falls upon him all the time, piercing pain (*dikšu*) touches him all the time, his saliva is much, he drinks [water a lot]: he has been overcome by sun-heat" (K. 6779 + I 20–21).[73] For this text, see above.
>
> "If a man's belly does not accept bread or beer, he repeatedly throws up blood with his spittle: that man has been overcome by sun-heat" (174:28–29). After this, the text continues with constipation (*esiltu*); the reverse discusses oath and mentions sun-heat or remittent (!) fever in this connection (rev. 25, 29–31).

BAM 2 146

The obverse is badly preserved, and speaks of a man suffering from sun-heat, inflamed belly, . . .[74]. Then follows a long passage (29–42) which we will discuss below. The last case of sun-heat follows: "If a man's fles[h (?) is (now) h[ot] (?), (now) cold, he eats bread, he drinks beer, and (*-ma*) he vomits ([*i*]*-ár-rù*), he becomes nauseated (*i-t*[*a*?*-n*]*a-áš*), above (*elēnu*) his flesh is cold, below (*šaplānu*) his bone is flaring-up: That man, he has been overcome by sun-heat, and (*-ma*) he has the *li'bu*-disease" (BAM 2 146:43–46).

---

72 Dupl. BAM 66 Rs. 6–7 and AMT 45,1:1–3? End: *tu-ta-na*[*-ṣar*]*-raš-ma* TI-*uṭ*.

73 F. Köcher, BAM 2 p. XX. K. 6779+ is AMT 48,3:6 + AMT 23,5:5, translated by R. C. Thompson, *RA* 26 (1929) 78f., (20)–(21).

74 An earlier version of lines 19–23 is KUB 37 2:18–23). As to KUB 37 2: I agree with R. Labat, *AfO* 17 (1954–56) 150, "je lirais plus volontiers: [*š. amîlu ṣêta*] *ḫamiṭ*".

We return to the preceding long description of symptoms, going from head to feet (BAM 2 146:29–42); it was excerpted on a separate tablet (BAM 2 145). It has as its conclusion the diagnosis, "That man has been overcome by sun-heat" (BAM 2 146:38, line lost in dupl. 145:17). "If a man is inflamed by sun-heat and (*-ma*)" also is the first symptom, which looks like a summary of all that follows.[75] However, Köcher's translation of this first line suggests that all symptoms are the consequence of sun-heat, a kind of sun-stroke: "[Wenn jemand] infolge der Sonnenglut überhitzt ist (wörtl. "ausgebrannt ist") und (*-ma*) sein Kopfhaar zu Berge steht, seine Gesichts (muskeln) fortwährend zucken, . . . (etc.).[76] The *-ma* "and" can also mean "so that". Medical specialists are invited to inform us about the consequences of sun-stroke; do the symptoms fit? The text has recently been translated by Köcher and we summarize the symptoms: hair stands up—vertigo (?)—flaring-up (fever) (*ṣarāḫu*) in innards (?)—fatigue (*tāniḫu*) in body—fever *la ḫaḫḫaš*—coughing up matter (*suālu*)—belly cramps—flowing saliva— . . . ing (*garāru*) belly—diarrhoea—flesh above cold, feet beneath flaring-up—turning over in sleep—blocking of windpipe—belching / cough (*gašû* / *ganāḫu*)—constant flaring-up belly fever. We add Köcher's translation in full:

> "[Wenn jemand] infolge der Sonnenglut überhitzt ist (wörtl. "ausgebrannt ist") und (*-ma*) sein Kopfhaar zu Berge steht, seine Gesichts (muskeln) fortwährend zucken, seine [Eingeweide?] immerzu brennend heiß sind, sein Körper ständig zunehmende Müdigkeit erfährt (mit) niedrigen Temperaturen; (wenn) er immerzu Hustenanfälle mit Schleim (auswurf) bekommt, sein Inneres fortwährend schmerzt, sein Speichel läuft, sein Leib sich immer wieder krümmt, er an *ridût* der Eingeweide leidet [diarrhoea?] und Kot entlehrt, seine oberen Körperpartien kalt, die un[te]ren (jedoch bis in) seine Gebeine (hinein) glühend heiß sind, er sich während seines Schlafes hin- und herwirft, seine Luftröhre ständig verstopft ist, er hustet, immer wieder brennende Hitze im Inneren ("Brennfieber") [*ṣiriḫti ummi libbi*] verspürt, (dann) ist dieser Mensch infolge der (übermäßigen) Sonnenglut überhitzt (wörtl. "ausgebrannt")".

[75] Sources: BAM 2 145:1 [U]D.DA TAB.B[A ..]; 146:29 [. . .]*-ma*. Cf. BAM 146:46, UD.D]A TAB.BA*-ma*.

[76] F. Köcher, in *Uruk. Die Gräber* (= AUWE 10) (1995) 213f.

Stefan Maul gave a translation of a very similar text.[77] We repeat his translation of "ein medizinischer Text aus Assur", describing symptoms of *ṣētu*:

> Wenn ein Mensch sehr ängstlich und nervös ist; wenn seine Augen ständig herumwandern und er unter Erschöpfung leidet; wenn seine Körpertemperatur nicht hoch ist, er aber häufig hustet, und während sein Inneres immer mehr drückt, Speichel zu fliessen beginnt; wenn seine Gedärme von der 'Durchfall-Krankheit' schmerzen und er an Durchfall leidet; wenn aussen sein Fleisch kalt ist während darunter seine Knochen vor Hitze brennen; wenn er aufgibt zu versuchen, sich schlafen zu legen, und während sich seine Luftröhre verstopft, er nach Atem schnappt und er 'Feuer-Brennen' oder 'Brennen des Inneren' an vielen Stellen hat—dieser Mann ist von dem *ṣētu*-Fieber befallen.

BAM 1 66

The *obverse* of this tablet gives a chronic disease, followed by prescriptions "in order that his illness does not last long" (*ana* GIG-*šu* NU GÍD.DA). We now have a parallel to the first lines of this text, the beginning of Chapter XXXI of the Diagnostic Handbook. Only a few lines have been published. Thanks to this new text we know that the disease is sun-heat; read: "If a man, sun-heat has inflamed him".[78] After this basic symptom follow additional symptoms occurring on the same day, and the prospects are given: "That man will be ill 3 days; in order that his illness does not last long, you shall (. . .)"; thus the Diagnostic Handbook. This Chapter XXXI, N. Heeßel, *Babylonisch-assyrische Diagnostik* (2000) 342–352, is most informative about sun-heat.

We now turn to BAM 66, sometimes supplementing it by the abstract of the diagnostic text.

> "[If a man, sun-heat has inflamed] him, he is cold on the same day: that man will be ill *3 days*; in order that his illness does not last long, you shall (. . .)" (BAM 66:1 and Ch. XXXI:1)
>
> "If ditto, blood in his nose has begun to flow on that same day: that man will be ill *25 days* (BAM: "*15 days*"); in order that his illness does not last long, you shall (. . .)" (BAM 66:7 and Ch. XXXI:9).

---

[77] Stefan M. Maul in *Ruperto Carola, Forschungsmagazin der Universität Heidelberg* 1/97 (1997), p. 18a.

[78] I. L. Finkel, *JCS* 46 (1994) 88b. Finkel gives two selected passages in transliteration. It looks as if his XXXI:1–2 = BAM 66:1–3, [XXXI:3–6 = BAM 66:4–6], XXXI:9–11 = BAM 66:7–9, XXXI:12–14 = BAM 66:10–12.—Nils Heeßel discovered that BAM 4 416 is the middle part of this Chapter XXXI.

"If a man, ditto, [. . . has no swea]t (?): that man will be ill *one month*; in order that his illness does not last long, you shall (. . .)" (BAM 66:10).

"If a man, ditto, his temples [. . . stand] up (?): that man will be ill *6 days*; in order that his illness does not last long, you shall (. . .)" (BAM 66:13).

"If a man, ditto, he is the one day ill, the other day healthy: that man will be ill *50 days*; in order that his illness does not last long, you shall (. . .)" (BAM 66:17)

"If a man, ditto, he has a flaring-up fever, *li'bu* [written KA-*'ba*], he drinks water a lot and (*u*) he [. . .] a lot, [that man] will be ill [*?? days*]; in order that his illness does not last long, you shall (. . .)" (BAM 66:21).

"If a man, ditto, always has a lot of sweat, the sweat like ..[. . .] water [. . .] is always dripping: a disease *that does not go away* has sei[zed] that man,[79] [it is overwhelming him; in order that his illness does not last long], you shall [. . .] diluted beer" (BAM 66:24). This is the end of the obverse of BAM 1 66 and an unknown number of lines is now lost.

A line at the beginning of another text, BAM 4 416, duplicates the case just discussed (BAM 66:24–28, dupl. BAM 4 416:4–7). Nils Heeßel has seen that this text is the middle part of Chapter XXXI of the Diagnostic Handbook; it continues the unpublished manuscript mentioned above. Our BAM 66 runs parallel to it.

BAM 4 416

"If, ditto, he always has a lot of sweat: that man [will be ill *??*] *day*[*s*], in order that his illness does not last long" (BAM 416:8–9).

"If, ditto, his face, like one who has drunk beer, [has] s[weat] a lot, [is . . ., . . .] ill: that man will be ill *21 days*; in order that his ill[ness does not last long]" (BAM 416:10–11).

"If, ditto, boils (*bubu'tu*) which like *ašû* [. . .], in order that his illness does not last long" (BAM 416 rev. 1–2).

"If, ditto, boils (*bubu'tu*) which like *ašû* . . . [. . .], in order that his illness does not last long" (BAM 416 rev. 3–4).

"If sun-heat has inflamed him, and his skin becomes red (*rašû*), and he scrat[ches himself . . .]: in order that his illness does not last long" (BAM 416 rev. 5–6).

"If, ditto, it overwhelms him *every day at a certain time*, [. . .], when it overwhelms him, [he gets (?)] a flaring-up fever, [his muscles hurt him], sweat falls upon him, and he comes to rest (*nâḫu*): that man [will be ill] 21 days; [in order that his illness does not last long]" (BAM 416

[79] GIG NU ZI DI[B-*su*]; restoration based on BAM 5 482 III 62–63.

rev. 8–10).[80] Nils Heeßel pointed out to me that this passage has a parallel elsewhere in the Diagnostic Handbook.[81]

Here ends this text BAM 4 416. We now return to BAM 66, *reverse*. The beginning is broken. Then:

"If a man, ditto, all kinds of [. . .]; in order that [his illness] does not last long, you shall (. . .)" (BAM 66 rev. 2).

Here follows a double ruling with the mark MAN, indicating the end of a "chapter".[82]

The following line must be an extract from a different text. One may say that what preceeded was taken from the Diagnostic Handbook, giving the prospects of sun-heat (length of disease) and adding a prescription. Now comes a section from a Therapeutic Handbook which gives no more than recipes for treating sun-heat. We indeed know that a chapter in that handbook began with this same line.[83] We are more interested in the concomitant symptoms. Note that now no more talk is of being "inflamed" by sun-heat, but of being "overcome" by sun-heat.

Text: BAM 66 rev. 4ff., dupl. AMT 14,7:1ff., dupl. AMT 45,1.

"If a man has been overcome by sun-heat, is ill of the standing up of the (veins on the) temples, it is difficult for him in . . . (LAM)" (BAM 66 rev.4, with catchline BAM 6 578 IV 47).

"If a man, ditto, has fever" (66 rev. 6, dupl. AMT 14,7:3; BAM 2 174:21).

"If a man, ditto, does not taste (var. accept) bread or beer" (66 rev. 8; var. BAM 2 174:23).

"If a man, ditto, cold (*ku-ṣú*), cold shivers (*ḫurbašu*) repeatedly fall upon him" (66 rev. 10).

"If a man, ditto, has fever, panic (?) (*ḫa-tu*) repeatedly falls upon him" (66 rev. 12).

"If a man, ditto, inflammation by sun-heat, all kinds of it" (66 rev. 14).

"If a man, ditto" (66 rev. 14)[84]

---

[80] We discussed some aspects of this passage and a parallel above, under *ummu* 2, b, 2, "Flaring-up fever", under BAM 2 174 rev. 29–31.

[81] TDP 154 rev. 15–16; dupl. SBTU II 181 no. 44 rev. 8 (Chapter XVI). That text has NE-*ma* (Labat: *ila'ib-ma*) instead of "[he gets (?)] a flaring-up fever". The diagnosis is *ḫajatti ṣēti*.

[82] M. Stol, NABU 1996/73.

[83] AMT 14,7:1–2; fully preserved in the catch-line in BAM 6 578 IV 47. Note that this catch-line has the unusual *ana* TI.BI instead of *ana* TI-*šú*, exactly as our BAM 66 rev. 10, 12, etc. does.

[84] Line 17 is largely lost. At the end of line 18 [. . .] GIG ma na šú *ṣi-na-aḫ-tu-ra*.

The plant *apruša* more than once is prescribed as the first one (rev. 6, 14) (cf. *ap-šur* in AMT 45,1). We find this plant in the pharmacological handbook as effective against fever.

2. *Isolated Passages about Sun-heat*

We have studied the few texts that discuss sun-heat in a systematic manner. We will now list descriptions of sun-heat scattered over other texts. We begin with the Diagnostic Handbook. As indicated above, its Tablet ("Chapter") XXXI has being "inflamed by sun-heat" as its theme by N. Heeßel (2000).

2.a. *In the Diagnostic Handbook* (*TDP*)

Tablet IX

> "If his face is full of *birdu*-marks: hand of his god; he will live. Ditto: he is inflamed by sun-heat (UD.DA TAB.BA): hand of the god of his father" (TDP 76:50). This text shows again that sun-heat can manifest itself on the skin.

Tablet XIV

> "If his urine is green/yellow, his disease will last long, ditto (= Hand because of his god?), he is inflamed by sun-heat (UD.DA TAB-*iṭ*); he will die" (TDP 136:40).

Tablet XVI

> "If he is ill 1 day, and his head hurts him: he is inflamed by sun-heat (UD.DA TAB.BA); the hand of the god of his father; he will die" (TDP 186:1, dupl. SBTU I 37:1).
>
> "If a man is ill 5 days, and on day 6 blood flows from his nose: his illness will be loosened; inflammation by sun-heat" (TDP 150:40).[85]
>
> "If he is 5 days, 10 days ill of a serious disease, and (GIG *danna* GIG-*ma*) he has diarrhoea (??) (*uštardima*), and blood flows constantly, 5 days, from his nose, and (*u*) it is stopped: his disease will be loosened; he is inflamed by sun-heat; he lives (UD.DA *ḫa-miṭ ba-liṭ* [?])" (TDP 150:44–45).[86]

---

[85] See J. V. Kinnier Wilson, *Journal of the Royal Society of Medicine* 89 (1996) 136b. I cannot believe in haemoptysis. Blood "flows" (*alāku*) from the nose and is ejected (*šalû, nadû*) from the mouth. Cuneiform writing does not distinguish between mouth and nose (both are written with the sign KA).

[86] AHw has a different rendering for *uštardi*, "(wenn der Kranke) weiterhin (krank) bleibt" (also in lines 42, 46, 47) AHw 968a *redû* Št², 2); also in M. Stol, *Epilepsy* 58:6, 8; SBTU I 46 no. 37:28, 29. *CAD* R 244 (15.): "to persist, to drag on".

"If it overwhelms and releases him every day at a certain moment, when it overwhelms him he is hot, and (NE-*ma*) his muscles hurt him, sweat falls upon him, and he comes to rest: a fit caused by sun-heat (LÁ-*ti* UD.DA)" (TDP 154:15–16).

"If he is ill many days, and red liquid flows from his anus: his illness will be loosened; he is inflamed by sun-heat (UD.DA TAB-*ma*), and he will live" (TDP 154:17–18, dupl. SBTU II 181 no. 44 Rs. 9).

Tablet XVII

"If he is ill all day, and is healthy at night: sun-heat (is) his disease" (TDP 164:74). The idea behind this line seem to be that the sun shines during the day and affects him only then.[87]

"If he is healthy all day, and at night he is ill: sun-heat (is) his disease; 27 days; hand of Ninurta" (TDP 164:75). "Sun-heat" can also strike at night, but only during the first 27 days of the month and not during the following moonless nights. So it is the moon that strikes. See our note 62.

"If, from the morning until the evening, malaria (?) (*di-ḫu*) begins in his body, and he gets a mild (?) illness (*sil'itu*) of the belly, his intestine stand(s) up, he belches (= throws up?) through the mouth, he vacates through the anus: a touch by sun-heat (TAG-*ti* UD.DA) which is not joined to his limbs. His disease (is) a mild (?) illness of 1 day" (TDP 168:100–103).

Tablet XVIII

"[If. . .] seizes him repeatedly: his illness is the illness of sun-heat (GIG-*su* GIG UD.DA)" (TDP 172 rev. 6). Lines on calculus follow, *muruṣ ṣēti* only appears here.

Tablet XXIII

"If he is ill, [and . . .] vomits gall, he is inflamed by sun-heat (UD.DA TAB.BA); the hand of the god of his father" (TDP 174:1).[88] Hand of Oath follows in line 2.

Tablet XXXI

"If sun-heat has inflamed him, and". The first line of this "chapter", according to the ancient catalogue.[89] The text remains largely unpublished. We discussed some lines in our survey of BAM 66.

---

[87] *Hippocratic Writings* (Penguin Classics) (1978) 100, *Epid.* I 24: "Nocturnal fever is not especially fatal but it is long drawn out. Diurnal fever is longer still and sometimes leads to consumption".

[88] With TDP 186:29, Planche XLVII, colophon; see H. Hunger, *ZA* 65 (1975) 64.

[89] I. L. Finkel, *Studies A. Sachs* (1989) 147 A 38 B 5'. BAM 4 416 is a published manuscript.

Pro memoria: *kiṣṣat ṣēti* in TDP 130:31, etc.; see below.

From an earlier version of the Diagnostic Handbook:
"If a sick man, his flesh is green/yellow all the time, the head [. . .]: that man, in his passing the sun-heat (??) (UD.DA *ina e-te-qí-šu*), if you make him drink beer [. . .]" (R. Labat, *Syria* 33 (1956) 124:13–14).

[. . .ṣ]*e-e-ti*, STT 1 89:211, with Stol, *Epilepsy* 98.

2.b. In the therapeutic texts

We now turn to passages in the therapeutic texts and we follow the body from head to feet.

"If the skull of a man is inflamed by sun-heat, and his eyes . . . (*barāru*)" (BAM 1 3 I 20, dupl. 480 II 19).

"[If the sk]ull [of a man] is inflamed by sun-heat, a[nd . . . his eyes are] . . . and (*ù*) are full of blood [. . .]" (BAM 5 480 II 21).

"[If the he]ad [of a man] is inflamed by sun-heat, and also (*-ma u*) his body hurts (*akālu*) him, his head is 'blown' (*nuppuḫ*) (BAM 5 480 III 17, dupl. 481:6).

"8 drugs, *ṭēpu*, if the eyes of a man are inflamed by sun-heat and (*u*) [are] . . .[..] (*ḫar*(?)- [..]", BAM 6 515 I 9.[90]

"If the eyes of a man do not see: That man is inflamed by sun-heat" (BAM 6 516 II 6).

"[If the he]ad of a man is inflamed by sun-heat, and the hair of his skull thins out [..]" (BAM 1 9:23). Duplicate has "hot" / "fever" instead of sun-heat: "If the he]ad of a man is hot, and the hair of his skull thins out: in order to [tear out] the fever of [his] head" (BAM 5 480 III 22).

"If a man has been overcome by sun-heat, [he is ill of standing up (veins on the) temple [SAG.KI], in . . . it is difficult for him]", AMT 14,7:1, dupl. BAM 1 66 Rs. 4.[91]

"If the breathing through the nose of a man is heavy: [he is ill of] *ṣinnaḫtiru*, inflammation by sun-heat (*ḫi-miṭ* UD.[DA])" (SBTU I 44:1); cf. sun-heat with *ṣi-na-aḫ-tu-ra* in BAM 1 66 rev. 18 (note 84).

[90] "To be inflamed" said of eyes, in an Old Babylonian letter: "My eyes were inflamed (*ittaḫmaṭā*) by continuous weeping" (AbB 13 175:14). Neo-Assyrian "He holds a fever in his eyes (*ḫunṭu* [*ina libbi ē*]*nāte uktil*)", SAA X 328:17–18; also in SAA X 243:5–6.

[91] This is the first line of a new tablet, "chapter", following the chapter on gall diseases. There our line is the catch-line, fully preserved (BAM 6 578 IV 47).

["If] the upper belly [of a man], his shoulders (?) hurt him, he coughs (*ganāḫu*): That man is ill of the lungs, he has been overcome by sun-heat" (BAM 6 564 II 14–15).

"[If] the chest [of a ma]n, his upper belly (!), his shoulders hurt him: [That man] has been overcome by sun-heat. If he coughs, he is ill [of the lung]s" (CTN IV 114:7–9).

"If a man has fever of the belly (NE ŠÀ) all the time, he has been overcome by sun-heat" (BAM 6 579 I 30).

"[If a man . . . to]gether with his spittle he throws (up) blood all the time: he is ill of 'belly knot' (*kiṣirte* ŠÀ); he has been overcome by sun-heat; his belly is ill of the interior (ŠÀ-*šú qer-bé-nam* GIG)" (BAM 6 575 IV 11). Six therapies follow. Much simpler is the next disease: "If a man throws up blood together with his spittle all the time, that man is ill of *ta-áš-ni-qa*" (IV 34).

"[If . . . his urine is] like the juice of cuscuta (*kasû*): that man has been con[quered] by sun-heat" (BAM 2 114:5).

"If the a man is weakened (?) (*unnut*) by *šāšitānu* and (*u*) repeatedly has an erection (*tebû*), his bladder is pressed: That man has been overcome by sun-heat" (BAM 1 111 II 15–17 [UD.DA KUR-*id*]; dupl. 159 I 15–16 [UD.DA DI.DI], cf. 396 I 14; CAD Š/2 172b).

"If the penis of a man is hot [. . .] He has been overcome by sun-heat" (BAM 1 112 II 6–7). The next cases say that the penis is blasted with wind (DIŠ NA GÌŠ-*šú* IM *iš-biṭ* [..], II 8–14).

"If a man has diminished (in strength) to go to a woman, either by old age, or by 'staff', or by inflammation by sun-heat, or by *niḫis narkabti*: in order to make him acquire potency so that (*-ma*) he goes to a woman" (AMT 88,3:1–3).[92]

Difficult:

DIŠ / *ana* UD.DA UGU BAD (?) [GI]G (?), BAM 3 316 IV 20 (after belly diseases). Dupl. BAM 318 III 32 seems to offer UGU BAD GIŠ GIG.

DIŠ / *ana* UD.DA UGU MAN ma (?) GIG, BAM 318 III 30.

As apodosis in liver omina: GIG.BI GIG-*uṣ* UD.DA GIG TI-*uṭ*, CT 31 36 rev. 14, with J. Nougayrol, *Semitica* 6 (1956) 14, "ce malade est atteint d'une fièvre oscillante: il guérira". Elsewhere: [G]IG UD.DA

[92] With R. D. Biggs, TCS 2 (1967) 52b; dupl. LKA 96 rev. 10–11 with Biggs, 62b.

GIG NA.BI ZI.GA, BAM 5 503 III 64 (an apodosis from liver omina and unusual in medical texts; M. Stol, *JEOL* 32 57).

3. *Some Aspects of Sun-heat*

3.a. One can be "full" of sun-heat:

"If the head of a man is full of 'wounds' [. . . .] he is full of inflammation by sun-heat" (AMT 105,1:26, catch-line)

"If the innards of a man are full of accumulation of wind and sun-heat" (BAM 1 52:72; 4 403 Rs. 7, catch-line)

"His belly is full of 'wounds': he has been overcome by sun-heat" (BAM 575 I 21, dupl. 52:63–4)

3.b. Sun-heat together with other diseases:

With "blast of wind".—"Inflammation by sun-heat" is often mentioned in one breath with the disease "blast of wind" (*šibiṭ šāri*).[93] The catch-line of a therapeutic text on sun-heat shows that the following tablet begins with "If a wind has blasted a man" (BAM 2 146:56). Both are found together in bilingual and lexical texts.[94] In the Diagnostic Handbook, the chapters on both follow each other (XXXI and XXXII). Köcher identifies this "blast of wind" as "Windpocken (Varizellen)".[95]

Within a group—There is one stock phrase in therapeutic texts summing up a group of the following diseases: inflammation by sun-heat, blast of wind, two kinds of paralysis (is one of them numbness?), a muscle disease (*šaššaṭu*), "hand of a ghost", "hand of an oath", sorcery, rectal disease, and "all kinds of illness".[96] Is this a standard list of all possible diseases?[97] The treatment is always rectal: either a clysma (*marḫaṣu*) is used, or the medication is "poured on his anus". Is it this treatment that unites them?[98]

---

[93] CT 51 142:12; BAM 6 579 II 54; IM 67692:261 = CTN IV 63 V 2–3, cited CAD Š/2 389a, (c).

[94] Sumerian ud.da tab im.ri.a = *ḫi-miṭ ṣe-e-ti* [*ši-biṭ ša-ri*], KAR 24 Rs. 22 with Ebeling, *AfO* 16 (1952–53) 297. Both in Antagal E 16–17 (MSL 17 [1985] 209; note that RA-*ti* Adad precedes here; the three also in the *tamītu* IM 67692 = CTN IV 63 V 2–3 cited in CAD Š/2 389a, (c).

[95] F. Köcher, in *Uruk. Die Gräber* (= AUWE 10) (1995) 214.

[96] See BAM 4 409 Rs. 23–24 with the modern translation by Köcher, *AUWE* 10 (1995) 210.

[97] M. Stol, *JEOL* 32 (1991–92) 49.

[98] Complete list of references for this group: 1. Clysma: BAM 2 189 I 6–12;

There is one medical text unique in naming the "surgeon" (*asû*) as the acting healer. He is given advice for treating . . ., muscle disease, loosening all diseases, paralysis, [blast] of wind, swollenness, fever (*ummu*), jaundice, inflammation by sun-heat, . . . (BAM 2 171:62, *ana ḫi-mì-iṭ* UD.DA *ka-liš-ma*).

3.c. Change of the disease

Sun-heat can "turn into" another ailment: "If sun-heat inflames a man and it turns into oath for him" (BAM 2 174 Rs. 25). We have seen that sun-heat, after a long time, can be(come) hand of ghost and that this change means that the disease becomes chronic.[99] The diagnosis "hand of ghost, sun-heat" can mean that this hand originates from sun-heat (TDP 192:34). Stol, *Epilepsy* 80f., explained this "hand of ghost, sun-heat" as the ghost of a man who had died through sun-heat, a real possibility in view of these words in another text, "or a ghost who has died through *ḫi-mi-i*[*ṭ ṣe*]*-ti*" (LKA 84:27). According to a unique late text, dated to the Seleucid period, "inflammation by sun-heat" originates in the stomach (*karšu*), (*napḫar*[?] *murṣu*) (SBTU I 43:19).

4. *Types of Sun-heat*

There are types of sun-heat. One text indeed speaks of "all (kinds of) sun-heat", UD.DA DÙ.A.BI (BAM 66 Rs. 14).

1. Best known is "inflammation by sun-heat" (*ḫimiṭ ṣēti*). Köcher seems to take this literally in translating *ṣēta ḫamiṭ* as "jemand (der) infolge der Sonnenglut überhitzt ist (wörtl. 'ausgebrannt ist')".[100] This word must have belonged to everyday language and is found already in Old Babylonian letters from Mari. We hear of "plants for *ḫi-*[*mi-iṭ*] *ṣé-e-tim*".[101] In other Mari letters, we see simple *ṣētum*. In one case, it seems to be a skin disease: "He is ill; under his ear a *ṣētum* has come out (*waṣûm*)"; the letter names this "a wound" (*simmum*).[102]

228:14–16; 229:9–11; 2. Pouring on anus, "1, 2, 3 times": BAM 1 52:36–37; 68:1–3; 2 168:18–19; 3 216:26–28; 3. Clysma and Pouring: BAM 3 226:7–11, with D. Goltz, *Studien zur altorientalischen und griechischen Heilkunde* (1974) 329f.; BAM 4 409 rev. 23–24. 4. Treatment broken off: BAM 1 69:1–9; 6 579 II 54–55, III 18–19.

[99] BAM 52:67; M. Stol, BiOr 54 (1997) 408.

[100] F. Köcher, in *Uruk. Die Gräber* (= AUWE 10) (1995) 213, on BAM 2 145:1.

[101] A. Finet, *AIPHOS* 14 (1957) 134 A. 2216:4, cf. 14f., 18f. (p. 135 note 1: "fièvre éruptive"). Perhaps also in a fragmentary letter: *ṣí-ib-tum* [. . .] *ḫi-mi-*[*iṭ ṣe-tim-ma*], AEM 1/1 299f. no. 136:10–11, summarized on p. 27.

[102] Finet, *AIPHOS* 14 (1957) 131 A. 140:8 = M. Birot, ARM 14 3 (cf. J.-M.

Other examples, less telling, are: "Three days I have been 'standing', and *ṣētum* has inflamed me; I am ill (*ṣētum iḫmuṭanni marṣāku*), I cannot come to my lord", AEM 1/1 563 no. 261:13. "As to me, I have been delayed up till now due to *ṣētu*" (AbB 12 11:6). An Old Babylonian medical text says that a man / his head "is inflamed by sun-heat" (*ṣe-e-tam* / *ṣe-tam ha-mi-iṭ*) (BAM 4 393:23 and rev. 22). To be inflamed by *ṣētu* seems to be the normal expression; so we may perhaps say that *ḫimiṭ ṣētim* = *ṣētum*. "Let my lord take care of his body in sun-heat" (ARM 10 11:12–14). Is it possible that the normal Assyrian word for fever *ḫunṭu* (studied above) is an abbreviation of this Old Babylonian *ḫimiṭ ṣēti*?

We add additional references for the Assyriological specialist.

In an Old Babylonian recipe: A. Cavigneaux, *Iraq* 55 (1993) 104 B 7 (*a-na ḫi-mi-iṭ ṣe-*[*e-tim*]). Bilingual texts offer UD.DA TAB.BA = *ḫimiṭ ṣēti* as a disease; CT 4 3:15 (OB), with A. Falkenstein, LSS NF I (1931) 95, MSL 9 (1967) 106, and R. Borger, BiOr 38 (1981) 629, on CAD M/2 103a. New manuscripts are TIM 9 56, CT 51 182. Fragmentary: *ṣētum* alone in TLB 2 21:24 (. . . *ṣe-e-tim*; OB diagn.), KUB 4 54:1 (BE LÚ *ṣe-e-tam* [. . .]).

In the Middle Babylonian of Ugarit it appears as *ḫa-ma-aṣ ṣe-ti*, *Ugaritica* V 31 no. 17:29 (among other physical problems); cf. the sandhi writing *ḫi-mi-ṣe-tim* (BAM 4 409 rev. 23).

An incantation begins: "He is hot by sun-heat (var. "inflammation by sun-heat") (ÉN *ki-i* UD.DA (var. TAB UD.DA) NE-*em* (var. *e-me-em*), BAM 2 147 Rs. 10, var. K. 2581:13, in K. van der Toorn, *Sin and sanction* Plate I). A commentary says *ḫi-miṭ* UD.DA *libbû imat mūtu imat šipṭu* KIMIN (SBTU I 36:7).

2. Hardly known is *kiṣṣat ṣēti* "gnawing by sun-heat".[103] The verb is *kasāsu*, or *kaṣāṣu*, perhaps "to gnaw". The disease *kissatu* is often associated with *kurartu* "carbuncle".

Durand, AEM 1/1 552).—Hippocrates, *Epid.* I 1, has a famous exposition of an epidemic disease in Thasos. One symptom was "swelling near the ears". M. Grmek devoted a chapter to this disease and diagnosed it as mumps. See Ralph Jackson, *Doctors and Diseases in the Roman Empire* (1988) 23.

[103] G. Wilhelm, *Medizinische Omina aus Ḫattuša in akkadischer Sprache* (= StBoT 36) (1994) 48 D 2:13 *ki-iṣ-ṣa-at ṣe-e-ti.* Also *ki-is-sat* [. . .], TDP 130:31; similar symptoms are diagnosed as *ki-is-sat* (!) UD.D[A], SBTU IV 152:102; according to the copy. Note that the commentary SBTU I 36:6–7 comments on TDP 128:30–31 (read against Hunger *ki-is-sat* U[D.DA]); it makes additional remarks on *ḫimiṭ* UD.DA.

3. *Ḫajjatti ṣēti.* According to some "fit by sun-stroke".[104] In STT 1 89:211, with Stol, *Epilepsy* 98 [. . . *ṣ*]*e-e-ti.*

4. "Mild (?) illness due to sun-heat" (*silʾitašu ša* UD.DA), Sm. 1644:6', cited CAD S 164a, (c).

5. Medicinal plants.

Plants used against "inflammation by sun-heat" (Ú TAB UD.DA) are branch of the tree *lipāru* (BAM 4 379 III 24), the plants *kazallu* (III 37), *laḫagu*, KADP 11 I 5 (Uruanna II 45), *šuqdānu*, [*ṣa*]*ṣumtu*, BAM 5 422 III 1–2; 423 I 7; dupls. CAD Š/3 332–3; also *tu-un*, BAM 4 379 I 27, dupl. CTN IV 195:26 (*tu un* Ú UD.DA *m*[*a* MU.NI).

Ú.LAL, "good for shivering fever (and) inflammation by sun-heat, and . . . ([*ana* .. *š*]*uruppê* TAB UD.DA *u* . . . SIG_5) (BAM 4 379 I 43, dupl. SBTU III 202 no. 106:18). In the short recipe BE 8 133: a stone, this Ú.LAL plant, and "fox grapes", against *ḫi-miṭ* UD.DA.

BAM 4 379 II 15: Plant *amuzennu*, *ana* ŠÀ.ZI.GA *ù* TAB.[. . .] ZI-*ḫi* SIG.

Note as plant name: Ú.BI Ú TAB UD.DA M[U.NI], STT 1 93:110.

BAM 1 1 I 49–58 ("vademecum"), a long list of plants for inflammation by sun-heat (Ú TAB UD.DA): *ṣaṣumtu*, *zē malāḫi*, *aprušа*, leaf of *amurdinnu*, *lipāru*, *ḫašû*, *šūmū*, *ararû*, *šuqdānu*, *pizzer*, *imḫur-lim.*

SBTU I 63:8, 32 plants, processed, "good for inflammation by sun-heat (TAB UD.DA), wind (IM), and kidneys (BIR.ME)".

BAM 1 1 I 42–44:

(42) PA *ašagi* Ú UD.DA
(43) NI.NE (*šūšu* ?) Ú *li-ʾ-bi*
(44) *ku-si-bu* Ú *ḫa-am*-ME (sic)

[104] M. Stol, *Epilepsy in Babylonia* (1993) 43. Written LÁ-*ti ṣēti.* Note that LÁ-*ti* is *naṣmatti* "poultice", in: (twelve drugs) LÁ-*ti ṣe-ti* in BAM 2 177:11–12. See P. Herrero, *Thérapeutique mésopotamienne* (1984) 101 (on top).

BETWEEN MAGIC AND MEDICINE—APROPOS OF AN OLD BABYLONIAN THERAPEUTIC TEXT AGAINST KURĀRUM DISEASE

Nathan Wasserman
The Hebrew University, Jerusalem

Human experience of encountering diseases is often described in bellicose terms. One could, therefore, paraphrase von Clausewitz' dictum on the relation of war and politics and say that medicine is nothing but the continuation of magic through other means. Indeed, the interdependence of magic and medicine in the Ancient World has been profusely emphasized by many scholars,[1] and no further general comments are needed here. I intend therefore in this paper to elaborate some aspects of the interwoven alliance of magic lore and medical texts, and to outline a few delicate contours of the interplay of those genres in the Old Babylonian period. In the next four sections the following topics will be discussed: 1) An analysis of two groups of Old Babylonian medical incantations; 2) The sequential order of diseases enumerated in Old Babylonian incantations and their relation to lexical lists; 3) The thematic correspondence between incantations against diseases and therapeutic texts; 4) Finally, a new Old Babylonian medical text is discussed in some detail.

1

As Table 1 demonstrates, there are nine Old Babylonian incantations dealing specifically with various diseases. Two other texts can be added. The first is a recently published text from Tell Haddad which lists therapeutic procedures against various diseases annotated

[1] See for instance, R. D. Biggs, "Medizin A", *RLA* 7 (1987–1990), 623–629, and "Medicine, Surgery, and Public Health in Ancient Mesopotamia", in: J. M. Sasson fed.). *Civilizations of the Ancient Near East*, Vol. III, 1995. 1911–1924. Cf. recently B. Böck, ""When You Perform the Ritual of 'Rubbing'": On Medicine and Magic in Ancient Mesopotamia", *JNES* 62 (2003), 1–16.

Table 1

Diseases Enumerated in OB Incantations and Related Texts

JCS 9,A/B	*YOS* 11,7	*YOS* 11,8	*Iraq* 55,104*	*YOS* 11,9	*YOS* 11,10**	*RA 88, 161*	*CT* 42,32	*MLVS* 11,2ff	*CT 4,3 and dupls.****
sikkatum[1]	*išātum*[1]	*sikkatum*[1]	*sikkatum*[1]	*sikkatum*[2]		*sikkatum*[1]		*di'um*	gug.gig.-ma=*sinnu*
išāṭum[2]	*sikkatum*[1]	*išātum*[2]		*išātum*[2]		*išātum*[2]		*ašûm*[5]	bu'.bu$_5$. gig.ma.= [. . .]
ašûm[5]		*miqtum*[3]		*miqtum*[3]	*miqtum*[3]	*miqtum*[3]		|	sa.ma.na= *sāmānu*[5]
ziqtum		*šanūdu*[4]	*šanūdu*[4]	*bé-*[*en*!*-nu*!]		*šanādum*[4]	(*Lamaštu*)	(*Lamaštu*)	mur.gig= *muruṣ hašê*
miqtum[3]		*ašûm*[5]	*ašûm*[5]	*šuruppû*[7]	*šuruppû*[7]	*ašûm*[5]	*pāšittu*	*ekketum*	ellag.gig= *muruṣ kalīti*
šanaḍu[4]		*sāmānum*[6]	*sāmānum*[6]	*sāmānum*[6]		*sāmānum*[6]	*ekk(m)tu*	*sikkatu*[1]	šà.gig= *muruṣ libbi*
sāmānum[6]		*epqennu*					*nišik kalbim*	*išāṭum*[2]	igi.sig$_7$.sig$_7$= *amurriqānu*
girgiššu		*šalattinum*					*šinni awīlūtim*	*šanādum*[4]	šà.mah= *esiltu*
ṣennitum/simmu		*girgiššum*	*girgiššum*				|	*šuruppû*[7]	šà.ta.ha.ar. gi$_4$=*ṣimirtu*
simmu matqum/ekketum							(*Kūbum*?)	(*Asakkum*	zú.muš= *pāšittu*
ekketum/nīṭum							*maštum*	& other demons)	kuš.kú.e= *kissatu*

(*continued on next page*)

Table 1 (*cont.*)

JCS 9,A/B	*YOS* 11,7	*YOS* 11,8	*Iraq* 55,104*	*YOS* 11,9	*YOS* 11,10**	*RA 88, 161*	*CT* 42,32	*MLVS* 11,2ff	*CT 4,3 and dupls.****
rištum							*rībum* (?)	*šibbum*	sa.ku.e= *ekketu*
nīṭum/sētum							*ešatum*	*muruṣ libbi*	sa.umbin
									ag.ag= *rišûtu* (x2)
šurppû[7] / *šagbānu*							?	*kīs libbi*	izi.šub.ba= *miqtu*[3] *išātum*[2]
*šagbānu/ša-*WI-*nu*								*di' qaqqadi*	gan.šub. ba=*garābu*
šaššaṭu/šuruppû[7]								*muruṣ zumri*	kak.šub.ba = *sikkatu*[1] (x2)
\ /*epqennu*								*irru ṣapru*	ud.da.táb= *himiṭ ṣēti*
\ /*būšānu*			*būšānum*					*rašbatu libbi*	kuš.bar.ra= *kibbu*
			simum matqum						tab.táb.e.
								dè=*hinṭu*	
			himiṭ ṣētim						gìr.im.šub. ba=*ziqtum*
									sa.sa.ad. nim=*šaššaṭu*
									íb.gig= *maškadum*
									háš.gig= *šanādu*[4]
									sag.gig=*di'u*
									sag.gá.ra=

(*continued on next page*)

Table 1 (*cont.*)

šuruppû[7] sag.[. . .]= *ra'ību* sag.du=*ašuš-* *tum qaqqadi* igi.nigin. ga=*ṣīdānu* [. . .] zag.kár.ra= *li'bu* *Utukku lemnu* *Asakku marṣu* *miqit Bēl ūri* & other demons

* *Iraq* 55. 104—therapeutic text mentioning incs. ** *YOS* 11.10—description of a demon mentioning diseases *** *CT* 4.3—OB sum. inc. with post-OB biling. dupls.

[disease name] **—a disease which makes part of the '*skeleton-list*' with its consecutive no. Cf. infra in table 2.

by magical instructions.[2] The second text, YOS 11, 10, delineates what seem to be the features of a demon, in which a pair of diseases is included. All eleven texts can be divided into two sub-groups according to the list of diseases enumerated in each of them. Some of these, as well as other motifs, will be discussed below.

Both groups represent a rather consistent inventory of diseases arranged along a basic sequence which will be called here the *skeleton-list* (see the diseases surrounded by boxes in Table 1 and summarized in Table 2). The diseases featuring in the first sub-group reappear in the second one, which consists of three incantations. Nonetheless, in the second sub-group other diseases predominate. One patent difference is the appearance of various demons in the second group: *Lamaštu, Asakkum, Muštabbabum, Kūbum, Bēl ūri*, and others. Furthermore, the way the two sub-groups treat the question of *pathogenesis*, the origin of various diseases, is totally different. According to the first group, a long list of diseases has descended from celestial sources.[3] They are said to afflict men and animals alike, an indication which might suggest that at least some of the diseases could be transmitted from sheep or cattle to human beings. Then follows the well known *mannam lušpur* topos[4] with the invocation of the seven and seven Daughters of Anu.[5] Most of these incantations conclude with the same list of diseases enumerated at the beginning.

Celestial allusion is also found in YOS 11, 10, the description of a demon mentioned above. In lines 4'–5' of this text, the heart of the creature described is equated with *miqtum* and *attalûm*. Later on, two other parts of its body are said to be *miqtum* and *šuruppû*.[6] Since

---

[2] A. Cavigneaux and F. Al-Rawi, *Iraq* 55, 104.

[3] *JCS* 9 (1955), 8, text A: 10 *ištu zi/sí-ku-ra-at šamê*, "from the ziqqurat of heaven", or, "from the closed-off regions (?) of heaven" (so W. Farber, *JNES* 49 (1990), 307 with n. 48); *JCS* 9, 10, text B: *ištu ṣerret šamê*, "from the lead-rope or probably better, the teat of heaven"; *YOS* 11,8 (= *JCS* 9, 11, text C): 5 *ištu kakkab* (MUL) *šamê*, "from the star of heaven". The recently published Mari incantation (A. Cavigneaux, *RA* 88, 1994, 155–161: rev. 11') reads: *ina zu-qú-ra-an šamê urdāma*, "des hauteurs du ciel".

[4] Cf. W. Farber, "*Mannam lušpur ana Enkidu*: Some New Thoughts about an Old Motif", *JNES* 49 (1990), 299–321.

[5] The Mari incantation (*RA* 88, 1994, 161: rev. 15') reads ^{d}n[in?-. . .].

[6] [*kitmā?*] 1' [*š*]*a-ap-ta-š*[*u-(ú)*] 2'[*ka?*]*-lu-ú pa-nu-šu-ú* 3'⸢GÚ? ⸣-BI *mi-ra-hu-um* SAG?-*šu-ḫú*⸣ 4'[*m*]*i-iq-tum a-ta-al-lu-u*[*m*](or: -*k*[*u*]) 5'[*l*]*i-ib-ba-š*[*u*]*-ú* 6'⸢KA(xX)⸣-*šu-ú mi-iq-tum* 7'*šu-ru-pu-um bu-da-šu*, "His lips are [enveloped], his face is (covered with) [ye]llow

Table 2

Minimal Sequence of Diseases Enumerated in OB Incantations:
The 'Skeleton-List'

sikkatum[1]
|
išātum[2]
|
miqtum[3]
|
šanādum[4]
|
ašûm[5]
|
sāmānum[6]
|
šuruppû[7]

in the first instance *miqtum* is attached to *attalûm*, "an eclipse", it seems to allude metaphorically to a "falling star". In the second time *miqtum* is connected with *šuruppû*, "shivering", a fact which indicates that this time it is taken literally, as a name of a disease.[7]

The whole issue of astral magic and celestial influence on diseases and remedies is wide and complex and has been treated in depth by E. Reiner,[8] M. Stol[9] and others. It will suffice here to comment briefly on one problem, that is, the question of the exact nature of the meteorological phenomenon which, I submit, could be held by the Babylonians as the origin of various diseases.

paste(?). His [*ne*]*ck*(?) is a little snake, a 'falling star', an 'eclipse' are his [h]eart, his . . . is a *miqtum*-disease, shivering is his shoulders". Restorations after *CT* 51, 142:16ff., a partial duplicate of *YOS* 11, 10. For the var. *mi-ra-hu-um* instead of *nīrahum*, *CAD* N/2, 259^{b}. References courtesy I. L. Finkel.

7 Observations of falling stars during lunar or solar eclipses are known from some passages from *Enūma Anu Enlil*. Most of them predict different ruinous results but, admittedly, not diseases; Cf. Ch. Virolleaud, *L'Astrologie chaldéene* (= *ACh.*), 1905–1912, Sin 27, 24; *ACh.*, Sin 28, 11; *ACh.*, Supp., 2, 21, 5, col. ii; *ACh.*, Sin, 28, 18; *ACh.*, Supp]., 22, 13; *ACh.*, Suppl., 2, 29, 15. See further, J. Kingston Bjorkman, *Meteors and Meteorites in the Ancient Near East*, Center for Meteorite Studies, Arizona State University, 1973, 100.

8 *Astral Magic in Babylonia*, Philadelphia, 1995, 59.

9 *Epilepsy*, 12–14.

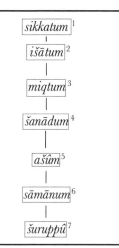

The simplest, almost self-evident explanation for the account of maladies descending from the skies—if not taken as entirely metaphorically—seems to be an impressive nocturnal shower of bolides and shooting stars which hit the ground and ignite fires. Rendering the relevant incantations as literally as possible, one may find that their whole setting bears the physical consequences of falling meteoric fireballs. Pertinent to this proposition is the comment of *YOS* 11, 8: 5–6: "from the star of heaven they (the diseases) have come down, here the earth has received them"—a possible indication that some kind of a celestial object has hit the ground. Note further the burning effects from which lambs and babies suffer, and the call in *YOS* 11, 8: 7–8 to the *girgiššum*-disease not to sojourn on earth but to return to heaven in the form of smoke and fog. And finally, if this suggestion holds true, the appeal to the Daughters of Anu to assist the ailing person by sprinkling water, thus extinguishing the inflammatory diseases, could now be understood as yet another indication in the same direction. Indeed, as was already noted,[10] the aid with which this healing team is supplicated consists primarily of an effective capacity to put out fire.

Contrary to the above, the three incantations comprising the second sub-group (*CT* 42, 32, *MLVS* II, 2ff. and *CT* 4, 3) do not concern themselves at all with the question of the aetiology of diseases. In this case maladies and demons seem to be ever-present, and as such must be constantly repulsed by a whole array of gods who are asked to cleanse the sick person, to cast spells and to drive away these nefarious elements. Since in this case the diseases go along with demonic creatures, it is clear that all the Igigi, or Enki and Asarluhi specifically, are summoned directly for this confrontation.

Summing up this point, we could say that since in the first subgroup of incantations the diseases are considered as a concrete natural outcome of an atmospheric phenomenon, the whole setting does not involve personal confrontation between malefactors and benevolent protagonists as in the second sub-group. Hence, the two subgroups belong to two distinct classes (*Gattungen*) of incantations, although some of the diseases they confront are the same.

[10] So already Farber, *JNES* 49, 302.

2

This discussion has considered the differences between the two subgroups of incantations. We may now turn to the sequential order of the diseases listed in them. Table 3 compares various lexical-lists with enumerations of diseases in incantations. The results of this examination are far from being conclusive. One sequence of diseases which clearly reflects a lexical list order is *sāmānu* → . . . *šakbānu* → *šaššaṭu* in *JCS* 9, 9 text A, found also in *Erimhuš* 264–268. Less indicative are a few short chains of diseases which appear in the lexical series but in another order. See, for instance, *šanādu* → . . . *ṣennitu* → . . . *šuruppû* in *JCS* 9, 9 text A, items which can be found in *Izi* E 166–175, or the string *pāšitum* → . . . *ekkimtum* → . . . *nišik kalbim* in *MLVS* II, 2ff. and *CT* 42, 32 which exist in an inverted order in the *OB list of Diseases* (= *MSL* 9, 77ff.:56, 99, 118).

It is hard to asses the value of such data, but it is clear that the order of the diseases enumerated in the incantations does not reflect the order of similar enumerations in lexical lists; or, at least, that the relation of enumerations of diseases in Old Babylonian incantations to different lexical lists is not consistent enough to be considered as significant.

Furthermore, no apparent organizing principle—be it an inner or extra-linguistic combinatory rule—can be found in the sequence of diseases enumerated in the incantations. In all but one case, I could not delineate any such ordering principle: neither a climactic or anticlimactic enumeration—from top to bottom or vice versa—of the afflicted parts of the body,[11] nor any other logical division into, say, inflammatory diseases, skin diseases, and diseases of inner organs. The possible division of perceptive or mental imbalances and somatic maladies was also abandoned, as was the eventual separation according to the prognosis of diseases to lethal and less grave ailments.[12]

[11] For the logical rule *a capite ad calcem* in medical compendia cf. D. Goltz, "Studien zur altorientalischen und griechieschen Heilkunde. Therapie—Arzneibereitung—Rezeptstruktur", *Sudhoffs Archiv. Zeitschrift für Wissenschafisgeschichte Beiheft* 16, Franz Steiner Verlag, Wiesbaden, 1974, 137f., 250 and 306f. For this principle in lexical lists, cf. Finkel and Civil, *MSL* 16, 1982, 23.

[12] Note D. Cadeli's remarks on the organizing principles operating in some tablets of the medical series *TDP*, cf. "Lorsque l'enfant paraît . . . malade", in B. Lion et al. (eds.), *Enfance et éducation dans le Proche-orient ancien* (= *Ktema* no. 22), Strasbourg, 1997, 11–33, esp. p. 13 with n. 18.

Table 3

Sequential Comparison of Enumerated Diseases in OB Incantations vs. Different Lexical Lists

<table>
<tr><td><u>JCS 9, A</u></td><td><u>Erimhuš I (MSL 17, 19)</u></td><td></td><td></td></tr>
<tr><td>sāmānu</td><td>264. sāmānu</td><td></td><td></td></tr>
<tr><td>| —</td><td></td><td></td><td></td></tr>
<tr><td>šakbānu</td><td>265. šakbānu</td><td></td><td></td></tr>
<tr><td>| —</td><td></td><td></td><td></td></tr>
<tr><td>šaššaṭu</td><td>268. šaššaṭu</td><td></td><td></td></tr>
<tr><td><u>CT 4, 3</u></td><td><u>Erimhuš I (MSL 17, 19)</u></td><td></td><td></td></tr>
<tr><td>šaššaṭu</td><td>267. ṣīdānu</td><td></td><td></td></tr>
<tr><td>maškadum</td><td>268. šaššaṭu</td><td></td><td></td></tr>
<tr><td>|</td><td></td><td></td><td></td></tr>
<tr><td>ṣīdānu</td><td>269. maškadum</td><td></td><td></td></tr>
<tr><td><u>MLVS II, 2ff. 3</u></td><td><u>Antagal e (MSL 17, 249)</u></td><td><u>CT 4, 3</u></td><td></td></tr>
<tr><td></td><td>4. muruṣ hašê</td><td>muruṣ hašê</td><td></td></tr>
<tr><td>muruṣ libbim</td><td>5. muruṣ libbim</td><td>muruṣ kalīti</td><td></td></tr>
<tr><td>kīs libbim</td><td>6. kīs libbim</td><td>muruṣ libbi</td><td></td></tr>
<tr><td><u>MLVS II, 2ff. / CT 42, 32</u></td><td><u>OB List of Diseases (MSL 9, 77ff.)</u></td><td><u>CT 4, 3</u></td><td></td></tr>
<tr><td>pāšittum</td><td>56. pāšittum</td><td>pāšittum</td><td></td></tr>
<tr><td></td><td></td><td>|</td><td></td></tr>
<tr><td>ekkimtum/ekketum</td><td>118. ekketum</td><td>ekketum</td><td></td></tr>
<tr><td>nišik kalbim (MLVS II, 2ff. Om.)</td><td>99. nišik kalbim</td><td></td><td></td></tr>
<tr><td><u>JCS 9, A/B</u></td><td><u>CT 4, 3</u></td><td><u>Antagal E (MSL 17, 212)</u></td><td></td></tr>
<tr><td>ekketum</td><td>ekketum</td><td>5'. ekketum</td><td></td></tr>
<tr><td>rišī/ūtum</td><td>rišūtum</td><td>6'. rišūtum</td><td></td></tr>
<tr><td><u>JCS 9, A/B</u></td><td><u>Izi E (MSL 13, 188)</u></td><td><u>MLVS II. 2ff.</u></td><td><u>CT 4, 3</u></td></tr>
<tr><td>šanādu</td><td>175. šannadu</td><td>šanādu</td><td>šanādu</td></tr>
<tr><td>|</td><td></td><td></td><td></td></tr>
<tr><td>ṣennitu (B om.)</td><td>166a. ṣennitu</td><td></td><td></td></tr>
<tr><td>šuruppû</td><td>173. šuruppû</td><td>šuruppû</td><td>di'u</td></tr>
<tr><td></td><td>170a–172a. di'u</td><td>di' qaqqadi</td><td>šuruppû</td></tr>
<tr><td><u>JCS 9, A/B</u></td><td><u>SB List of Diseases (MSL 9, 92ff.)</u></td><td></td><td><u>CT 4, 3</u></td></tr>
<tr><td>ziqtum</td><td>214. ziqtum</td><td></td><td>ziqtum</td></tr>
<tr><td>|</td><td></td><td></td><td></td></tr>
<tr><td>šanādu</td><td>78. šanādu</td><td></td><td>šaššaṭu</td></tr>
<tr><td>sāmanu</td><td>216. sāmānu</td><td></td><td>|</td></tr>
<tr><td>nīṭu</td><td>161. nīṭu</td><td></td><td></td></tr>
<tr><td>|</td><td></td><td></td><td></td></tr>
</table>

(*continued on next page*)

Table 3 (*cont.*)

JCS 9, A/B	*SB List of Diseases* (*MSL* 9, 92ff.)	*CT* 4, 3
šaššaṭu	79. *šaššaṭu*	*šanādu*
(B om.)		

YOS 11, 8	*Nigga* (*MSL* 13, 122)	*JCS* 9, A	CT 4, 3
sāmānum	267. *sāmānum*	*sāmānum*	*sāmānum*
│	│	│	
šalattinu	282. *šalatinnu*		
	│		
	266. *šaššaṭum*	*šaššaṭum*	*šaššaṭum*

JCS 9, A	*Kagal* B (*MSL* 13, 236)	*SB List of Diseases* (*MSL* 9, 92ff.)
sāmānum	214. *sam*[*ānum*]	78. *šaššaṭum*
│		
šaššaṭum	215. *šaššaṭum*	216. *sāmānum*

JCS 9, A/B	*Pract.Voc.Assur*	*CT* 4, 3	*Comm. Aa* VIII/2 (*MSL 14, 505*)	*Comm. Aa* II/2, B (*MSL 14, 275*)	*Malku* IV
sāmānu	999. *simmu*	*simmu*			
│	│	│			
simmu	1001. *sāmānu*	*sāmānu*	*simmu*	*epqenum*	66. *epqenum*
│					
šakbānu			= *šakbānu*		
│					
epqenu				= *simmu*	= *simmu*

The reason for this shortcoming might be our insufficient comprehension of the various unidentified diseases. It is possible, however, that an elusive rule based on some aetiological, therapeutic or mytho-magical principle lies behind this order. Some hidden mnemonic technique might also be involved here. A new interpretation of the sequence of diseases in the relevant incantations was advanced by Th. Kämmerer.[13] According to this view, the ailments listed in the incantations do not designate different diseases, but different stages or symptoms of one single disease: pox. Though intriguing and innovative, I find it hard to accept this suggestion. Most of these ailments are well known from many other texts (incantations, therapeutic texts and lexical lists) to be independent diseases, each with its own typical characteristics. I can see, therefore, no reason to consider these lexemes here in a different way. Kämmerer's idea should,

[13] "Die erste Pockendiagnose stammt aus Babylon", *UF* 27 (1995), 129–168.

nevertheless, be taken into future consideration. Applied less sweepingly, it may give an important clue to the reasoning behind some *sections* of such enumerations of diseases.

Restricted as they may be, the results presented above are not futile and some conclusions can be arrived at with their help. An important point pertinent to this discussion is the colophon of *Esagil-kīn-apli* published by I. L. Finkel in *Sachs' Memorial Volume*,[14] which supplies us with a crucial piece of information regarding the editorial process of the medical series SA.GIG. According to the colophon, it was *Esagil-kīn-apli*, the *ummânu* of *Adad-apla-iddina*, a descendant of a long line of sages, who arranged the passages of the series *ištu muhhi adi šēpāti, a capite ad calcem*, thus producing the canonized version of the series. This is *Esagil-kīn-apli*'s own statement, but there is no reason not to take his testimony at face value. Yet this descending order is operative in other, non-medical Old Babylonian literary texts. Thus *Esagil-kīn-apli*'s arrangement of the medical material was not a total editorial innovation, but rather an application of an already known organizing principle to the large body of medical series. It is not impossible that this principle has only replaced a previous constituent order, in most cases not yet detected.

Moreover, the fact that Old Babylonian disease incantations are not aligned by a clear lexical arrangement might indicate that contemporary medical material had developed separately from lexical tradition or, more cautiously, without apparent dependency of the former on the latter. This statement gains further weight once it is recognized that lists of other items enumerated in Old Babylonian incantations, such as snakes, domesticated and wild animals, colours and geographical names, do occasionally follow the order of the lexical series.[15]

Although chains of diseases in Old Babylonian incantations do not show a conspicuous ordering principle, they are by no means erratic. As was previously mentioned, a basic sequence of illnesses, here labelled the *skeleton-list*, can be extracted from the different enumerations (see Table 2). Without committing oneself to over-precise medical identifications, some short remarks will not be out of place. The

[14] I. L. Finkel, "Adad-apla-iddina, Esagil-kīn-apli, and the Series SA.GIG", in: E. Leichty et al. (eds.), *A Scientific Humanist. Studies in Memory of Abraham Sachs*, Philadelphia, 1988, 143–159, esp. 148f.

[15] The relationship between lexical lists and items enumerated in magical texts is too vast to be tackled here. I intend to deal with this subject in a separate study.

first illness in the list is *sikkatum*, which designates a kind of pox or pimples. The fact that this disease is usually listed first and is widely documented (not only in medical texts) should indicate that this was a fairly common disease.[16] Next comes *išātum*, generally meaning "inflammation" or "fever".[17] The next disease of the *skeleton-list* is *miqtum*, a disease whose main symptom is "falling", that is, serious fits or convulsions. This disease designates probably a specific form of epilepsy[18] or hyperthermic convulsions known especially in sick *šnd'* children.[19] As for *šanādum*, still unidentified, the Syriac cognate (ܫܢܕܐ), "torment, torture", offers a possible derivation for the name of this sickness. The following member of the *skeleton-list* is *ašûm*, which is usually found after *šanādum*. It seems to afflict the patient's general perception (head and vision). It remains unclear whether the disease mentioned in a Mari letter (*ARMT* III, 64:11) spelled *ha-šu-um* should be connected to the former disease.[20] As for the *sāmānu* disease, the last component of the *skeleton-list* to be treated here, Kinnier Wilson has recently proposed to identify it as a "fungal skin infection known as *mycetoma*".[21]

---

[16] Cf. the extensive discussion of this disease in Th. Kämmerer, *UF* 27 (1995), 129–168.

[17] Prof. J. Naveh has suggested (private communication) to identify *išātum* as malaria. The latter proposal is supported by the appearance of *šuruppû*, "shivering", at the end of the list. A parallel pair of diseases, אשתה and עריתה, "fire and coldness", is attested in the Babylonian Talmud (*Shabbat* 66b–67a), and in Aramaic amulets and magic bowls (cf. J. Naveh, "A Recently Discovered Palestinian Jewish Aramaic Amulet", in M. Sokoloff (ed.), *Arameans, Aramaic and the Aramaic Literary Tradition*, Ramat Gan, 1983, 83:2; J. Naveh and Sh. Shaked, *Amulets and Magic Bowls*, Jerusalem, 1985, 46:12; Naveh and Shaked, *ibid.*, 50:22. Naveh and Shaked, *Magic Spells and Formulae*, Jerusalem, 1993, 36f. See also J. Naveh, "Illness and Amulets in Antiquity, in: Ofra Rimon (ed.), *Illness and Healing in Ancient Tunes*, University of Haifa, 1996, 26*f.). This proposal should, though, be carefully examined. The fact that in Akkadian texts, unlike in Aramaic, this pair of diseases is not attached merismatically should be counted against it. Furthermore, there is no conclusive evidence that malaria and the mosquitoes which cause it were already present in Mesopotamia at that time. Another identification for malaria which was proposed by *CAD* D, 166 and accepted by some scholars (cf. M. Stol, *Epilepsy*, 38) is *di'um*, for which see also M. Stol in this volume.

[18] Stol, *Epilepsy*, 9.

[19] Cf. D. Cadeli. "Lorsque l'enfant paraît . . . malade" (note 12 above), 23.

[20] For this letter see now, J.-M. Durand, *Les documents épistolaires du palais de Mari* Tome I (= Littératures anciennes du Proche-Orient 16), Éd. du Cerf, Paris, 1997, no. 175. This disease is rendered there by the general term "*indisposition*". See also D. Cadeli, "Lorsque l'enfant paraît . . . malade" (note 12 above), 28, n. 128.

[21] J. V. Kinnier Wilson, "The *sāmānu* disease in Babylonian Medicine", *JNES* 53 (1994), 111–115.

Hence the *skeleton-list* consists of a type of pox, some kind of a fever, epilepsy, *šanādu*-disease, *ašûm*-disease, fungal(?) skin disease and "shivering". The Old Babylonian scribes did not follow it strictly, but this minimal list of ailments can be generally seen at the core of many texts of the period which enumerate diseases. Again, the existence of a rationale behind this order, be it medical, sequential or mnemonic, could not be positively confirmed. In fact, one may argue that the very diversity of this scaled-down list is its *raison d'être*; a kernel of many other possible diseases. Resuming for a moment the issue of interconnections between disease enumerations in incantations and lexical series, it is noteworthy that this minimal list of diseases encapsulated in many incantations has virtually no trace in lexical series.

3

Before examining the thematic contacts between Old Babylonian incantations and medical texts in the Old Babylonian period, one has to keep in mind that only a small number of therapeutic and diagnostic texts are known from the Old Babylonian period.[22] The reason for this paucity of documentation could simply be chance, and/or the fact that another genre, namely incantations, occupied productively this rubric in the mental system of the time. One way or another, one should not forget that a discovery of even a small amount of new material might enlarge or change our understanding by many degrees. A case in point is the *kurārum*-text which is discussed below.

[22] Old Babylonian therapeutic texts known to me are: *YOS* 11, 28; *YOS* 11, 29; *RA* 66, 141–143; *Iraq* 55, 104—all of which combine incantations with therapeutic instructions. *BAM* 393 was unique insofar as it was considered to be the sole example of a large multi-sectioned tablet listing various therapeutic instructions from the Old Babylonian period. Nonetheless, after discussing the matter with I. L. Finkel, it is not impossible that this text is in fact a *Neo* Babylonian archaized copy of an Old Babylonian original. I. L. Finkel has also kindly communicated to me his transliteration of UET 6/3, 895, another Old Babylonian multi-sectioned therapeutic text, which will be published by him together with other medical material from Ur. The sole Old Babylonian example of a diagnostic text which I am aware of is *TLB* II, 21. Note, further, the few Old Babylonian physiognomic texts: Sippar tablet Si. 33 [= Kraus, *AfO Beih* 3, 1939, no. 62, cf., *MVAG* 40/2, 1935, 57]; *YOS* 10, 54; *YOS* 10, 55 and VAT 7525 [= F. Kocher and A. L. Oppenheim, *AfO* 18 (1957/58), 62–77].

With this in mind, the thematic agreement between medical texts and incantations in the Old Babylonian period can now be understood with the help of Table 4. A thematically-corresponding incantation can be attached to many diseases mentioned in therapeutic texts. This relationship in itself is not surprising, yet the degree of correspondence merits our attention. This situation demonstrates the compatibility of the verbal-magical procedures and the practical-therapeutic prescriptions. It remains to be investigated whether such an intimate thematic concurrence can also be found in later, first-millennium sources.

Table 4

Thematic Correspondence between Therapeutic Texts and OB Incantations

Therapeutic Texts	Incantations	Remarks
1. sorcery – *BAM* 393:1–3; rv. 13–14	*PBS* 1/2, 122	
2. scorpion-bite- *BAM* 393:19–20	*YOS* 1.1; *YOS* 11, 4:11–22: *RA* 66,141(?); *RA* 88, 155–6	*RA* 141: inc. followed by therap. instructions.
3. dog-bite- *BAM* 393: rv 5–8	*CT* 42, 32:10; *OECT* 11,4; *ZA* 71,62: rv. 13–19; *VS* 17,8; *Studies Pope*, 85; *ZA* 75, 182; *TIM* 9,73; *OBTI* 302; BM 79938 (unpubl.)	more unpubl. incs. in Mari. Rabies mentioned in OB letters, LE § 56/7
4. *awurriqānum* (jaundice) *BAM* 393:4–7	– *UET* 5,85; *YOS* 11,14:7–12; *CT* 4, 3:10	
5. toothache (tooth-worm) – *BAM* 393:8–13: rv. 9–10; rv. 9–10; *YOS* 11, 29: 19–22	*CT* 42, 32:10; *YOS* 11,4: 1–10; *YOS* 11,12:31–7	*YOS* 11.4: inc. followed by therap.
6. headache (unspecific) – *BAM* 393: rv. 2–4	*BiOr* 18,71:22 (*di'um*)	
7. *sītum* (infection/sunstroke)	*JCS* 9,10 B:6 letters	passim in OB
– *BAM* 393:23–26; *Iraq* 55, 104 B:7'–9'. *BAM* 393: rv. 22–25: head-fever and *YOS* 11, 28:1–2: mouth-fever.	*JCS* 9,10 B:6	passim in OB letters

(continued on next page)

Table 4 (*cont.*)

Therapeutic Texts	Incantations	Remarks
8. *libbim* (internal disease) – *BAM* 393:27–28; rv. 11–12; rv. 26–27	*BiOr* 18,71:20–21; *VS* 17,9	
9. *sikkatum* (pox / pimples) – *Iraq* 55, 104 A: [broken]	*JCS* 9, 9 A:1,21; *JCS* 9, 10 B:1, 19; *YOS* 11, 7:3; *YOS* 11, 8:1, 14; *YOS* 11, 9:1; *BiOr* 18, 71:13; *RA* 88, 161:10'	
10. *ašûm*- *Iraq* 55, 104 A: 4'–6'	*JCS* 9, 9 A:2, 23; *JCS* 9, 10 B: 2; *YOS* 11, 8:2; *BiOr* 18, 71:6; *RA* 88, 161:10'	
11. *miqtum* (epilepsy) – *YOS* 11, 29:1–7	*JCS* 9, 9 A:3, 23; *JCS* 9, 10 B:2, 20; *YOS* 11,8:1.14; (*YOS* 11, 10:6'); *YOS* 11, 9:1; *RA* 88, 161:10'	
12. *šanādum*- *Iraq* 55, 104 A:3'–6'	(*JCS* 9,9 A:4); *JCS* 9, 10 B:3; *YOS* 11,8:1, 14; *BiOr* 18, 71:14; *RA* 88, 161:10'	
13. *sāmānum* (myctome, fungi) – *Iraq* 55, 104 A:7'–8'	*JCS* 9,9 A:4; *JCS* 9, 10 B:3; *YOS* 11,8:2,15; *YOS* 11, 9:2,9,12.16; *RA* 88, 161:10'	
14. *girgiššum* (skin disease) – *BAM* 393:14–18; *Iraq* 55, 104: B 1'–2'; *UET* 6/3,895: 27–30	*JCS* 9, 9 A:5. 25; *JCS* 9,10 B:4, 22; *YOS* 11,8:4,7,17	
15. *simmum* (/*matqum*) – *Iraq* 55. 104 B:4–6'; *UET* 6/3,895: 39–41	*JCS* 9, 8 A:6; *JCS* 9, 10 B:4	passim in OB letters, CH §§ 215, 218
16. *būšānum* (scurvy?) – *Iraq* 55. 104 B: 3'	*JCS* 9, 10 B:9	
17. Eye disease- *BAM* 393:21–22	*YOS* 11,5:1–8 (eye-worm); *JNES* 14, 15A (*merhum* – ergot)	eye surgery mentioned in CH §§215, 218

(*continued on next page*)

Table 4 (*cont.*)

Therapeutic Texts	Incantations	Remarks
18. *sagbānum*- *UET* 6/3,895: 14–26	*JCS* 9,9 A:8; *JCS* 9, 10B:7	
19. -/-	*maškadum* *YOS* 11, 14; A 633 (unpubl.)	
20. *baskiltum* (haemorrhoids?) *YOS* 11, 28:3–6: *YOS* 11,29:8–11	-/-	
21. *kurārum* (ringworm, fungi) – *RA* 90, 00:0	-/-	
22. *kullārum* – *UET* 6/3,895: 1–4	-/-	
23. *garāštum* – *UET* 6/3,895: 5–9	-/-	
24, *pûm bašlum* (burnt mouth?) *UET* 6/3,895: 10–13	-/-	cf. no. 7 (*YOS* 11, 28:1–2)
25. *dalihtum ša* ZA-AB *-ri-im-* *UET* 6/3,895: 22–26	-/-	
26. *serretum* – *UET* 6/3,895: 31–34	-/-	
27. foot disease – *BAM* 393: rv. 19–21	-/-	passim in OB letters. CH §221
28. anal disease – *BAM* 393: rv. 15–18	-/-	

4

At this point, it seems appropriate to introduce to the discussion the Old Babylonian therapeutic text against the *kurārum*-disease.[23] Since its publication I had the opportunity to collate the text once again with M. J. Geller, and to benefit from helpful comments from other colleagues. Here follows an improved edition and translation of this text. Some unsolved problems remain.

87.56.847

Obv.

1 [*šum-ma*] ⸢*a*⸣-⸢*wi*⸣-⸢*lum*⸣ ⸢peš⸣./gíg
2 ⸢gig$^{?}$⸣-⸢*ru*⸣ -⸢*uṣ*⸣
3 geštin-bil-lá° *ši-mi-ta-am*$^{!?}$
4 *ši-zi-ib a-ta-ni-*⸢*im*$^{?}$⸣
5 *ù mu-sú-uk-ka-tim*
6 *i-na* ^{na4}bur *i-li-ip-pí*
7 ì-eren ì-giš ì-sag
8 *ù* NA$_4$°-HAL *a-na li-ib-bi-im*
9 *i-na-ad-di-i-ma*

Rev.

10 21 *ha-aṣ-ba-a-tim*
11 ⸢*ú*°-*ša*⸣-*ap*°-*pa*°(over erasure)-*at*°-*ma*°
12 *i-na mu-uh-hi-im i-ša-ak-ka-am-ma*
13 síg gi$_6$ *a-na i-ša-a-tim*
14 *i-ša-ar-ra-*^{ap}*-am-ma*
15 *ù ša-ra-*⸢*at i*⸣*-me-ri-im*
16 *ša ku-ra-ra-am mar-ṣú*
17 *i-ša-ar-*<*ra*>*-am-ma*
18 *qá-aq-qá-ra-am*$^{!}$(Text: GA) *ú-ul i-la-ap-/pa-at*
19 *šu-ta-ak-ti-im*
20 [*ki*]-⸢*ma*⸣ *i-ga-am-ma-ru*
21 [*ša*$^{?}$*-am*$^{?}$]*-na pa-ni-ka ta-pa-aš-ša-/aš-ma*
22 [gig? *ul*?] ⸢*i*⸣*-tu-ur-ra-ku-ma*

---

[23] N. Wasserman, "An Old Babylonian Medical Text Against the *Kurārum* Disease", *RA* 90 (1996), 1–5; for copy and photos see *RA* 91 (1997), 31–32.

[1][If a m]an [is affected with *kur*]*ārum*; [6]he (= the healer?) will *mix*(?) [3]vinegar, *beetroot*, [4]milk of a she-ass and of an impure- woman [6]in a stone bowl, [9](and) pour [7]cedar oil, (regular) oil, fine oil [8]and . . ., [11](and) he will shatter [10]21 shreds [12](and) place them (as plaster) on the head. [14](Then) he will (throw and) burn [13]black wool into the fire, [16](and) the one who is affected with *kurārum* [17]will (also throw and) burn [15]hair of a donkey. [18]He (= the patient) will not touch the ground. [19]Cover (yourself) well. [20][As] soon as he (= the patient) finishes [21]you should rub your face so that [22][the sickness will not] return to you.

Some short philological notes are required here.

Line 3: geštin-bil-lá° *ši-mi-ta-am*[!?]. Collating this line again, M. J. Geller and the present author were able to detect a minute lá sign adjoining the geštin-bil compound. The following *ši-mi-ta-am*[!?] might be a by-form of *šumuttu*, "(a red plant, possibly beetroot)", *CAD* Š/3, 301 and *AHw* 1276[a] (suggestion E. Weissert).

Line 6: *i-li-ip-pí*: Prof. Werner Mayer has pointed out to me (private letter 23/5/98) that this form is probably a verbal form and not a preposition as I took it to be in the first edition. A corroboration to this suggestion is the prepositional phrase *a-na li-ib-bi-im* spelled out fully in line 8, as well as the fact that the text carefully maintains the mimation. A probable derivation for this verb is *lebûm* or *lepûm*, both hitherto unknown in Akkadian. The sense of the phrase demands a verb whose meaning is presumably close to *balālum*, "to mix". Arabic *laffa*, Hebrew/Aramaic *lf(l)f*, and Akkadian *lapāpum* "to to wrap up, roll up, fold up; to wind, coil, spool"[24] may be suggested as possible cognates. Note that Akkadian *lapāpum* and its derivative *lippum*, "tampon" is commonly used in medical texts.[25]

Line 8: In the first edition I have misread the second sign which still puzzles me. A reading gišimmar is technically not impossible. Epigraphically, though, NA_4 seems to represent this sign best. Understanding this sign with the next sign, HAL (or didli) evades me as well. (Perhaps a badly written šinig?)

Line 11: As proposed by E. Weissert, ⸢*ú*°-*ša*⸣-*ap*°-*pa*°(over erasure)-*at*°-*ma*° is to be understood as a form of *papātum*, "in kleine Stücke schlagen" *AHw* 824[a] (the Š stem is attested for the first time). In

[24] Cf. H. Wehr, *Arabic-English Dictionary*, 871, s.v. *laffa*, and *CAD* L, 82.

[25] Cf. D. Glotz, *Studien zur altorienialischen und griechischen Heilkunde. Therapie - Arzneibereitung—Rezeptstruktur*, Wiesbaden, 1974, 72.

Akkadian this verb is rarely documented in Middle- and Neo-Assyrian, and this is its first attestation in Babylonian known to me. In Arabic, Syriac and Hebrew, however, this verb (in the by-forms of *ptpt* or *ptt*) is quite well attested and generally means "to break (edibles, shreds, egg-shells etc.) into small pieces". (Job 2:7–8 may not be irrelevant here.)

Lines 14, 17: I render now both *i-ša-ar-ra-*^{ap}*-am-ma* (l. 14) and *i-ša-ar-<ra>-am-ma* (l. 17) as forms of *šarāpum*. (suggestion W. Mayer). The former is morphophonemically written whereas the latter gives the actual pronunciation of the form.

Line 18: For *qá-aq-qá-ra-am*$^{!}$ (Text: GA) *ú-ul i-la-ap-/pa-at* see the parallel expression in Küchler, *Beiträge zur Kenntnis der assyrisch-babylonischen Medizin*, pl. 1: i 16 cited in *CAD* Q, 115b, 2'.

Line 21: The restoration [*ša*$^{?}$*-am*$^{?}$]*-na* was proposed by W. Mayer, improving on my previous suggestion. Note, however, that as a rule in our text mimation is carefully kept, hence one rather expects [*šam*]*nam*.

As for the text in general, it is important to mark the following points: first, the inconsistency (found in other similar texts as well) in which Is. Mu. 87.56.847 refers to the parties involved. The third-person voice is used to both the healer (ll. 3–14) and the sick person (*ša kurāram marṣu* in ll. 15–18). The dual involvement of the healer and the patient in the curing procedure is clear in lines 13–17, where both sides are respectively called to throw wool and hair into the fire. Then, however, towards its end the text switches to second-person instructive voice referring to the healer, whereas the third-person voice is retained for the patient (ll. 19–22). Another point is the absence of magical formulae, incantation elements, or indirect reference to their recitation. This phenomenon is found in other Old Babylonian therapeutic texts as well. And lastly, as can be seen in Table 4, this text belongs to those therapeutic texts which do not have, so far, a thematically-matching incantation.

Is. Mu. 87.56.847 can supply, however, a missing editorial link of short, single-sectioned Old Babylonian texts, which eventually were gathered—already by the Old Babylonian scribes—to multi-sectioned medical compendia of therapeutic or diagnostic texts, such as *BAM* 393,[26] or *TLB* II, 21.

[26] For the possibility that *BAM* 393 is actually a *Neo Babylonian* copy of an Old Babylonian original, cf. note 20 above.

Looking for a contextual framework for this text, one quickly finds out that most of the pertinent sources dealing with the *kurārum*-disease are post-Old Babylonian.[27] In fact, the closest text—chronologically and thematically speaking—is the large tablet from Susa published by Labat in 1972 as *MDP* 57, VIII. The intriguing group of literary texts from Susa is probably to be dated to the very end of the Old Babylonian period, or to the beginning of the Middle Babylonian period, roughly around 1500 BCE.[28] It is not impossible that our text also dates to this period, although there are no corroborative factors to this suggestion.

What, then, is the *kurārum*-disease? The corpus of texts dealing with this disease is quite instructive in this respect: the clearest pathological symptom of *kurārum* is deep abscesses or pustules which show up mostly on the patient's face or head. They have the potential to spread from the spot of origin in other directions (*ṭuhhudum*—literally, "to flourish, to thrive")[29] and a sufferer might be afflicted with up to four such pustules at a time. The disease affects mainly male adults.

Relying on this data, P. B. Adamson has identified *kurārum* as some kind of ringworm disease, caused, probably, by the fungus *Trichophyton*.[30] He had further commented that "this species of fungus in man tends to be self-curative and is not highly infective to other people".[31] It should be pointed out that according to our text *kurārum* has clear contagious characteristics which were manifestly known to the ancient practitioners, for the text ends with a sober recommendation to the healer to wash his face in order to avoid further contamination. The instruction to throw black wool and hair

---

[27] To the references listed in *CAD* K, 556 add also: *BAM* I, 3:44; 33:1; 34:5 (= J. Nougayrol, *RA* 73 (1979), 69); for *BAM* II, 156: 25–27 cf. K. Deller, *NABU* 1990/3; *BAM* IV, 379: 18; *BAM* V, 422: ii' 12'; 494: iii 21'. 24', 42', 55', 66'; *BAM* VI, 515: ii 36; R. Labat, *RA* 53 (1959), 8:42 and n. 5. I am grateful to Prof. M. Stol who has kindly sent me numerous references for the *kurārum* disease from his files.

[28] Farber, "Zur Orthographie von EAE 22: Neue Lesungen und Versuch einer Deutung" in Galter H. (ed.), *Die Rolle der Astronomie in den Kulturen Mesopotamiens*, Graz, 1993, 249.

[29] "To bloom" is a common metaphor in many modern and ancient languages for the spreading-out of bud-like pimples or pustules; cf. N. Lewis, *The Book of Babel. Words and the Way We See Things*, Penguin, 1995, 49–53.

[30] P.B. Adamson, "Anatomical and Pathological Terms in Akkadian: Part III", *JRAS* 1981, 125–132.

[31] Adamson, *ibid.*, 125.

of a donkey into the fire may also be a prophylactic gesture of the literal burning of cloths and belongings of an infected person, a preventive measure well known from Mesopotamian[32] and other sources.[33]

Final remarks concerning the etymology of the *kurārum*-disease may be offered. An object made of skin with the same name is mentioned in an administrative text from Mari.[34] J.-M. Durand has suggested interpreting the *kurārum*-disease as a secondary meaning of this *lemma*, connecting the two words with *karrum*, as in "knob, pommel". Further support to his proposition comes from the fact that *sikkatum*, "peg, nail", has undergone the same semantic process, that is, a utensil which secondarily denotes a specific name of a disease.[35] As for the root, Durand has proposed *karārum*, "to set, to place an object, to throw, to cast an object". Resisting the temptation of etymological acrobatics, it is important to note that virtually all of the Old Babylonian references to this disease use explicitly voiced /g/ not /k/.[36] The respective roots *garārum* or *qarārum* exist in both Akkadian and cognate Semitic languages. It is not improbable, therefore, that we are dealing actually with a disease named *g/qurārum*.[37]

Bibliography

Adamson, P.B., "Anatomical and Pathological Terms in Akkadian: Part III", *JRAS* 1981, 125–132.

Biggs, R.D., "Medizin A", in: RLA 7 (1987–1990), 623–629.

Biggs, R.D., "Medicine, Surgery, and Public Health in Ancient Mesopotamia", in: J. M. Sasson (ed.), *Civilizations of the Ancient Near East*, Vol. III, 1995, 1911–1924.

Böck, B., ""When You Perform the Ritual of 'Rubbing'": On Medicine and Magic in Ancient Mesopotamia", *JNES* 62 (2003), 1–16.

D. Cadeli, "Lorsque l'enfant paraît . . . malade", in B. Lion et al. (eds.), *Enfance et éducation dans le Proche-orient ancien* (= *Ktema* no. 22), Strasbourg, 1997, 11–33.

32 See for instance the Mari letters *MARI* 3 (1984), 145f., *ARM* XXVI/1, p. 547, and the Susa medical text *MDP* 57, XI, iv:13'–14'.

33 Cf. e.g., the biblical example in Leviticus 13:52.

34 *ARMT* XXI (1983), 306 and p. 376.

35 Another step in this semantic development is furnished by a Mari letter in which *sikkatum* denotes a vegetal term for "bud", or "shoot" of a fig-tree; cf. B. Lafont, "Techniques arboricoles à l'époque amorrite: transport et acclimation de fuguiers à Mari", *FM* III, Paris, 1997, 263–268, esp. 266. The meaning of *sikkatum* in this text is close to its meaning as a physiognomic phenomenon.

36 As in lú.gig.peš=*ša gu-ra-ri-im*; OB Lú A 398 and the examples collected s.v. *kuraštu*. *CAD* K. 556f.

37 So also *AHw*, 510a: *k/gurāru* and Adamson, *ibid.*

Cavigneaux, A. and Al-Rawi, F.N.H., "New Sumerian Literary Texts from Tell Hadid (Ancient Meturan): A First Survey", *Iraq* 55, (1993), 91–105.
Cavigneaux, A., "Magica Mariana", *RA* 88, 1994, 155–161.
Durand, J.-M., *Les documents épistolaires du palais de Mari*, Tome I (= Littératures anciennes du Proche-Orient 16), Éd. du Cerf, Paris, 1997.
Farber, W., "*Mannam Lušpur ana Enkidu*: Some New Thoughts about an Old Motif", *JNES* 49 (1990), 299–321.
Farber, W., "Zur Orthographie von EAE 22: Neue Lesungen und Versuch einer Deutung" in Galter H. (ed.), *Die Rolle der Astronomie in den Kulturen Mesopotamiens, Graz*, 1993, 247–257.
Finkel, I. L., "Adad-apla-iddina, Esagil-kīn-apli, and the Series SA.GIG", in: E. Leichty et al. (eds.), *A Scientific Humanist. Studies in Memory of Abraham Sachs*, Philadelphia, 1988, 143–159.
Goltz, D., "Studien zur altorientalischen und griechieschen Heilkunde. Therapie—Arzneibereitung—Rezeptstruktur", *Sudhoffs Archiv. Zeitschrift für Wissenschaftsgeschichte, Beiheft* 16, Franz Steiner Verlag, Wiesbaden, 1974, 137ff.
Kämmer, T., "Die erste Pockendiagnose stammt aus Babylon", *UF* 27 (1995), 129–168.
Kingston Bjorkman, J., *Meteors and Meteorites in the Ancient Near East*, Center for Meteorite Studies, Arizona State University, 1973.
Kinnier Wilson, J.V., "The *sāmānu* disease in Babylonian Medicine", *JNES* 53 (1994), 111–115.
Lewis, N., *The Book of Babel. Words and the Way We See Things*, Penguin, 1995, 49–53.
Naveh, J., "A Recently Discovered Palestinian Jewish Aramaic Amulet", in M. Sokoloff (ed.), *Arameans, Aramaic and the Aramaic Literary Tradition*, Ramat Gan, 1983, 81–88.
Naveh, J., and Shaked, Sh., *Amulets and Magic Bowls*, The Magnes Press, The Hebrew University, Jerusalem, 1985.
Naveh, J., and Shaked, Sh., *Magic Spells and Formulae*, The Magnes Press, The Hebrew University, Jerusalem, 1993.
Naveh, J., "Illness and Amulets in Antiquity", in: O. Rimon (ed.), *Illness and Healing in Ancient Times*, University of Haifa, 1996, 24*–28*.
Stol, M., *Epilepsy in Babylonia*, Styx Publications, Groningen, 1993.
Reiner, E., *Astral Magic in Babylonia* (= Transactions of the American Philosophical Society, 85/4), Philadelphia, 1995.
Virolleaud, Ch., *L'Astrologie Chaldéenne*, Librairie Paul Geuthner, Paris, 1905–1912.
Wasserman, N., "An Old-Babylonian Medical Text Against the *Kurārum* Disease", *RA* 90 (1996), 1–5; *RA* 91 (1997), 31–32 (photo and copy).

INFANTILE AND CHILDHOOD CONVULSIONS, AND SA.GIG XXIX

J. V. Kinnier Wilson
University of Cambridge

Introduction

The discovery of new texts and a Commentary of Tablet XXIX of the diagnostic series *Sakikku* or Sa.gig—a series well represented in this volume—was reported in 1988 in a familiar study.[1] Further information with a transliteration and translation of the first entry of the Tablet was provided by Marten Stol in his study of 1993,[2] although he declined to take the matter further owing to the difficulties and fragmentary nature of the text. In some defiance of the difficulties the present study feels able to discuss the first three entries of the Tablet, and has been helped in the interpretation by the proposal which heads this paper. The BM sources of the tablet are as given in the first reference, note 29; a copy and edition of the full tablet has been prepared by N.P. Heeßel as part of a larger study on the later Tablets of Sa.gig: *Babylonisch- Assyrisches Diagnostik*, Ugarit-Verlag, Münster (2000): editions 318–338, copies 462–465.

Transliteration

1. *šumma Bēl-ūri* (^{d}LUGAL ÙR.RA) *itti-šu*(KI.BI) *alid*(Ù.TU) *ina šēpē-šú*(GÌR^{II}-*šú*) *bīt abi-šú*(É AD-*šú*) *issappah*(BIR-*ah*) *ana la sapāh*(NU BIR-*ah*) *bīt abi-šú*
2. *kīma kūbi*(^{d}KÙ.BI) *tuš-na-al-šu-ma lumun-šu*(HUL.BI) *it-ta-bal itta-šu* (GISKIM.BI) *kīma* ⸢*iballuṭu?*⸣ (⸢AL?⸣.TI)
3. *i-bak-ki i-<i-za-ár>-za-ár ù im-ta-nam-ga-ag*

---

[1] I. L. Finkel, 'Adad-apla-iddina, Esagil-kin-apli, and the series Sa.gig,' in E. Leichty, M. Ellis and P. Gerardi (eds.), *A Scientific Humanist: Studies in Memory of Abraham Sachs*, Philadelphia, p. 147 and note 29.

[2] *Epilepsy in Babylonia*, Cuneiform Monographs 2, Groningen, p. 88.

4. *šumma ina* MU 3 <KAM>[a] *imqut-su*(ŠUB-*su*)[b] *ina rēši-šu*(SAG.BA)-*ma ultabbar*(TIL)[c] *a-na la lubburi?-šu*(NU TIL-*šu*)
5. *šakirâ* (Ú ŠAKIRA) *šá ina* UD ⌜30.KAM⌝ *innasihu*(ZI) *tasâk*(SÚD) *ina mê*(A) *nāri*(ÍD) *tuballal*(HE.HE) *taptanaššas-su*(ŠÉŠ-*su*)-*ma iballuṭ*(DIN)
6. *šumma ina* MU 7.KAM *imqut-su*(ŠUB-*su*) *ina šatti-šu*(MU.BI)[d] *ultabbar*(TIL) *a-na la luburri?-šu*(NU TIL-*šu*) *annâ*(NE) *attalê*(AN.TA.LÙ) *ina* UD 30.KAM[e]
7. *ina mê*(A) *nāri*(ÍD) *tuballal*(HE.HE) *taptanaššas-su*(ŠÉŠ-*su*)-*ma iballuṭ* (AL.TI)

a) Probably, if not quite necessarily, to be so restored as in line 6 and elsewhere on the tablet
b) Followed by *ul? ta*, regarded uncertainly as a faulty anticipation of *ultabbar* (to have been written *ul-ta-ab-bar*)
c) To be so read after the *ul-tab-bar* of lines 8 and 29
d) Preferred to *šatti šiāti* which could also be read
e) For the reading at this point cf. Commentary

Translation

(1) If Bēl-ūri (or, Lugal-urra) is present (with the child) from birth (lit.: 'has been born with him'), at the foot of his bed his father's household will disperse (in terror). That the household of his father should not disperse (2) you shall (pretend to) bury him as though he were a still-born child and the evil will be removed. The sign 'when he recovers, (3) (the child) will begin to cry', should be looked for; (during the convulsion) he will twist and 'stiffen and relax' (his limbs).
(4) If he (Bēl-ūri) falls upon him in the third year, he may remain for a long time at the head of his bed. That he should not so remain, (5) a *šakirû*-plant which has been uprooted on the thirtieth day (i.e., the day of the moon's disappearance) you shall bray, mix with river water and anoint him regularly therewith. So he will recover.
(6) If he falls upon him in the seventh year, throughout that year (Bēl-ūri) may remain (at the head of his bed). That he should not so remain, the same (plant), (uprooted) at an eclipse or on the thirtieth day (of the month), (you shall bray), mix with river water and anoint him regularly therewith. So he will recover.

Commentary

It is well known that convulsions in infants and young children form a special category in neurological disorders. The nervous system at this age is relatively immature, and brain irritation, however caused, may send signals to the nerves which cause contracture of various kinds in the responding muscles. In fact such convulsions 'vary in severity from localised twitching (often seen in the newborn) to major seizures,'[3] and this statement would accord with the offered translation of line 1: 'If Bēl-ūri is present (with the child) from birth.' With 'major seizures' one enters a field which belongs equally to epilepsy, and later entries on the tablet which relate to attacks of the thirtieth year and beyond are certainly concerned with that condition.

With the young as our only concern in this study, it may be said that infantile and childhood convulsions have many causes of which two may be mentioned here. The first is birth injury with intra-cranial damage, this being the more likely to occur following a difficult or prolonged labour.[4] The second cause is a rise in temperature following an infection, the resulting state being then known as febrile convulsions. Since age is of concern in this paper we may note (from the textbooks) that the first episode of such convulsions occurs generally between the ages of two and three, a point which may perhaps relate to the choice of 'three years' in the second entry of our texts. In the majority of cases the convulsions cease after the age of five years; in a case study of 110 children 'the latest age of onset was 8 years.'[5]

Two further points relate the texts to the interpretation proposed. Firstly, it is a feature of the entries that they prescribe the action to be taken to avoid the persistence of the condition into a further period. To explain the allusion one may note that, while convulsions may occur as a single event, they are liable to recur with the return of a high temperature; the attacks 'are physically exhausting,

[3] R. G. Mitchell, 'Diseases of Infancy and Childhood,' in W. N. Mann and M. H. Lessof (eds.), *Conybeare's Textbook of Medicine*, 15th. edit., Edinburgh and London, 1970, p. 158.

[4] D. B. Jelliffe, 'The Newborn and premature Infant,' in H. C. Trowell and D. B. Jelliffe, *Diseases of Children in the Subtropics and Tropics*, London, 1958, p. 99.

[5] J. G. Millichap, *Febrile Convulsions*, New York, 1968, p. 23.

and one convulsion predisposes to another.'[6] Secondly, the specific 'sign' of the first entry that 'when he recovers, (the child) will begin to cry,' may be found also in the medical literature: 'On recovering from a convulsion, the child will often cry and then fall asleep.'[7]

A few notes may be added on specific points raised by the text.

1–3. As was noted also by Stol, the commentary BM 38375 explains the ideograms KI.BI Ù.TU in line 1 as *it-ti-šú a-lid*,[8] thereby dispelling the long uncertainty as to the meaning of these signs. In the same line *ina šēpē-šu*, supposedly 'at the foot of his bed,'[9] has been interpreted in the light of *ina rēši-šu*, 'at the head of his bed,' in line 4; and the words 'in terror', *sc.*, at the demon's presence, have been added to give point to the threatened dispersing, or disbanding, of the father's household. In line 3 the offened translation would seem altogether appropriate to the diagnosis. 'In a "typical" febrile convulsion the child's body suddenly stiffens, and then the muscles of his body, arms and legs clench, relax and clench again so that he jerks and shudders.'[10]

4–5. The plant *šakirû* of line 5 is best regarded as unidentified at the present time, cf. CAD Š/1 167f. There are many uncertainties. It could, however, be mentioned that, in the Ur 'maintenance' texts,[11] the line

30 ŠAKIR.SAR.M[EŠ *ša*] 7 [M]U.MEŠ (No. 51, obv. 8) is likely to mean, '30 *šakirru*-vessels of (seasonal) vegetables (SAR.MEŠ = NISSA.MEŠ, Akk. *arqu*) for 7 years,' and therefore not to provide a reference for the *šakirû*-plant.[12]

6–7. For the astrological allusions in this, as also the previous, entry the standard authority is Erica Reiner, *Astral Magic in Babylonia*

---

[6] J. Chandy, 'Convulsive Disorders', in H.C. Trowell and D.B. Jelliffe, *Diseases of Children in the Subtropics and Tropics*, London, 1958, p. 264.

[7] R. G. Mitchell, *op. cit.*, p. 158.

[8] See I. L. Finkel, 'On TDP Tablets XXIX and XXXI, and the nature of Sa.gig,' *Journal of Cuneiform Studies* 46, 1994, p. 87.

[9] For additional references see M. Stol, *Epilepsy*, p. 89 and note 122.

[10] Penelope Leach, *Baby and Child: from birth to age five*, London, new edit., 1989, p. 507.

[11] O. R. Gurney, *The Middle Babylonian Legal and Economic Texts from Ur*, London, 1983, Nos. 51–54.

[12] Cf. also for this interpretation the '[1 DUG.]GAL .[. . . .]. 1 ŠAKIR.SAR' of Text No. 52, obv. 10.

(Philadelphia, 1995).[13] It would remain to comment on the apparent hiatus in the text at the end of line 6. No error is recognised in the absence of *ina* before *attalê* in the phrase AN.TA.LÙ *ina* UD 30.KAM, since this could be explained as an example of the ellipse of the second preposition,—not uncommon, it is believed, with *ina, ana* and *ša.*[14] However, one is faced also with the problem of whether, or not, to restore the signs ZI and SÚD, supposedly *innasihu tasâk*, after UD 30.KAM, as in line 5. The signs have not been restored for the reason that deficiencies do occur in the 'instruction' sections of the prescriptions. The (mental) supplying of *talaš*, 'you shall kneed,' at the end of prescription No. 3 in the 'Stroke and facial palsy' paper of this volume, would be a case in point. A further example may be seen in AMT 74,1, col. ii, where in prescriptions for foot trouble involving 'pomegranate skins', line 16 has *taqallu*, 'you shall roast', line 21 has *tasâk*, 'you shall bray', whereas both procedures would seem necessary on general considerations as well as in the light of iii, 16: 'pomegranate skins you shall dry and bray', *tabbal tasâk.* If to be upheld as a principle, it could be that only in closely parallel texts were such deficiencies allowable.

---

[13] Cf. especially pp. 134f., 'Moonless nights are . . . particularly appropriate for gathering herbs,' and the text cited (BAM 580, v, 5'ff.).

[14] As, for example, KAR 61, 8: *lu hašhūri lu ana nurmê šipta . . . tanaddi*, 'Either (over) an apple or a pomegranate you will recite . . . the incantation.'

ON STROKE AND FACIAL PALSY IN BABYLONIAN TEXTS

J. V. Kinnier Wilson and E. H. Reynolds
King's College London

PART I

I *The Sources*

Many years ago, the second writer of this paper recognised that Tablet XXVI of Labat's *Traité akkadien de diagnostics et pronostics médicaux*, despite the apparent, and mistaken, association with 'contusion' or 'bruising', was in fact concerned with stroke. He expressed the hope that, at some future time, it might be possible for the writers to produce a joint paper on stroke, on the same general lines as for the then emerging paper on epilepsy.[1]

The present study is the result of this new collaboration. Following the evidence of the catalogues,[2] the tablet in question is cited as No. XXVII, not XXVI, a figure accepted in the latest edition of M. Stol.[3] This latter work has already taken the study some distance forward; however, a more detailed medical analysis is here provided, and further note will be taken of K 2418+, a reconstructed tablet of the Therapeutic series, *šumma muhhašu*.[4] Many of the pieces of this

[1] J. V. Kinnier Wilson and E. H. Reynolds, 'Translation and Analysis of a cuneiform text forming part of a Babylonian treatise on Epilepsy,' *Medical History* 34/2 (1990), pp. 185–198.

[2] ND 4358 + 4366 and BM 41237, on which see in the last instance I. J. Finkel, '*Adad-apla-iddina, Esagil-kin-apli*, and the series SA.GIG,' in E. Leichty, M. Ellis and P. Gerardi (eds,), *A Scientific Humanist: Studies in Memory of Abraham Sachs*, Philadelphia, 1988, pp. 143–159; also, by the same writer, 'On TDP Tablets XXIX and XXXI, and the nature of SA.GIG,' *JCS* 46 (1994), pp. 87–88.

[3] *Epilepsy in Babylonia*, Cuneiform Monographs 2, Styx Publications, Groningen, 1993 (hereafter abbreviated as *Epilepsy* and 'CM 2'), pp. 74ff.; also, by the same writer, 'Diagnosis and therapy in Babylonian medicine,' *JEOL* 32 (1993), 51 with note 52.

[4] Suggested as a convenient abbreviation for the full title of *šumma amēlu muhhašu umma ukâl*,—and without prejudice to the use of "UGU", as coined by Köcher, to indicate the sub-series with the same title.

tablet were copied in R. C. Thompson's AMT,[5]—details are as cited below, in Section IV—but in its present form much is owed to joins made subsequently by Franz Köcher. Although as yet the tablet has not been recopied for the BAM series, something of its nature will be seen from the photograph of the reverse which is included with this account (fig. 1).

A curious feature of the tablet may be mentioned at this point. As may be seen on the photograph, the colophon fails to indicate—supposedly by a scribal error—the series and sub-series to which it belongs and its position within it; the catch-line is followed at once by the library subscript beginning 'Palace of Ashurbanipal.' In fact from a manuscript of Köcher's which reconstructs first lines of the corpus based on new fragments from Ashur,[6] one learns that the tablet belonged to the fifth sub-series of the work, beginning *šumma amēlu labān-šu ikkal-šu*, 'If a man's neck tendons hurt him.' It was the fifth of the six tablets comprising this series.

Help in restoring certain prescriptions on the tablet is afforded by BAM 132–136 and 138, and by SBTU I, 46,[7] a text which describes itself as the '10th *pirsu*' of the larger corpus. Relevant also, although a different order is followed, are the three fragments of OECT XI, Nos. 72–74.[8] The sources for Tablet XXVII of the diagnostic series (*Sakikku* XXVII) are documented by M. Stol, *Epilepsy in Babylonia*, p. 74. They are the two Louvre tablets, AO 6680 and A 3441, published by R. Labat in TDP II, plates XLVIII to LI, and text No. 89 of E. von Weiher, SBTU III, lines 16–62.

II *Initial Considerations*

In this section we seek firstly to define our subject and to declare essential terminology. What, therefore, one may say about stroke is

---

[5] *Assyrian Medical Texts from the originals in The British Museum*, Oxford, 1923.

[6] Published by G. Beckman and B. R. Foster, 'Assyrian scholarly Texts in the Yale Babylonian Collection,' in E. Leichty, M. Ellis and P. Gerardi (eds.), *A Scientific Humanist: Studies in Memory of Abraham Sachs*, Philadelphia, 1988, pp. 1–26.

[7] H. Hunger, *Spätbabylonische Texte aus Uruk*, I, Ausgrabungen der Deutschen Forschungsgemeinschaft in Uruk-Warka, Bd. 9, Berlin, 1976.

[8] O. R. Gurney, *Literary and Miscellaneous Texts in the Ashmolean Museum*, Oxford Editions of Cuneiform Texts, Vol. XI, Oxford, 1989. Acknowledgement is made to Dr I. L. Finkel for drawing our attention to this source.

that it is a cerebrovascular disease which follows either from a release of blood into the brain (cerebral or intracranial haemorrhage), or else from a thrombosis or embolism which impedes the flow of blood to the brain, resulting in cerebral ischaemia (restriction of bloodflow) or cerebral infarct (localised death of brain tissue). When the cause of the stroke is from haemorrhage a severe, even an intense, headache leads often to a period of unconsciousness or 'coma'; this may continue for some hours, less commonly for a day or more. Laboured breathing may be noticed at this time, and there is an accompanying paralysis of the muscles of one side of the body—hemiparesis if partial, hemiplegia in the case of a complete paralysis. Commonly the mouth is affected, and if consciousness is regained some impairment of speech may be evident,—'dysphasia' if the lesion is in the dominant hemisphere of the brain, 'dysarthria' if paralysis affects the actual mechanisms of speech. Other symptoms may ensue and locally persist; they include a slowing of movement and difficulty in walking from affected muscles becoming stiff or 'rigid'. A loss of balance at this time may lead also to falls and injury.[9] Stroke accordingly is a serious condition, recovery—or otherwise—depending much on the site and severity of the haemorrhage (when so caused) and being seldom complete. In the ischaemic condition the mortality rate is lower and there is 'a far wider range of severity.'[10]

It should be mentioned that the documents include also a reference to facial palsy. This is a largely benign condition having an aetiology different from that of stroke, but it is understandably included in a stroke context. The matter is discussed further below, under 'Selected Prescriptions.'

We turn next to the Akkadian terminology, where it is now generally recognised that a verb *mašādu*, and its derivative noun *mišittu*, were the essential terms denoting stroke and (flaccid) paralysis in ancient Mesopotamia. The dictionaries[11] and Marten Stol[12] have well understood the matter, although it is here believed that the precise medical term for stroke in Akkadian was *šipir mišitti*, perhaps literally

[9] Cf., *int. al.*, A. Forster and J. Young, 'Incidence and consequences of falls due to stroke: a systematic enquiry,' *British Medical Journal* 311 (1995), pp. 83–86. Two further references are cited below, under note 63.

[10] I. M. S. Wilkinson, *Essential Neurology*, 2nd. edit., Oxford, 1993, p. 63.

[11] CAD M/1 351 and M/2, 125; AHw 623, 3 (*mašādu* as "schlagen, von Schlaganfall"), and 660–661.

[12] *Epilepsy in Babylonia*, pp. 74ff.

'attack of paralysis' following G. Meier's "Anfall" for *šipru* in *ZA* 45, 208. A convincing example occurs in the first entry of *Sakikku* XXVII (see below, in Section VI), and importantly, in the therapeutic tablet, *mišittu* is associated with specific parts of the body, namely, the cheek, neck, hip, trunk, arm and leg,[13] and in such instances 'paralysis' is appropriate while 'stroke' is not. It is to continue, rather than to support, the above proposal that two further references may be brought forward at this point. They are respectively AMT 77,5: 4, + K 11127, 7, and AMT 77,1: 11, which read:

> *šumma šipir* (KIN) *mi-šit-ti šá mehri*(GABA.RI) *lapit*(TAG) . . ., and
> *šumma šipir* (KIN) *mi-šit-ti šá arkati*(EGIR) *lapit*(TAG).

These lines supposedly concern a stroke 'of (or, from) the front' and a stroke 'of (or, from) the back,' but it is not certain what is precisely meant. Ideas that have been considered are (1) that the terms relate to frontal and occipital headaches as focal events in the condition and of differential importance; (2) that they refer to front and back parts of the body as unprotected areas in bathroom falls, on which cf. Stol, CM 2, 76;[14] and (3), as here preferred, that they have a temporal significance and refer to strokes of sudden or slow onset.[15] Less disputable by comparison would be the entry of AMT 78,1: 5 and 6, and SBTU I 46, 33:

> *ana šipir* (KIN) *mi-šit-tú šá pâ-šú uṣabbitu*(DIB.DIB-*tu*$_4$)
> 'For a stroke which has permanently seized his (the patient's) mouth,'

'permanently' being here a rendering of the intensive D-stem of the verb *ṣabātu*, 'to seize.'

We may inject here a note on the term '(flaccid) paralysis' as thus used to define *mišittu* in the above paragraph. The Akkadian for 'flaccidity'—a limp or relaxed state of the muscles—was probably *rimûtu*, lit. 'looseness', from *ramû*, 'to be loose.' In many texts *rimûtu* is associated with *šimmatu* meaning 'paralysis', and, interpreted as a

[13] Cf., with Stol, *op. cit.*, p. 75, AMT 79,1, respectively lines 6, 9, 11, 17, 21 and 24.

[14] And as discussed further below in the Commentary to *Sakikku* XXVII, lines 12–13.

[15] For the adverb *mihrā* meaning 'directly' (or, in effect, 'suddenly') one may consult CAD M/2 59, 3. The opposite concept for *ša arkati* would follow from the argument that a straggler on a line of march, or an animal who falls behind in a moving herd, may certainly be regarded as 'slow'.

hendiadys, the resulting 'paralysis-and-flaccidity' will often then describe hemiplegia. From this position one may newly understand the phrase *ši-pir šim-mat ri-mu-ti u sagalli*(SA.GAL) of KAR 44, rev. 9. It will mean: 'Treatments[16] for hemiplegia and paraplegia,' for *sagallu* as the latter term is neatly defined by BAM 130, 19–21:

19 *šumma amēlu šer᾽ān pēmi*(ÚR)-*šú ka-la-šu-ma tab-ku*
20 *tebâ*(ZI-*a*) *a-tál-lu-ka la i-le-᾽i*
21 *sa-gal-lum iṣbat*(DIB)-*su*

> 'If the leg tendons of a man are all without strength
> and he cannot stand up or walk about,
> paraplegia has seized him.'

By comparison, and as far as is known, the combination of *mišittu* with *rimûtu* finds only a single example in our texts, the somewhat difficult phrasing being: *ana amēli ši-pìr mi-šit-ti šu-up-šu-hi u ri-mu-t*[*i*].[17] The text is discussed further below, under 'Selected Prescriptions' (No. 3).

We look for a moment to the beginnings of our subject, it being in 1950, in his translation of the Babylonian Chronicle, that A. L. Oppenheim,[18] wrote of the fourth year of Mushezib-Marduk of Babylon:

> In the month of Nisanu, the 15th day, Menanu, king of Elam, suffered a stroke [*mi-šit-tum i-mé-šid-su*],[19] his mouth was paralysed, he was unable to speak. In the month of Addaru, the 7th day, Menanu, king of Elam, died.

For the same event described as a historical statement one may refer also to J. A. Brinkman:[20]

> In Nisan, the first month of 689, Khumban-nimena, the Elamite king, suffered a stroke and lingered incapacitated for almost eleven months. During this interval of dislocation in Elam, the city of Babylon fell to the Assyrians.

The incident was recorded also in a letter to Ashurbanipal from

---

[16] For *šipru* in this sense cf. CAD Š/3 83–84, under 7; AHw 1246, 6e.
[17] Text from BAM 138 ii, 9–10, with AMT 82,2: 7.
[18] In J. B. Pritchard (ed.), *Ancient Near Eastern Texts*, 1st. edit., p. 302.
[19] *Imešid* of the text, transliterated as *i-mi!-šid* in AHw 623, is taken to be a 'durative' present, I/1, from an /e/ verb *mešēdu*, to which also the stative *mé-ši-id*, cited below, must likewise belong.
[20] *Cambridge Ancient History* III/2, 1991, p. 38.

Nabû-bēl-shūmāte of Babylon: 'I have heard that the king of Elam has had a stroke (*mé-ši-id*), and many cities are rebelling against him.'[21]

A further *mišittu*-text may be mentioned here. This is SBTU I, 43, 16, reading:

KIMIN(= *ultu pī*) *mi-šit-ti*

The text as a whole has been discussed by both Hunger[22] and Köcher,[23] and if the cited line has been properly understood, and according to the 'physical' theory of disease etymology proposed by Köcher, it would seem that, at some period, *mišittu* was deemed to originate 'from the mouth' or to have some such connection. So far as early ideas go one may note the near parallel of classical Arabic where the term for 'stroke' was *sukta(h)*, from the verb *sakata*, 'to be silent'.[24] These findings lead directly to the following Section.

III *Kadibbidû*

It will be the aim of this Section to show how central a part mouth paralysis or 'mouth seizure', Sum. ka-dib-bi-da, Akk. *kadibbidû* or *ṣibit pī*, played in the description and treatment of stroke in ancient Mesopotamia. The references are all taken from column iii of the therapeutic tablet, K 2418 +, and are presented initially under five headings.

1. The two parallel prescriptions of iii 19 and 25 respectively are introduced as follows:

   šumma amēlu pâ-šú šapat-su ana imitti / ana šumēli / kup-pu-ul-ma da-ba-ba la [*i-le-ʾi*],
   'If the mouth of a man and one of his lips are twisted to the right (or, secondly, to the left) and he is unable to speak.'

2. Lower down on the column at iii, 36, and as already mentioned in the previous Section, the protasis of the entry reads:

[21] R. F. Harper, *Assyrian and Babylonian Letters*, Chicago, 1892–1914, No. 839, lines 9–10.

[22] SBTU I, pp. 50 and 51, note to line 13.

[23] 'Spätbabylonische medizinische Texte aus Uruk,' in C. Habrich, F. Marguth and J. H. Wolf (eds.), *Medizinische Diagnostik in Geschichte und Gegenwart*, Munich, 1978, pp. 22–25.

[24] An extension of meaning not shared by the Akk. *sakātu*, 'to be silent.'

ana šipir mi-šit-tú šá pâ-šú uṣabbitu(DIB.DIB-*tu*$_4$)
'For a stroke which has permanently seized his (the patient's) mouth.'

3. At iii, 40ff., the prescriptions concern *kadibbidû*, beginning:

šumma amēlu pâ-šú kadibbidâ(KA.DIB.BI.DA) *iši*(TUK-[*ši*?])
If the mouth of a man has 'mouth seizure.'

4. Ten further prescriptions for *kadibbidû* follow the above, the style of the protasis then changing at iii, 58, to:

ana kadibbidê pašāri(BÚR-*ri*)
'to release (the hold of) "mouth seizure"'.

5. Finally, as the bottom of the column is reached (iii, 61f.), the prescriptions are prophylactic:

ana kadibbidê amēli la ṭehê(NU TE-*e*)
'That "mouth seizure" should not (again) approach a man.'

It may be of interest at this point if we attempt an edition of a Sumerian medical incantation on ka-dib-bi-da found in col iv, lines 14'–16' of our text. Copies of the text will be found in AMT 76,5: 14–16, (+) 79,4: 5–7, but it is well exemplified elsewhere, the additional sources—owed gratefully to I. L. Finkel—being BAM 28, 13–16; BAM 533, 16–21; BAM 534, iv, 5–9;[25] AMT 23,2: 1–4; and OECT XI, 72 rev. 7f. As commonly, the incantation invokes the divine power of Asalluhi, son of Enki, whose cult-centre was at Eridu on the ancient 'Abzu'(-lake) of southern Mesopotamia. For clarity we offer an idealised text, presented in five lines:

én: èš abzu nì-nam mú-a ^{d}En-ki lugal abzu-ke$_4$
^{d}Asal-lú-hi ka-dib-bi-da[26] ku$_5$-ru-da lugal hé-gál
ka-dib-bi-da ku$_5$-ru-da ka-dib-bi-da hul-gál zi-ku$_5$-ru-da
^{d}Asal-lú-hi mu$_7$-mu$_7$ abzu-a-ke$_4$[27] ka-kešda-bi duh-ù-da
ka-dib-bi-da ku$_5$-ru-da tu$_6$ ÉN
'In the abode of the Abzu which produced all that there is, (thus declared) Enki, the king of the Abzu:

[25] This source, K 3484, has now been joined to K 8792 (information from I. L. Finkel).

[26] The sign *mah* copied (strangely) on AMT 79,4: 5 after *-da* at this point does not appear on the tablet (collated).

[27] On BAM 534 iv, 8, the sign *ke*$_4$ appears somewhat as *šà*, which may explain the error of 533 obv., where ⌜*a*⌝ is found written at the end of line 20 and [*k*]e$_4$—or [*š*]*à*—at the beginning of line 21.

> "Asalluhi shall be master of the life-threatening *kadibbida*!"
> '(So) life-threatening *kadibbida*, O evil *kadibbida* that would cut off the breath of life, Asalluhi, the exorcist of the Abzu, can release the spell (you have cast)! Life-threatening *kadibbida*!'

The above text is certainly old, and indeed, is doubtless to be interpreted in terms of that 'I-thou' relationship between man and natural phenomena first clearly expounded by Jacobsen a half century ago.[28] To that world even diseases belonged; they had their own wills and 'personality', and might then submit to a stronger will. But here, as elsewhere, one must be careful from a modern standpoint not to give *kadibbida* too restrictive a meaning. Aphasia, as the basic term, had other causes apart from stroke; mutism and aphonia may also have had their place;[29] and for 'mouth seizure', written *pâ-šú ṣabit*, in epilepsy (*Sakikku* XXVI, rev. 16), Reynolds explained that 'post-ictal silence may be due to severe dysphasia or dysarthria, drowsiness or psychological or physical exhaustion.'[30]

One further text is of relevance in the context of 'mouth seizure.' In S. Parpola's *Letters from Assyrian and Babylonian Scholars*,[31] No. 327, a text edited by the author under the title 'List of Remedies', 'side 1' of the tablet includes the phrase:

> *ka-par pi-i nap-šal-*[*ti ša*] *kadib*[*bidê*] (KA.DIB.[BI.DA]),
> 'Mouth rubbing and ointme[nt for] 'mouth sei[zure].'

The place of 'rubbing' and massage in the ancient treatment of paralysis has been discussed in basic studies by F. Köcher and I. L. Finkel.[32] The same will be evident from a brief study of the prescriptions.

IV *Treatment and Selected Prescriptions*

The several imperfections of the reverse of the stroke tablet, K 2418+, will be clear from the photograph, although no edition of the tablet

---

[28] In H. and H. A. Frankfort, J. A. Wilson and Th. Jacobsen (eds.), *The Intellectual Adventure of Ancient Man*, Chicago, 1946, republished as *Before Philosophy*, Pelican Books, London, 1949, pp. 142f.

[29] Cf. J. V. Kinnier Wilson, 'An Introduction to Babylonian Psychiatry,' *Studies in honor of Benno Landsberger*, AS 16, Chicago, 1965, p. 292.

[30] *Medical History*, 34/2, 1990, p. 197.

[31] Published in the series *State Archives of Assyria*, Vol. X, Helsinki, 1993.

[32] Respectively 'Die Ritualtafel der magisch-medizinischen Tafelserie "Einreibung"', *AfO* XXI, 1966, 13–20, and '*Muššu'u, qutāru*, and the scribe Tanittu-Bel,' *Aula Orientalis* 9, 1991 (Miguel Civil Festschrift), 91–104.

is attempted in these pages. We offer in its place an economically transcribed text,[33] with translation and discussion of five prescriptions which are either complete or nearly so and may be thought representative of the collection. The main source, as introduced in Section I, consists of the following pieces: K 2418 + 2465 + Rm 141 (AMT 77,1 and 2; 78,1; 79,1) + 2458 (AMT 82,2) + 2488 (AMT 76,5) + 5893 + 9140 (AMT 77,5) + 10174 (AMT 79,4) + 11127 + Sm 1397 (AMT 28,7) + Rm 2,143 (AMT 24,1).

Such other texts as have been used in support of, or to restore, the individual prescriptions are as indicated in each case. A partly relevant text which does not feature in the following selections is BAM 398, discussed by Köcher in the Catalogue entry of Bd. IV, p. xxix.

1 *Prescription for Mouth Paralysis* (kadibbidû)

Texts: A: K 2418+, rev. iii, 41–42, copies: AMT 78,1: 10–11 with 28,7: 7–8
B: K 6025, 11–13, copy: AMT 23,2.

41 *šumma amēlu pâ-šú*[a] *kadibbidâ*(KA.DIB.BI.DA) *iši*(TUK-*ši*) *sah-lé-e ina mê būrti*(A PÚ) *tasâk* MUN AL.ÚS.SA[b] *ṭābāti*(A.GEŠTIN.NA) *ana l*[*ibbi*]

42 *haṣba*(ŠIKA) *tanaddi*(ŠUB)[c] *ina kakkabi*(UL) *tuš-bat ina še-rim ubān-šú rabīti* [*i*]*-kar-rik*[d] *ba-lu*[e] *pa-tan pâ-šú ik-ta-na-par*[f] [*ma iballuṭ*]

a) From A; B: *-šu*
b) From A, the Akk. reading being uncertain; B: KAŠ AL.ÚS.SA = *billatu* (exceptionally written with the AL prefix)
c) Text of A; B seemingly replaces the whole phrase with *tu-ta-rap*, on which see AHw 1325, under *tarāpu* D
d) From A; B: *tuš-ta-kar-rak*
e) So A; B: *la*
f) Text of A; B: *tak-ta-na-*[*par*]

Translation, Text A: (41) If the mouth of a man has 'mouth seizure', [cre]ss seed you will grind into well water,[34] fish brine and vinegar

[33] That is, without indication of common ideograms where the reading of the signs composing these could not be in doubt.

[34] In col. iv, 5', 'well water from the temple of Marduk,' *mê būrti šá bīt* ^{d}*Marduk*, was specified in a similar use.

(42) 'spoon' into it with a potsherd, and leave overnight under the stars. In the morning he (the patient) shall dip his (unaffected?) thu[mb] into (the mixture) and rub his mouth constantly (therewith) before eating. [So he will recover].

Translation, Text B: (11) If the mouth of a man has 'mouth seizure', cress seed [you will grind] (12) [into well water], matured beer and vinegar you will pour (over it) [and leave overnight] under the s[tars]. (13) [In the morning] you will have (the patient) dip his (unaffected?) thumb into (the mixture) and you will rub his mouth constantly (therewith) before eating. [So he will recover].

Notes: The two versions of the above text have much in common, but it has been thought necessary to provide two translations since there are important differences in the instructions. Both use the verb *kitappuru*, 'to rub constantly (or, frequently)' in the treatment of the mouth condition, thus linking the text closely to the *kapār pī* of the previous Section. However, the first, and perhaps the older, of the two versions directs that the patient should perform this operation himself; in the second version it is the *asû*, or 'physician', who controls the rubbing. The prescription would have been appropriate, and massage has still its place in the modern treatment of paralysis. Additionally, the application of vinegar which is astringent, as also the salt of the brine in text A—salt being a sialogue—may have been useful in the attempt to stimulate mouth movement.

It should be mentioned that a closely similar prescription to that of text A occurs in col. iii, 48f., of K 2418+ (copies are as given in AMT 78,1: 17–18 and 28,7: 14–15). The same ingredients are there prescribed, but interestingly they are now followed by the instruction: *la tu-qar-rab la šu-ku-lu*, 'you shall not serve (these) at a meal; they must not be given for eating.' As to the translation 'fish brine', the ideogram MUN.AL.ÚS.SA, somewhat on the analogy of the Sum. mun-gazi, is considered to be a compound expression consisting of MUN = *ṭabtu*, 'salt', and AL.ÚS.SA = *šiqqu*, 'fish sauce.' The Old Babylonian origins of the text are clear from this reference.[35]

[35] Following A. L. Oppenheim, *Ancient Mesopotamia*, Chicago, 1964, p. 46: 'Fish ... were used on a large scale as food ... only up to the middle of the second millennium B.C.'

2 *Prescription for Paresis in an Upper Limb*
Texts: A: K 2418+, obv. i, 11–12, copy: AMT 77,1: 11–12
B: VAT 13891, BAM 132, 3'–6' (the line-numbering follows this text).

3' *šumma šipir*(KIN) *mi-šit-ti šá arkati*(EGIR) *lapit*(TAG) 1/2 qa *zēr kitê*(GADA) *teṭên*(ÀR-*en*)
4' *ina* [A] [KUG].GA[a] *ina* DUG *diqāri*(UTÚL) *tu*[*šabšal*(ŠEG$_6$-*šal*)]
5' *ba-ah-ru-su ina maški teṭerri ištu uppi a*[*hi*(MUD Á)]
6' [*adi ubā*]*nāte*([ŠU.S]I.MEŠ)-*šú*[b] *taṣammid-ma ina ṭu*[*p-pi-šu tapaṭṭar*][c]

a) Free restoration, with GA supposedly preceded by an anticipatory *ina*
b) Free restoration, suggested *per exclusionem*
c) Restored after AMT 77,5: 9, lower down in the same col., *ina ṭup-pi-šú* DU[H-*ár*]

Translation: (3') If a man has been slightly paralysed (lit.: 'touched') in a stroke of gradual onset (*ša arkati*), grind 1/2 *qû* of flax seed, (4') boil with [pure wa]ter in a clay cook-pot, (5') spread hot onto a skin and bind on(to the patient) from his shoulder so[cket] (6') to his [fing]ers. [You may remove (the bandage)] during this (treatment).

Notes: Despite the difficulty of *ša arkati* discussed above in Section II, the text seems likely to have concerned a paresis of the arm in a case of ischaemic stroke. Such slight, or incomplete, paralysis would fit the verb *lapātu*, and also the early removal of the bandage (if so correctly understood) will mean that the paralysis was recognised as being possibly of short duration. The proposed treatment by hot poultice has many parallels in our texts and so also in those next described. The flax seed, or linseed, would have yielded mucilage and oil in the boiling process.

3 *Prescription for Hemiplegia*

Texts: A: K 2418+, rev. iii, 9–10, copy: AMT 82,2: rev! iii, 9–10
B: VAT 10645, BAM 138, ii, 9–15

9 [a]*ana amēli*(LÚ) *ši-pìr mi-šit-t*[*i*] *šu-up-šu-hi u ri-mu-t*[*i*][a] *sah-lé-e*[b] *qalâti*(ŠE.SA.A) *la na-pa-a-t*[*i*][c] *bīnu*(GIŠ.ŠINIG) *ta-haš-šal*
10 *itti qēm kunāši*(ZÍZ.ÀM) *taballal ina šikāri tu-šab-šal* [NÍG].-LÁ.MEŠ-*ma*[d] *iballuṭ*(TI-*u*[*ṭ*])

a-a) Text as given on B; A: *ana* KIMIN
b) From A; B: ZÀ.HI.LI.ŠAR
c) From A; B: *na-pa-te*
d) Restored after the parallel text of BAM 138, ii, 8; no reading can be suggested

Translation: (9) That a man may be relieved of a stroke with hemiplegia, cress (or, cardamom) seed, unsifted husked (lit.: roasted) barley-flour and (dried out) tamarisk (leaves) you shall crush, (10) mix with flour of emmer-wheat and boil in beer; (knead), make into poultices, and he will recover.

Notes: That the prescription is for the condition stated has been anticipated in Section II where the combination of *šimmatu*, 'paralysis', and *rimûtu*, 'flaccidity', was briefly discussed. *Mišittu* with *rimûtu* is here taken to have the same meaning of 'hemiplegia', although rules governing the use of the 'construct state' in Semitic languages have separated *rimûtu* from *mišittu* in the phrase concerned. It is of interest, and of support, that the previous prescription of K 2418+ (iii, 4, cf. AMT 82,2: 4), begins:

> *šumma amēlu mi-šit-tú ma-<šid-ma>*[36] *qāt-su u šēp-šú ta-bi-i*[*k*]
> 'If a man has suffered a stroke and is without strength in his hand and foot (on one side).'

If 'hand and foot' may here serve for 'arm and leg',—and *šēpu* in particular seems occasionally to be so used,—a 'diagnosis' of hemiplegia would be clear accordingly.

The treatment requires that dry, coarse materials be made into hot poultices for the affected limbs. Such procedure forms no part of modern treatment; but when morale is low, and with anxiety, perhaps, as a secondary concern, some visible and well-tried practice—such as poulticing—may well of itself have proved comforting and been of therapeutic value. As a brief note on the procedure, it will be seen that the instruction to 'knead' the poultice materials in line 10 has been placed within brackets. The insertion, based on the *ta-la-aš*, 'you shall knead', found in a similar position after *tušabsal* in BAM 138, ii, 8, is made only for the clarity of modern reading. No error is supposed.

---

[36] Signs supposedly omitted by haplography.

4 *Prescription for Mobility Problems after Stroke*

Texts: A: K 2418+, iv, 27–32, copy: AMT 79,1: 11–16
B: VAT 13770, BAM 136, ii, 3'–10'

27 *šumma amēlu mi-šit-ti qabli*(MURUB$_4$) *maruṣ a-tál-lu-kám*[a] *la ile'i*[b] *qablā-āú ki-iṣ-ra-t*[i X X (X)][c]

28 GIŠ *bi-nu maštakal*(Ú ÌN.ÚŠ) *qān šalāli*(GI.ŠUL.HE) *suhuššu*(GIŠ.GIŠIMMAR.TUR) *tubbal*(HAD.A) *tahaššal tanappi itti* [X X *taballal ina* X X]

29 *ina tangussi tara-bak ina maški teṭerri*(SUR-*ri*) *taṣammid-ma* UD 3 KÁM *la tapaṭṭar*(NU DUH) *ina* UD 4 [KÁM xxx]

30 *nappī*(SIM)[d] *qēm ha-ru-*[*b*]*i qadūt šikani*(IM.GÚ.EN.NA) *ina isqūqi taballal ina* KAŠ SAG [*tara-bak* (. . . . .)]

31 *ina mê*(A) *šunê*(GIŠ ŠE.NÁ.A) *sek-ru-ti tu-maš-šá-a'-šú ina himē*[*ti tapaššas*(ŠÉŠ)-*su*][e]

32 *ina maški teṭerri ba-ah-ru-us-su* [*taṣammid-ma* . . . . .]

a From A; B: *-ka*
b Text of A: NU ZU; B: *la i-*[*le-'i*]
c A form of *rakāsu* or *kaṣāru* is perhaps to be restored
d For this reading cf. in the Notes following
e For such restoration cf. BAM 124, ii, 20f., etc., also SBTU I, 46, 4

Translation: (27) If a man is suffering from paralysis of the hip (muscle) and he is not able to walk about, his hips [being bound(?)] at(?) the joints, (28) tamarisk (leaves), cyperus grass, and (leaf-blades) of *šalālu*-reed and dwarf date palm you shall dry out, crush, sift, [mix] with [. . . . . .], decoct (29) [with beer(?)] in a copper kettle, spread onto a skin, bind on.

Do not take off for three days. On the fourth day [. . . . . .], (30) sievefuls(?) of carob flour and river silt you will mix with bran, [decoct] in freshly-brewed beer, [and, in the meantime(?)] (31) rubbing him with *Vitex*-water of long standing, and [anointing him] with leban, (32) spread onto a skin and bind on hot [. . . . . .].

Notes: The above interesting text, despite the lacunae and uncertainties, belongs necessarily to the history of neurophysiology. In the cases observed there was a serious degree of muscular dysfunction, it being actually in doubt whether 'he is not able to walk about' means 'he is not able to walk (at all).' In any event one may diagnose the case as one of spastic(?) rigidity of a paralysed hip (and leg) in hemiplegia. At the end of the prescription there is space for a restored *iballuṭ*, '(so) he will recover,' if this should be thought appropriate. But the prognosis cannot have been good.

As to the 'dispensing', the difficult SIM of line 30, seemingly a noun, has been interpreted in the light of the word *nap-pi-i* [. . . . . .], AMT 53,1: iii, 9, likewise found at the beginning of a sentence. Probably it was a measure, 'sieveful', relating to *nappû*, Ass. *nappiʾu*(?), 'sieve', and the verb SIM = *napû*, 'to sift.' Otherwise the adj. *sekru* of line 31 deserves comment. Given as 'warm abgestanden (von Flüssigkeiten)' in AHw 1036, and simply as 'heated', CAD S 217, the term seems rather to apply to water, etc., that is 'long standing' and so 'distilled' (in the sense that particles or impurities held in suspension have been allowed to settle by standing), and to have had no semantic connection with heat. This might appear to be so in the several instructions of the type *ina tinūri tesekker*, cited by CAD S 213, which are considered to mean '(the stated materials) you heat in an oven.' However, a translation '(the materials) you will allow to stand in an oven' is also suitable, and, in AMT 92,4: 1, is even assisted by the additional *kal ūmi*, 'all day long', and the following *ina kakkabi tuūbât*, 'you will let (them) stand under the stars.' A further argument in the matter is the point that the Sumerian for *sekru* is u_4-zal-le, from the verb u_4-zal, 'to pass, of time.'[37]

Regarding the plant names of the text, the series *bīnu, maštakal, qān šalāli* and *suhuššu* of line 28 is otherwise well known. They were 'used for their power to clean in the magical sense,'[38] and are principally found together outside of the medical texts, namely, in the *mīs pī* rituals, in *namburbi* rituals, in *Šurpu*, and elsewhere.[39] We seek here to advance understanding on *maštakal*. This plant is listed in Hh XVII, 131, in the same section as unu.gi = *suʾādu*, line 130a, and if the latter was a species of Cyperus grass as suggested by CAD

---

[37] For this equation cf. Hh XXIII, iii, 33', as found in MSL XI, 1974, p. 73. The unsatisfactory 'heated hot' for *sekrūti bahrūti* in CAD S 217, is a further argument for change.

[38] B. Landsberger, *The Date Palm and its By-products according to the Cuneiform Sources*, AfO Beih. 17, Graz, 1967, p. 14; cf. also F. Köcher, 'Ein Text medizinischen Inhalts aus dem neubabylonischen Grab 405,' in R. M. Boehmer, F. Pedde and B. Salje (eds.), *Uruk: die Gräber*, Mainz am Rhein, 1995, 211, note to line 6': *maštakal* as *šammi tēlilte*, "Pflanze der rituellen Reinigung."

[39] For the relevant texts cf. CAD S 352, under *suhuššu*, or M/1 391f., under *maštakal*, and AHw 127, 630, 898 (*qanû*, I 4a), and 1055.

S 339 on the basis of the Syr. *suʿda* and Arabic *suʿd* with such meaning, one could accordingly believe that the Akk. *maštakal* was of similar or related meaning. *Cyperus rotundus* in particular 'occurs all over Iraq in moister regions.'[40] The edible tubers of its root system is the meaning perhaps required in the text following.

5 *Prescription for Facial Palsy*

Texts: A: K 2418+, iv, 11–13, copies: AMT 76,5: 11–13 and 79,4: 1–4
B: K 8685, AMT 77,8: 4'–8'
C: W. 22307/14, SBTU I, 46, 16–20, copy: p. 142
D: 1924.1819, OECT XI, 72, Obv. 1'–3'

11 *šumma amēlu mi-šit-ṭi*[a] *pa-ni i-šu*[b] *īn-šú i-ṣap-par ur-ra u mu-šá *ip*(text: *ur*)*-ta-na-at-t*[*i*][d]
12 *la it-ta-na-a-a-al ina dišpi*(LÀL)[e] *himēti*(Ì.NUN.NA) *pānī*(IGI.MEŠ)-*šú ka-a-a-nam-ma*[f] *muš-šu-du*[g]
13 *la i-kal-la*[h] *maštakal*(Ú ÌN.ÚŠ)[i] *ba-lu pa-tan itanakkal*[j]*-ma iballuṭ*

a) So A; B: *-ṭú*
b) So A; C: *-šú*
c) Following C; A: GE_6, B: G[E_6]
d) Suggested reading, cf. further in the notes following
e) So A and C; B: uncertain signs, not easily readable (cf. copy)
f) From A; omitted on C; B: broken
g) So A and B; C: *-da*
h) Following A; C: *i-kal-li*
i) So A and C; D: Ú IN.NU.[ÚŠ]; B: broken
j) B and C: KÚ.KÚ; A: NAG.MEŠ, considered less satisfactory.

Translation: (11) If a man has facial palsy, his (affected) eye deviates from the other and day and night remains open so that he cannot lie down to sleep, (12) he should not cease constantly to rub his face with honey and leban (13) and should gnaw *maštakal* (root) when not eating at mealtimes. So he will recover.

Notes: From the given symptoms a diagnosis of facial palsy, and possibly of Bell's palsy—so named after the Scottish anatomist, John

---

[40] H. L. Chakravarty, *Plant Wealth of Iraq: A Dictionary of Economic Plants* I, Baghdad, 1976, p. 184.

Bell, 1763–1820—is not in doubt. In this condition there is a one-sided paralysis of muscles supplied by the seventh, or facial, nerve and the patient cannot close the eye on the affected side. The name of *lagophthalmos* is given to this condition; the term derives in its first element from the Greek *lagōs*, 'hare', there being a popular belief that the hare sleeps with its eyes open.

Facial palsy has no relation to stroke, although to an observer, weakness about the mouth and speech difficulty might well suggest the possibility of connection. There is, however, no hemiparesis or hemiplegia, and indeed, a good recovery is usual within a matter of weeks or months. As to what currently may be done, massage by the patient of the paralysed muscles and facial exercises (before a mirror) are not essentially very different from the prescription of line 12. The proposed eating, interpreted as 'gnawing', of *maštakal*—possibly the small, hard tubers of *Cyperus rotundus* as anticipated in the previous *Notes*—may likewise have been directed towards the exercise of weakened mouth muscles.[41]

It should be mentioned that there is a problem regarding the end verb in line 11, which in text C has become corrupted into *ur-ga-at-tú*. While the commentary SBTU I, 47, 10, struggles to defend this reading (see further in Hunger's edition, p. 58), the correction to *ur-ta-at-tú*, translated "er wach ist", does not seem tenable either. Otherwise, for the previous verb *iṣappar* of line 11, it will be seen that *ṣapāru*, elsewhere 'to squint (of the eyes)', has been given a meaning appropriate to Bell's palsy where the affected eyeball rolls upward and slightly outward when an attempt is made to close the eye. For the interest of the matter one may add that this *ṣapāru* belongs clearly with the *par*-verbs of 'separation and dispersion', as *parāsu, paṭāru.*

[41] For further study references may be made to C. C. Townsend and Evan Guest (eds.), *Flora of Iraq* VIII, Baghdad, 1985, pp. 333ff., under 'Cyperus L.'; H. L. Chakravarty, *Plant Wealth of Iraq*, pp. 182ff. (cf. previous note); and D. Hooper and H. Field, *Useful Plants and Drugs of Iran and Iraq*, Field Museum of Natural History, Botanical Series IX/3, Chicago, 1937, pp. 111–112. Following the proposal made it is relevant that the plant *sikillu* or *usikillu*, a known synonym of *maštakal*, had the same twofold application in medicine, namely, bound in leaf-form onto a patient's forehead as in AMT 14,2: 6, and eaten alone, for a stomach complaint, as in BAM 574, ii, 9. To mention one further part it was perhaps the fibre of the 'fibrous root system' of the plant—thus Lise Manniche of *Cyperus esculentus* in *An Ancient Egyptian Herbal*, London, 1989, p. 98,—that best explains the meaning of *sikillu* when this was to be twisted (*talappap*) between the beads of a necklace in magical use. Wool was similarly used in many parallel texts.

parāru, šapāru, parāʾu, etc., cf. further in W. von Soden, *Grundriss der akkadischen Grammatik* (Rome, 1952 and 3rd. edit., 1995), § 73, 1), b.

Other Components of Babylonian Stroke Therapy

The above prescriptions will have shown that the central measures used in the ancient treatment of stroke were massage and poulticing. A brief statement may be added here of the several other procedures which were tried, the list concerning simple *šammu u šiptu* texts (where one or more 'drugs' or other ingredients are used with an accompanying incantation), mouth washes, fumigation and phylacteries.

A single text may be considered under the first of these categories, this being K 2418+, iv, 19–21 (copy in AMT 79,1: iv, 3–5). The instruction is that honey and leban are to be rubbed on the affected mouth, the fragmentary incantation, which is remarkable for the abundance of its *a*-vowels, beginning:

u_4-da-ta hé-en-duh-a lal-ì-nun-na
ka—ba—*d[ib-ba hé-en-duh-a],
'From today may they open, may (this) honey and leban [open the seiz]ed mouth.'

It will be recalled that 'honey and leban' (paralleled, it may be said, by the 'honey and curds' of II Sam. xvii. 29; Job xx. 17, etc., in the translation of the *New English Bible*), occurs again in our material, as commonly also elsewhere, in the treatment for facial palsy, prescription No. 5, line 12. We remain with the mouth to consider the import of *mašqâte*, Ass. *mašqiāte*. There are two references in the texts, firstly, K 2418+, iii, 52 (copy in AMT 78,1: iii, 22), which summarises the three previous lines as *3 maš-qá-a-tum*, and secondly, AMT 23,2: 10, a partial duplicate, where the summary reads, [*2*] *maš-ka*(sic)*-a-tú*. While 'potions' or 'enemas' may be appropriate elsewhere, the *mašqâte* of present concern were almost certainly 'mouth washes', a term which could be added to the dictionary entries. The evidence is that, in both references, the *mašqâte* are found centrally in the long list of prescriptions concerned with *kadibbidû* and thus undoubtedly relate to that condition. Secondly, in both stroke and Bell's palsy food particles may become lodged in the mouth owing to the flaccid paralysis of the cheek muscles on the affected side; there is usually a problem also with salivation.

Fumigation as the third of the 'other components of Babylonian stroke therapy' must, for the moment, await the publication of relevant texts. However, the phrase *qutāru ša mišitti*, 'fumigation for (flaccid) paralysis', has been noticed briefly by I. L. Finkel in the Civil Festschrift, p. 103,—for the full reference cf. above, under note 32.

Finally, phylacteries, *mêlū ša mišitti*, are mentioned in BAM 135, 10'. The composition of three *mêlū* are given, the first of these, lines 2'–3', consisting of three stones,—*anzahhu*-glass, 'hate stone', and *pindû*, see further, in a careful study, Anais Schuster, *Die Steinbeschreibungsserie* abnu šikinšu, Heidelberg, 1996, pp. 28, 38 and 48. A group of *4 abnē mišitti* are found in BAM 372, iii, 11f., and in 376, iii, 6f.,—the same references are given in Stol, *Epilepsy*, p. 109, note 97. Exceptionally two fish eyes might be used in the control of stroke, of the *purādu* fish alone as in AMT 82,2: iii, 1–3, and of the *arsuppu* and *purādu*, as in AMT 78,1: 6–9 + 28,7: 3–6, with 23,2: 14–17. The eyes, in the usual way, were to be placed in a skin round the patient's neck,—but not until the 'fourth-day'. On the preceding days they were to be embedded in salt (*ina ṭabti tušnâl*). The period seems likely to have represented the maximum allowed time for the demon to have left the possessed body in haemorrhagic stroke.

It is intriguing that, in the last line of the tablet (copy in AMT 79,1: 30), the name of Tiāmat (written *Ti-amat*) is somehow linked with the '8 bandages' of the prescriptions, but no convincing explanation can be offered at the present time. It should be mentioned otherwise that the details of an impressive 'medicine', where, on the authority of the 'Seven Sages', '17 tested plants' (*17 šammū latkūtu*) are to be taken as an infusion for *kadibbidû*, or applied dry to the mouth for *kadibbidû* as one of several mental disorders, have been published by Erle Leichty in the Sachs Festschrift, pp. 261ff.—the editorial details are as given in note 6. It is possible that only the first part of the prescription would have been related to stroke.

PART II

V *The Relevance of Ludlul, Tablet II*

In introducing the Second Part of the present study, attention may firstly be drawn to an essential distinction. The First Part concerned stroke; Part II to a large extent will concern the demons of stroke. That these existed at all has not previously been mentioned. There has indeed been no reason to do so while the *asû*, or 'physician', has been mainly of concern. But the *āšipu*, a more learned(?) man, had by contrast a clear interest in nosology, or 'the classification of disease'; and gods, demons and ghosts had their place in his research.

The translation of Section VI, as also the studies already mentioned of Labat and Stol, will reveal at once this aspect of the stroke concept, and the *alû*-demon in particular has been studied by Geller[42] and Stol[43] in recent work. But an additional source for the investigation of stroke in this way, and one which exclusively names the *alû* as the demon responsible, is *Ludlul bēl nēmeqi*, or 'The poem of the Righteous Sufferer.' This long and interesting document has been approached and analysed in different ways,[44] but that the Sufferer's ailments included a stroke-like condition, which he in fact describes in some detail, has not previously been suggested. Thus initially in II, 71–74, following Lambert's edition, we read:

> '(Thereupon) the *alû*-demon enfolded me as with a garment,
> 'The deep sleep (of coma) enmeshed me like a net.
>
> 'Staring were my eyes, but they could not see,
> 'Open were my ears, but they could not hear.'

At this time a total paralysis, here seen more as confabulation than as quadriplegia, assailed him (75–76):

> 'Flaccidity (*rimûtu*) seized all of my body,
> 'Paralysis (*mišittu*) descended on my flesh.'

Seemingly also the three following lines (77–79) emphasize the Sufferer's complete immobility during the period of coma, so that 'Even my feet forgot how to move.' The following couplet is more difficult, but if to be restored:

> [*mi?-i*]*h?-ṣu šuk-šu-du ú-nap-paq ma-aq-t*[*i-i*]*š*
> [*a-a iš*]*-du-ud mu-tu i-te-rim pa-ni-ia*

---

[42] *Forerunners to Udug-hul: Sumerian exorcistic Incantations*, Freiburger altorientalische Studien, Bd. 12, Stuttgart, 1985, pp. 80–82, lines 857ff.

[43] *Epilepsy in Babylonia*, pp. 41–42.

[44] The standard edition is that of W. G. Lambert, *Babylonian Wisdom Literature*, Oxford, 1960, chap. 2. It has been discussed poetically, with a new translation of Tablet II, by Erica Reiner, *'Your thwarts in pieces, your mooring rope cut': poetry from Babylonia and Assyria*, Ann Arbor, Mich., 1985, pp. 101–118. For a medical interpretation cf. J. V. Kinnier Wilson, 'An Introduction to Babylonian psychiatry', *AS* 16, Chicago, 1965, pp. 296f., the document being there presented as the autobiography of a paranoid schizophrenic.

'While the attack was overcoming (me) I gasped for breath like an epileptic,[45]
'(Nay), [had he not de]layed, death would have "covered my face,"'

the reference would be to the laboured, or stertorous, breathing of a stroke patient during coma. In lines 84–85 the Sufferer's loss of speech is remarked:

'A snare was laid on my mouth,
'And a bolt barred my lips.'

And finally, following an allusion to eating difficulty (line 87), one reads of the tastelessness of the offered food (88–89):

'When grain was served, I ate it as stinkweed;
'Beer, the very life of man, became distasteful to me.'

Even this statement may be newly understood. The condition is known medically as 'ageusia', from the Gk. *geusia*, 'taste,' with alpha privative. Such loss of taste occurs commonly in Bell's palsy and then affects the anterior two-thirds of the tongue (which is innervated by the seventh nerve). It is not *per se* a symptom of stroke, but we have previously had occasion to associate the two conditions, see above in Section IV, Prescription 5.

VI *Tablet XXVII of the Diagnostic Series: A New Translation*

The following translation and Commentary of *Sakikku* XXVII concludes the present statement on stroke. The translation is based textually on the edition of Stol in CM 2, and while accordingly it has been thought unnecessary to repeat the text in this account, certain technical or 'key' words from the original have occasionally been provided and may assist understanding. Actually, not all of Tablet XXVII is concerned with stroke. This condition is clearly the subject of the first section of the Tablet, lines 1–13, as so recognised by Stol; it will be shown that the third section, involving the *Alû*-demon, relates also to stroke as does much of the last (lines 26–36). However, three entries concern epilepsy. One or two of the remainder have proved difficult to assess accurately.

As with our previous paper on 'epilepsy' we have replaced the rule-lines which occur in the text with modern summaries. These

[45] So proposed on the basis of *miqtu*, 'epilepsy', *maqtu* being properly the past part. of the verb *maqātu*, 'to fall.'

lines divide the Tablet into five sections. Each ascribes the stated symptoms to a specific agent, and these, with relevant line numbers placed in brackets, are:

Rābiṣū, or 'lurker'-demons (9–13, to which *Sakikku* XIV, iv, 3'–4', may be added, see further after line 13),

Lemnu demons[46] (14–19),
The *Alû*-demon (20–23),
The river-demon (24–25),
Ghosts, as individually specified (26–36).

The additional point may be made that the symbol '*R*', for 'Redactor', has again been used where a variant reading has been introduced into the given text. Examples of this editing occur in lines 4 and 34.

Introductory Entries with Prognosis: Symptoms Attributed to Lurker-demons

1. If a man is suffering from facial paralysis (*mišitti pāni*) and half of his body is (also) paralysed (*išammam-šu*), it is 'stroke' (*šipir mišitti*).[47]

2–3. If he has had a stroke and is recovering but still suffers from frontal headache and is much afraid, for one ye[ar (the demon's)] possession will not be relaxed.[48]

4. If he has had a stroke and is still suffering from frontal headache, he is subject to a demon; he will die.—*R*: he is subject to a *lemnu* demon; he will die.

5–7. If he has had a stroke and has been stricken (*mahiṣ*) on either his right or his left side, if in the event that his shoulder socket has not been dislocated (by a fall) (*uppi ahi-šu la paṭir*) he can stretch out his fingers, raise and stretch out the (affected) hand, flex and stretch out the (affected) foot (*šēp-šu ikannan u itarraṣ*), and does not refuse food and drink, in three <days> he will recover.

8. If it is with difficulty that he flexes the (affected) hand or foot he has had a stroke, but he will recover.

---

[46] Written HUL, for which the expected reading *lemnu* has been established by Stol, CM 2, p. 77 (there translated as 'Evil').

[47] Either *šipir mišitti*, 'it is stroke' as suggested, or *sipir mišitti maruṣ*, 'he is ill with stroke,' which has also manuscript support, appear to be the readings offered at this point,—see further in the Commentary.

[48] On the basis of the single text TDP II, pl. XLVIII, cf. in this account, fig. 1 Labat read the line as *m*[*u?-ki*]*l(?) rēši-šu(?) la pa-ṭir*, which was followed by Stol but without the question marks. For the present account there is still a case for uncertainty and, with the text as copied being analysed differently, a reading M[U] 1.[K]ÁM ⌜DIB⌝-*s*[*u*] *la pa-ṭir* is suggested, and forms the basis of the given translation.

9. If his right side is without strength (*tabkat*), the paralysis (*mišittu*) has been inflicted by a (lurking) *rābiṣu*-demon; he will recover.

10. If the whole of his right side is without strength, the paralysis has been inflicted by a (lurking) *rābiṣu*-demon; he has been gradually stricken (*arkatam mahiṣ*).[49]

11. If his left side is without strength (it is a symptom of) the hand of Shulak.

12–13. If the whole of his left side is without strength and he was suddenly stricken (*mihra mahiṣ*),—hand of Shulak, the (lurking) demon of the bathroom. The *āšipu* should not make a prognosis for his recovery.[50]

A translation of Sakikku XIV iv, 3'–4'[51] *may be inserted at this point:*

13a. If (being stricken on the right side) he drags his right foot (*šēp-šú ša imitti imaššar*), and his mouth remains contorted (*pâ-šú ṣu(n)dur*), the paralysis is from a (lurking) *rābiṣu*-demon. He will live on for a time and will then die.

Symptoms Relating to a Lemnu Demon

14–15. If (after an epileptic attack) the features of a man's face (*simat pāni-šu*) are gradually changing back (to normal) (*ittanakker*), his eyes wander about (*ittanaprarā*), and blood, bespattering his lip(s) and chin, flows uncontrollably from his mouth, a *lemnu* demon has possessed that man.

16–17. If a man falls forward as he walks along,[52] his eyes remain wide open and are not able to turn, and he cannot of himself[53] move either his hands or his feet, a *lemnu* demon has possessed that man; it is as if epilepsy had been poured out upon him (*kīma miqtu/antašubbû uš-tar-*hu-šu*).[54]

---

[49] On the problems of this phrase, as also of the following *mihra mahiṣ* (line 12), cf. above in Section II with note 15.

[50] Further examples of this statement in the medical texts are documented in AHw 920, under *qību*, 3, and in CAD Q 249b, cf. also M. Stol, CM 2, 94, with note 13, and 'Diagnosis and therapy in Babylonian medicine,' *JEOL* 32, p. 56.

[51] Text of TDP 142, 3', as restored by TDP 238, 63.

[52] A 'variant' reading, *šumma amēlu sūqa*(E.SÍR) *ina alāki-šú*, 'If a man as he walks along a street,' is provided by col. i, 3, of a Nimrud text, ND 4368. The relevance of this text for the *lemnu* section of the Tablet is explained in the Commentary, notes to line 14f.

[53] Following Labat, 'de lui-même', and supposing that the text is describing the patient's inability to perform voluntary movements. Stol: 'he does not move his hands, feet (or) himself.'

[54] Copy *uš-tar-ri-šú*, seemingly from *šurrû*, 'to begin', and thus Stol, CM 2, 77.

18. If epilepsy frequently pours out upon him (*miqtu/antašubbû irtenehhi-šu*), whereupon he cannot of himself move either his hands or feet, a *lemnu* demon has possessed that man.

19. [If a man, being alt]ogether forgetful,[55] keeps throwing off his garment and putting it on again, and wanders aimlessly about; if also he has severely bruised his eyes (perhaps a misinterpretation of ecchymoses around the eyes), a *lemnu* demon is possessing that man.

Symptoms Attributed to an Alû-demon

20. [If, when he is smi]ting him,[56] (the demon) draws back but later he (the patient) becomes hot (*ēm*), loses consciousness (*ramān-šu la idê*) and holds his eyes in a fixed stare, it is the hand of an evil *alû*-demon.

21–22. [If] (the demon) frequently possesses him (*iṣṣanabbat-su*) [as for] (a possession involving) coma (*lit.*: 'sleep'),[57] (at which time) his limbs are without strength (*iššappakā*), his ears ring and his mouth is seized so that he cannot speak, it is the hand of an evil *alû*-demon.

23. If (the demon) frequently possesses him as for (a possession involving) coma (*lit.*; 'sleep'), and whenever he possesses him (*enūma iṣbatu-šu*) his ears ring and his mouth is seized so that he cannot speak, it is the hand of an evil *alû*-demon.

Symptoms Attributed to a River-demon

24. If, while bathing, *he is all right (restoring <*šalim*>), but on coming out of the river he staggers (dizzily) from side to side and falls down, a (lurking) demon of the river has smitten him.

25. If, when coming up from the water, his body shivers (with cold) (*ihmi-šu*), and he staggers (dizzily) from side to side and falls down, a (lurking) demon of the river has smitten him.

However, in the equivalent position the Nimrud text has *ir-te-ni-hi-šú* from *rehû*, 'to pour out,' and, interpreted as a subjunctive III/2 (with passive significance), the suggested *uš-tar-*hu-šú* differs only by a single wedge from *uš-tar-ri-šú*. Collation might settle the matter.

55 A proposed reading of [*ṭa-a*]*b ma-ṣi-ma* in SBTU III, No. 89, 6, and of [*ṭ*]*āb*(DÙG) *ma-ši-ma* in TDP II, pl. XLVIII, 19, is here advanced as a solution to the initial difficulties of this line. The thought, more freely translated, would be: '[if a man, not know]ing at all what he is doing.'

56 A reading [*šumma enūma*(UD) *i*]*mahhaṣu*([S]ÌG.MEŠ-*ṣu*)-*šú* is suggested uncertainly for the beginning of the line.

57 Akk. [*kīma*] *šitti*, a reading confirmed by the parallel phrase of line 23. As interpreted (cf. further in the Commentary), the phrase is taken to mean that coma (*šittu*) was not a feature of the condition being described.

Symptoms Attributed to Ghosts

26. If he remains motionless and deathly silent (*iprur-ma ušharrir*), ghosts are persec[uting] the sick man (*ired*[*dû-š*]*u* (⌈UŠ-*šú*⌉)).

27–28. If, being finally abandoned (by the demon), he asks repeatedly for water, and then, when his (body)-heat is again stable(?) (*mithar*) and the pulses of his hands beat normally (*šerʾān qātē-šu illakū*), he groans incessantly from the beginning of the night to the middle of the (morning) watch, it is (a symptom of) the hand of a ghost.

29–31. If a state of depression falls upon him, he begs (for help) to everyone whom he sees and his limbs every day are hot and sweaty (*umma u zuʾta ūmišam-ma iraššī*); if at times he has a great craving (for food), and until they bring it to him he trembles with rage (?) (*libba i-ha-*⌈*al*⌉),[58] but then when they do bring it to him he only looks at it but does not eat it—hand of a ghost who has [not], through the hole [made for him, received food offerings].[59]

32–34. If his skin (or, epidermis)[60] is pricking him, his ears ring, he keeps straightening out(?) the hairs of his body (*šārat zumri-šu uštanazzaz*), and (thinks that) his whole body is crawling as if lice were there, but when he brings his hand (to scratch them) there are none—*R*: (so) he does not scratch any more—it is the hand of a ghost.[61]

35–36. If the staff of Sin (the moon god) has been laid against his (rigid) leg, but when he tries to bend or stretch it out he howls (with pain) (*irammum*) and saliva flows from (the corner of) his mouth,—a ghost wandering in the steppeland has seized him.[62]

---

[58] The previous reading has been *libbu i-ha-*⌈*hu*⌉, translated by Labat as 'il vomit', and by Stol 'he is disgusted,' but even if justifiable neither seems correct on grounds of sense. The proposed *libba i-ha-*⌈*al*⌉ takes the verb to be *hiālu* or *hâlu*, documented by CAD H 54f. and AHw 342, and discussed importantly by Landsberger, MSL IX 85.

[59] If *ina a-p*[*i-šú*] may be read. The practice of placing food offerings (*kispū*) in a hole (*apu*) in the ground to appease the spirits of the departed was well established in ancient Mesopotamia.

[60] Akk. *tuqnu*, here regarded as a metathesized form of *qutnu*, a 'thin skin' that might cover certain parts of the human or animal body (cf. Dictionaries).

[61] Some textual corruption at the end of the entry appears to be in part a faulty anticipation of the line following. It is here omitted.

[62] An additional source for the entry is found in BAM 471, ii, 21–22, as thus noted by Köcher in the Inhaltsübersicht to Bd. V, and Stol, CM 2, 81, note 97.

VII *Commentary*

1. It will be recalled that the opening line of the previous Tablet on epilepsy, as reconstructed by the writers, was a general statement on the place of demons and ghosts in differing aspects of the disease. Line 1 of the present Tablet seems equally to have been of general significance, facial weakness and hemiplegia being singled out as pathognomonic of the condition of 'stroke'. The word translated as 'half of his body' with reference to the hemiplegia is *talammu*, discussed briefly in the previous study, p. 195 with note 50; of relevance also is STT I, 89, 48, where a contrast is made between the right and left halves of the body (*ta-lam imitti-šú, ta-lam šumēli-šú*). On AO 6680 (cf. in this paper, fig. 2), the reading of the last sign of the line may have been *m*[*aruṣ*], 'he is ill', in accordance with the GIG of the catch-line of BM 47753, seen thus on M. J. Geller's copy, *apud* Stol, *Epilepsy*, Pl. 2. However, the catch-line of the duplicate text as given in STT I, 91, rev. 87', omits *maruṣ*, as also does K 2418+ (copy in AMT 77,1: 1) which, strangely, cites initial lines of the diagnostic text. The precise choice is as presented in note 47.

2–4. Residual headache persisting upon a return to consciousness is well known in stroke attacks. This will often, following haemorrhage, have been as the result of raised intracranial pressure, but there are many possibilities. For the *lemnu*-demon of line 4, if rightly so interpreted, cf. further below, in lines 14–19.

On a philological matter it may be said that the idea of a sick person being 'subject to a demon' represents a new understanding of the Akk. *mukīl rēši-*(*šu*) *naṭālu*. The phrase was otherwise interpreted in *Med. Hist.* 34/2, 187, with notes 12 and 13. The new proposal owes something to the verb *dagālu*, which has the two meanings of 'to look at' (as *naṭālu*) and 'to be subject to'; it is considered less satisfactory to suppose that 'in a dreamy state the patient believes he sees the attacking demon', Stol, *Epilepsy*, p. 59.

5–7. The reference to recovery within three days—which, in modern terms, may have meant two days owing to the Semitic custom of 'counting both ends'—suggests that a 'reversible' ischaemic event (which cannot further be determined), was the condition seen and carefully noted by the ancient observer. The 'transient ischaemic attack' of still shorter duration was possibly referred to in lines 21–23 of the Tablet, as discussed below.

8. The 'difficulty' experienced in the making of limb movements may have been an indication of early rigidity, more seriously seen in the entry of lines 35–36.

9. With the exception otherwise of the inserted text '13a', the prognoses cease with this line. There are five altogether. In lines 4 and 13a the prognosis is 'he will die'; in lines 5–9 it is premised that 'he will live', or 'recover'. The pattern is intriguing, and not easy of explanation. With the conspicuous silence on the matter of lines 10–36 one perhaps senses that the difficulty of predicting the outcome of a stroke attack from presenting symptoms was known even in Babylon.

12–13. Shulak (or, Shulag), 'the lurking-demon of the bathroom', has been discussed by Stol, *op. cit.*, p. 76, who cites also an interesting parallel from the Babylonian Talmud. In fact, stroke and bathrooms are not disassociated, if mainly in connection with hip fracture following a fall.[63] Such was not obviously the case in the present instance, but Shulak's association with the hip—or at least with the *rapaštu* (ÚR.KUN), a part adjacent to the hip and usually translated 'loins', or 'pelvis'—is known from TDP 108, 17: [*šumma ina rap*]*ašti-šu mahiṣ qāt* ᵈ*Šu-lak*, 'If he has been injured in the loins, (it is a symptom of) the hand of Shulak.'

13a. The few but certain examples of *mašāru* in the specific sense of 'to drag (the feet)', are documented in CAD M/1, 359, 2a, and by AHw 624, *mašāru* G, 3. What was involved by the entry may be visualised from a modern description: '. . . the gait of the patient is characteristic. In walking he leans to the sound side and swings round the affected limb from the hip, the foot scraping the ground as it is raised and advanced.'[64] The entry will relate to the recovery phase of a stroke attack.

14–15. As presented in the offered translation, and in marked contrast to the concern of the previous section, the symptoms of these lines refer seemingly to the recovery stage of a major epileptic attack. The eyes are beginning to move again; colour is returning to a less vivid and congested face; and the blood issuing from

[63] Cf. specifically H. C. White, 'Post-stroke hip fracture,' *Archives of Orthopaedic and Trauma Surgery*, 107 (1988), pp. 345–347; also S. G. B. Kirker, *Neurophysiological Studies of hip muscle function in posture and gait after Stroke*, MD thesis, submitted to Dublin University, 1997, p. 18.

[64] Gordon Macpherson (ed.), *Black's Medical Dictionary*, 37th edit., London, 1992, p. 438.

the mouth we would interpret as arising from a badly bitten tongue or cheek sustained during the clonic phase of the seizure.[65] Since also there is no mention of any of the initial symptoms, it is possible to think that, in the original case, the person concerned fell alone and there were no witnesses.

It should be mentioned (with Stol, *Epilepsy*, p. 77), that lines 14–18 of our text are paralleled in part by a Nimrud text, ND 4368 (i. 3ff.), to which attention has been drawn in notes 52 and 54. This text was published (by KW) in *Iraq* XVIII, 1956, pl. XXV (copy), and Vol. XIX, 1957, pp. 40–49 (edition). An association with the present Tablet XXVII of the diagnostic series was there noted, but since prescriptions were provided with the individual observations, the text was thought to belong to a 'companion series' to *Sakikku*, see in the second reference, p. 45. It is now better regarded as forming part of the first edition of *Sakikku*, along with two other texts,[66] and indeed the first ten lines of K 2418+. The proposal has the support of Tablet XXVIII of *Sakikku* (cf. TDP 192, 37ff., and Stol, *Epilepsy*, pp. 82–85), which contain a number of prescriptions similar in both style and content to those found on ND 4368.

16–17. Probably to be regarded as an observation regarding stroke as this may overtake a man in some public place. That in the Nimrud text this was specified as 'in the street', *cf.* note 52, recalls the Sumerian texts published by Geller[67] where demons are often declared to be sila-a šu bar-ra-àm, 'let loose in the street(s).' While in line 17 *kīma* is regarded as a conjunction—the tense of the verb following being taken as subjunctive—it is clear, with Stol pp. 77ff., that the case is being 'likened' or compared to epilepsy, so that epilepsy itself is not primarily of concern.

18. Clearly related to the preceding entry and employing the same phrase: *qātē-šu u šēpē-šu ramān-šu la unaš*, '(having fallen), he does not (or, cannot) of himself move either hands or feet,' the entry may concern tonic epilepsy, although information is sparse, and it is not clear, in any instance, for how long the lack of movement should

---

[65] A reference to 'blood flowing from the mouth' in a similar case is found in Tablet XXVI, obv. 26, cf. the writers' note on this line in *Med. Hist.*, 34/2, p. 195.

[66] The essential references are to M. Stol, 'Diagnosis and therapy in Babylonian medicine,' *JEOL* 32 (1991–92), p. 43, and to the same writer's *Epilepsy in Babylonia*, chap. V, 'A second Diagnostic text.'

[67] *Forerunners to Udug-hul: Sumerian exorcistic Incantations*, Stuttgart, 1985, *e.g.*, lines 170–173.

be deemed to apply. Tonic epilepsy, for whatever reason, is not mentioned in Tablet XXVI in the company of the other varieties.

19. While stroke patients, in recovering, may be also confused, this line relates definitely to the post-ictal confusion of an epileptic, one of the automatisms that are mentioned having already found a place in Tablet XXVI of the series (rev. 19–20).

20–23. The *alû* demon's concern with stroke has been suggested above in Section V. The present section would appear to bear out the association although uncertainties remain. In line 20 the word *ēm*, 'he becomes hot', may be regarded as of significance in that bodily exertion or stress may often precipitate a stroke attack. The second and third entries, and despite the difficulty of deciding how precisely they should be distinguished,[68] refer probably, as one may think, to the transient ischaemic attack, or 'TIA'. Such episodes are of short duration, lasting minutes or hours; they may recur, so that the 'iterative' tense of *iṣṣanabbat,* confirmed by the following *enūma iṣbatu-šu,* 'whenever (the demon) seizes him,' is satisfied accordingly. The ischaemic attack is of several kinds depending on the brain area involved, but, if the translation does not deceive, the limb weakness (no side being specified), the loss of speech (as dysarthria), and the ear noise or tinnitus, suggest that the ischaemia was in the vertebro-basilar territory, or, in other terms, in the blood vessels which run through the bones of the neck.

There has been a *crux interpretum* in the middle of line 20. Labat, followed by Stol, there read ÉN = *šiptu,* 'incantation', but the same strokes, in the same position, could produce IGI.BAR = *naplusu,* 'to look'.[69] In association with the following *īnē-šu izqup* this is surely preferable.

24–25. It is clear that the original person of line 24 who staggered and fell after bathing in a river may not necessarily have had a stroke,—one would have expected some reference to hemiplegia or paralysis if this had been the case. One might consider the possibility of a heart attack or angina, but some reference to chest pain would then have been expected. An alternative suggestion[70] would be to suppose that the person concerned simply fell in a faint, his

---

[68] In *Med. Hist.* 34/2, pp. 190 and 192, the term 'paired entries' was used to describe such texts, which are numerous in the Diagnostic series.

[69] As, indeed, suggested as an alternative reading by Labat in TDP 190, note 337.

[70] Proposed by Dr S. G. B. Kirker (Cambridge).

blood pressure falling rapidly as he made his way to the bank, but being maintained at a normal level in the river by the weight of the water against his body.

A note may be offered on the verb *hamû* in line 25. Historically there have been two approaches to understanding. The first is that the concern of the verb is with the muscles and so means "lähmen", AHw 319, or with an extended figurative sense, 'to paralyse, immobilise, stun,' as CAD H, 72. The second relates *hamû* to the skin, and specifically to *cutis anserina* or 'goose-flesh', Germ. "Gänsehaut,"[71] so that the essential meaning is 'to shiver', whether from cold, fear or in awe (of something).[72] The latter sense is clearly required in the context of our passage.

26. The 'ghost diseases', *qāt eṭemmi*, and in its several varieties *ṣibit eṭemmi*, will require no introduction in these pages. Salient texts have been transliterated and translated by Köcher in a familiar study;[73] the symptomatology of the group has also been examined by M. J. Geller.[74] The relevance of these notes is that the final Section of Tablet XXVII concerns states or conditions which were believed to have been caused by ghosts. They are of different kinds, the first concerning a patient who is 'motionless and deathly silent.' As usual, one would wish to have further details, but as given the symptoms are suggestive of either a profound emotional depression, or of post-ictal stupor if the primary condition was that of epilepsy.

27–28. The initial *uzzub* of line 27, which applies (it is thought) to a patient when 'finally abandoned (by the demon),' may suitably explain at least three of the remaining four entries of the Tablet. The argument will be that they describe sequelae to stroke (or other) attacks,[75] the 'groaning' throughout the night of the present entry being an example of such development from an early 'post-possession'

---

[71] Proposed by B. Landsberger, *Die Welt des Orients* III (1964), p. 50, and accepted by F. R. Kraus, *ZA* 77 (1987), 198, line 11, with note, p. 199, and M. Stol, CM 2, 79, line 25.

[72] Cf. Landsberger, *op. cit.*, pp. 52–54, note 28 a–d, also *RA* 62 (1968), 114, note 59.

[73] 'Spätbabylonische medizinische Texte aus Uruk,' in C. Habrich, F. Marguth and J. H. Wolf (eds.), *Medizinische Diagnostik in Geschichte und Gegenwart*, Munich, 1978, pp. 25–32.

[74] 'A Recipe against ŠU.GIDIM,' *AfO* Beih. 19, 1982, pp. 192ff.

[75] Even as the concluding entries of the previous Tablet XXVI describe epileptic sequelae, including automatisms and post-ictal confusion.

phase. We are not informed as to the cause of the groaning—and this, of course, may attend upon 'distress' of any kind. However, at least one possibility is that the groaning was symptomatic of the continuing headache which may follow an attack of stroke or epilepsy, the patient being too disorientated, or still too weak, to articulate his problem to another person.

29–31. Depression and anxiety are thought to characterise the situation of these lines. They may occur after many illnesses, including stroke, being then classified as 'secondary affective disorders'. In detail *ašuštu* is certainly 'depression' (line 29); anxiety has been mentioned since the notice of daily sweating in the same line may be readily so interpreted. Loss of appetite (line 31) may occur following both stroke and anxiety, but there was a psychological aspect to the matter which cannot easily be penetrated on the information given.

32–34. We are reasonably certain that no account of lice-hunting in the body occurs in modern descriptions of stroke. However, sensory symptoms including paraesthesiae, both unilateral and bilateral, occur in the form of cerebral ischaemia discussed above, lines 20–23, and might arguably have given rise to the actions observed. Paraesthesia, as commonly described, is a 'pins and needles' sensation felt in the skin; in this connection the *uzaqqat-su* of the text, from *zaqātu*, 'to sting' or 'prick', would be appropriate accordingly. The Redactor's comment, '(so) he does not scratch any more', is also instructive—although probably incorrect. As we conceive of the matter, the scratching would have continued. The symptom of ear noise or tinnitus (line 32) is also relevant to the condition, if not always present.

35–36. The last entry of the Tablet would seem unmistakeably to relate to stroke, and concerns, as we propose, the rigidity or contracture of paralysed limbs in hemiplegia. Regular massage of the muscles may do much to allay suffering and improve the circulation, but there is a price to pay for the neglect of this. Indeed, how far the spasticity has advanced in the specific case of the text may be seen from the fact that the sufferer 'howls (in pain)' in the effort to flex his paralysed leg. 'The slightest jarring of fixed joints may cause severe pain' writes a modern textbook of this condition.[76]

[76] D. Brinton in J. Conybeare and W. N. Mann (eds), *Textbook of Medicine*, 12th edit., Edinburgh and London, 1957, p. 629, and similarly in later editions.

It may be added that the 'staff of Sin' mentioned in line 35 is to be accepted factually as an instrument of healing. Stol in his own commentary recalls that 'The prophet Elisha ordered his servant Gehazi to lay his staff on the face of a child that had died of sun-stroke, 2 Kings 4: 29 and 31.'[77]

[77] It may be said in conclusion that the above paper in various drafts has been read by Drs. Alan Barratt, Stephen Kirker, Irving Finkel and Markham Geller, and stands in much debt to all of these persons for their helpful counsel and comment.
Since the above was written the authors have published a summary paper for a medical readership in a neurological journal (Reynolds, E. H., Kinnier Wilson, J. V., 'Stroke in Babylonia', *Archives of Neurology* 2004; 61: 597–601). While much relates to the present paper, it was newly suggested (p. 600) that the 'staff of Sin' as above discussed was possibly 'a crutch provided for the patient's (paralysed) leg.' Since Sin was the name of the moon god, it was considered that the crutch may have had 'an attachment in the shape of a crescent to fit under the armpit.'

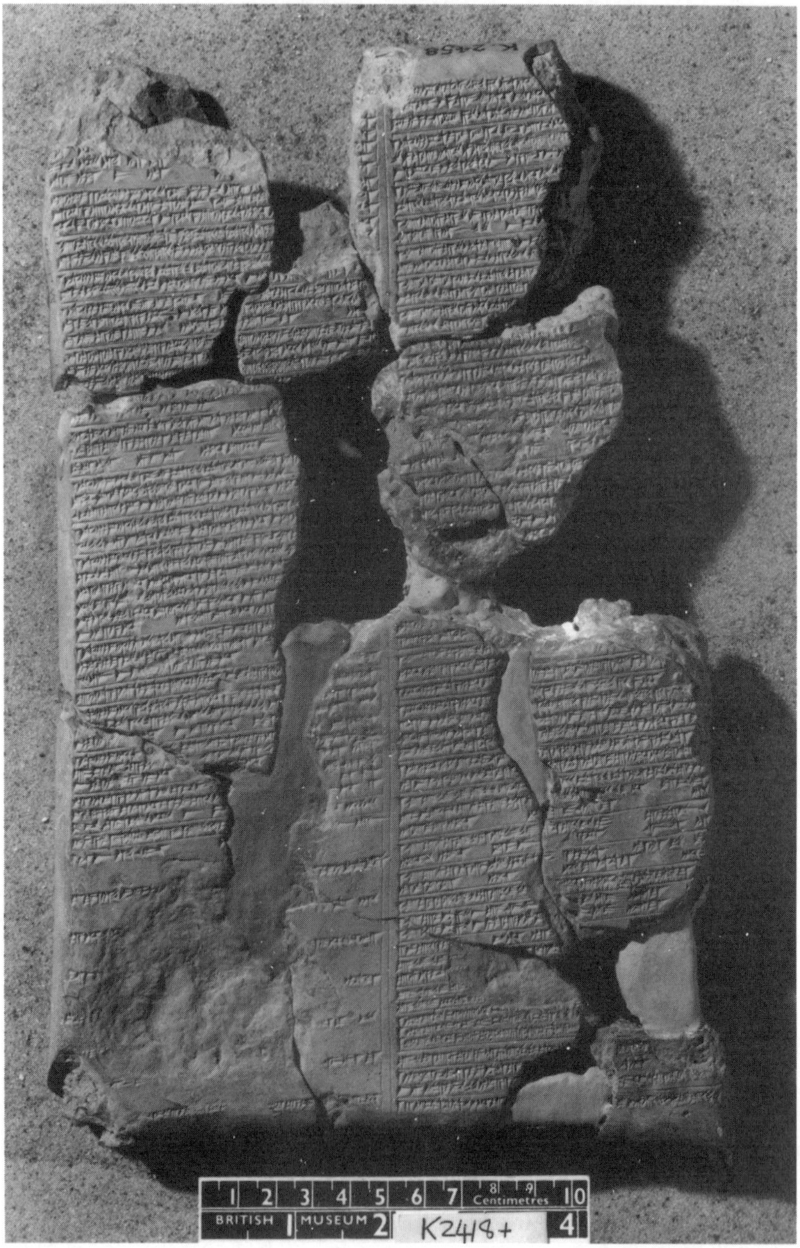

Fig. 1. Reverse of the 'Stroke Tablet', K 2418+, from the 'Therapeutic Series' of medical texts. Reproduced by courtesy of the Trustees of The British Museum.

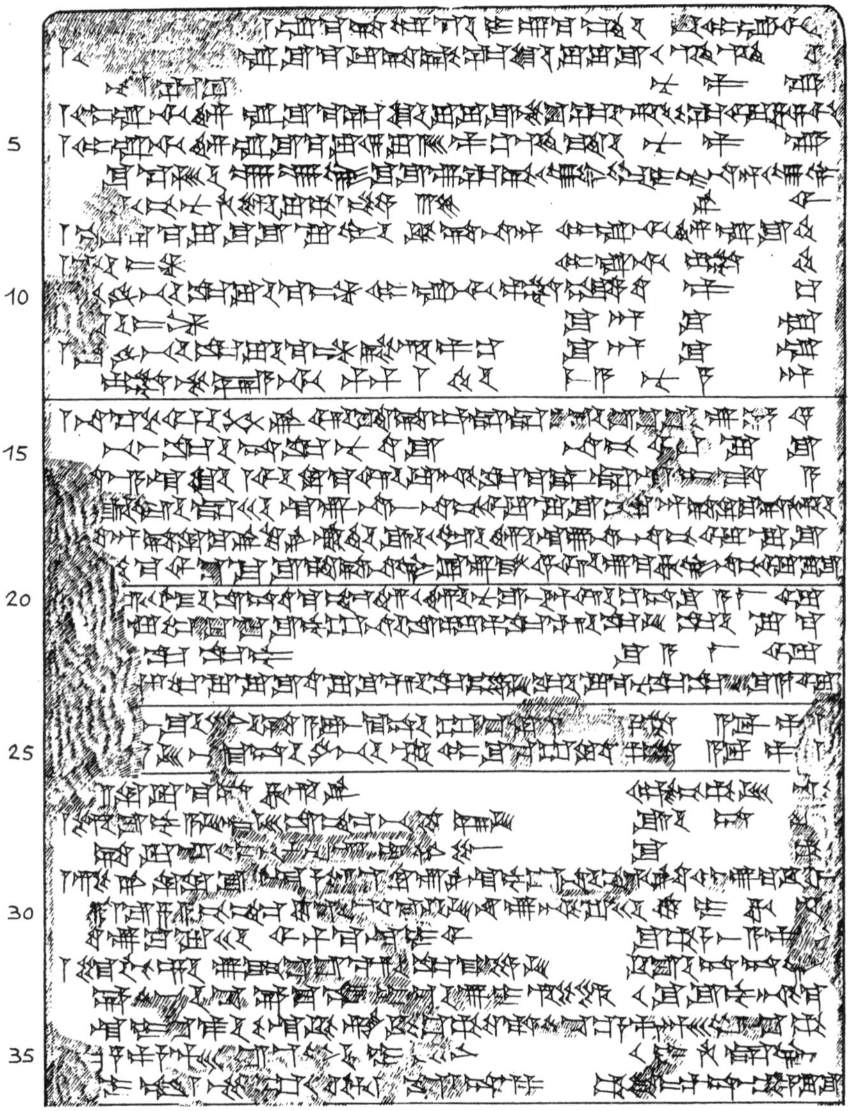

Fig. 2. Copy by the late René Labat of the Obverse of A0 6680, a text from the 'Diagnostic Series' concerning stroke. Reproduced by courtesy of Brill NV of Leiden.

HITTITE RITUALS AGAINST THREATS AND OTHER DISEASES AND THEIR RELATIONSHIP TO THE MESOPOTAMIAN TRADITIONS*

V. Haas
Freie Universität, Berlin

I deliberated for some time with which topic a Hittitologist would best serve the ends of these proceedings, and finally decided that a synopsis on the Hittite incantation literature or healing rituals with its diverse traditions and most of all, its close affiliation with the Babylonian art of incantation, would make most sense. With this paper I intend to explain the importance of Hittite ritual and incantation literature or, in the spirit of this the theme of this volume, of Hittite magical science of healing for the study of Akkadian ritual literature as a whole.

According to Hittite belief, any divergence from a state of normality, be it on an individual level, in a social group, or in nature, is viewed as a threat and can only be repelled through a ritual act. Such threats are primarily disorders either of a physical, or more important, a mental nature. Moreover, there are negative omens, criminal acts, family troubles, economic, military and natural disasters like droughts or severe storms. From a perspective of the ritual, all such distressing events are alike in that they represent a serious disruption of the normal state of affairs. The task of the ritual is hence to reinstate normality.

Troubled normality is conceived of as a state of constraint, whereas normality as one of ease. In this sense the following terms *lauwar* "to be loose" and *ḫamenkuwar* "to be attached" are diametrically opposed to each other in a magical dualism.

An individual in a state of attachment or bewitchment is doomed to suffer psychosomatic disorders, of which the subjective symptoms are usually described as fear of "evil gossip of the community" (EME *pangauwaš*), "burden of the soul" (*ištanzanaš impa-*), "constriction of

* Translated from German by Paul Larsen.

the body" (*tuekkaš taššiyatar*), a state of being pinned down (*taruwant*), of confinement, or strong excitement. As though in a state of captivity the bewitched is "like a sheep in a pen, like a bull in a shed, like a dog in a kennel, like a pig in a pigsty". This condition of suspension leads to a sleepless condition, evil dreams,[1] fear and nightmares "as if someone keeps seeing a deadly ghost night after night"; it also leads to ill-fated omens like "evil" and "hideous birds", to impotence, miscarriages, and even paralysis, blindness and various diseases of the head. This state inflicted by witchcraft is thus transferred to the sorcerer, in which it is stated that "the witchcraft shall be like a head scarf and shall be pressed to his head . . . shall act like a belt, and tie him up".[2]

The cathartic ritual which tries to release the patient from the described condition effectuates in the first place the abilities of self-healing. Accordingly diverse is the application of one and the same ritual for the alleviation of the spell.

The remarkably large amount of magical rituals in comparison to the rest of the Hittite epigraphic corpus exemplifies how common such psychosomatic disorders were. An idea of the magnitude of the corpus embracing Hittite, Hittite-Hattian, Hittite-Luvian and Hittite-Hurrian rituals, is obtained from a glance at Laroche's *Catalogue des Textes Hittites*.[3]

A classification of the ritual literature from Boğazköy is best carried out according to the various priestly classes involved in the performing of such rituals. Therefore one may differentiate between the following prominent categories: first of all, there are cathartic rituals which are usually linked to the sphere of the AZU-priest[4] as opposed to the rituals carried out by the female magician ^{MUNUS}ŠU.GI, who as a rule is mentioned by name. These rituals usually counteract witchcraft. Following the recitals contained in the rituals, we must distinguish rituals from a Hattian, Luvian, and Hurrian setting on the one hand, from ones with a Babylonian background on the other. Closely related to the ŠU.GI-rituals from the Hattian

---

[1] KUB 5.7, edition K. van der Toorn 1985, 125–33.

[2] Cf. V. Haas 1980–1983, 241.

[3] E. Laroche 1971.

[4] Their function rather seems to correspond with the Babylonian (*w*)*āšipu*-priests than the *barû*-priests represented by sumerogram AZU.

environment are rituals of the priest designated as "man of the weather god" (LÚ ᴰU/IŠKUR), since it may occur that he carries out his rituals in conjunction with the ŠU.GI-magician.[5] Some ŠU.GI-rituals from the Luvian milieu are closely connected to the rituals of the ᴸᵁ́MUŠEN.DÙ-man[6] which protect against evil bearing omens. The ŠU.GI-magician and the MUŠEN.DÙ-man also carry out some of their rituals together. Correspondingly, the ŠU.GI-magician cooperates with the AZU-priest. Moreover, there is a close relationship between ŠU.GI-rituals from the Luvian environment and ones related to "Hierodulen" (MUNUSSUḪUR.LÁ).[7] The SUḪUR.LÁ Kuwatalla performs ŠU.GI-rituals on her own.[8] The midwife MUNUS*ḫaš(ša)nupalla*,[9] who also often performs in the presence of a ŠU.GI-magician, carries out pregnancy or birth rituals. The *patili*-priests[10] whose rituals are similar to the ones of the AZU-priests are primarily cathartic in nature. Their rituals take place exclusively in the ante-room of the temple, the so called *šinapši*-room, and inside the gate house.[11] Medical rituals are subject to the duties of the LÚA.ZU-healers.[12]

The different groups of ritual practitioners, partly situated within high-ranking circles of society,[13] seem to have founded some kind of guilds or schools insofar as the techniques according to which their rituals were performed differ from each other. Thus the well documented charm performed carried out with red wool previously dipped in oil is only carried out by the AZU-priests.[14] The existence of such

[5] For example CTH 732. A Middle Hittite letter from Ortaköy (Šappinuwa) states that the "man of the weather god" and the ŠU.GI-magician no longer are to perform their common ritual near the river outside the city.

[6] The rituals of the MUŠEN.DÙ-men: CTH 398 "Rituel de Huwarlu, l'oiseleur", CTH 425 "Das Ritual des Maddunani". See also KBo 23.8 on the instructions relating to an evil forecast from a bird omen while travelling.

[7] This relationship is so close that one of the rituals of the "Hierodule" Kuwatalla (KUB 35.43) over long passages is virtually identical to another ritual by ŠU.GI Tunnawi (KUB 7.53+12.58), F. Starke 1985, 143–147. Accordingly, the ŠU.GI-magician named Tunnawi is assisted by a MUNUSSUḪUR.LÁ (KUB 7.53+12.58 obv. ii 65 ff.).

[8] F. Starke 1985, 72–104.

[9] Cf. G. M. Beckman 1983, 232–35.

[10] Cf. ibid., 235–38.

[11] Cf. V. Haas 1980–1983, 242 and ChS I/9, 5–6.

[12] Cf. C. Burde 1974, 1–11.

[13] In the case of SUḪUR.LÁ Kuwatalla, the author of a lengthy ritual, we are dealing with a donation certificate by Arnuwanda-Ašmunikkal, KBo 15.7 rev. 47 sq., cf. H. Otten 1980–1983, 398.

[14] E.g. KBo 23.1 obv. i 9–18.

schools is moreover indicated by the rituals of the ŠU.GI-magician Zuwi, who in her own turn relies on the ritual techniques of the "man of the weather god" in uttering the words: "When I treat an individual according to the way of the man of the weather god".[15] Along the same lines, the colophon of two rituals carried out by the magician Ḫebattarakki discloses that, "they were performed according to the Hattian way".[16] The *mantalli*-rituals finally can be performed "in the way of Ḫattuša or Arzawa."[17]

Gurney defined a point of origin when he indicated that the Hittite plague rituals were by authors who came from the land of Arzawa: the ritual against an epidemic in the army (CTH 425) can be traced back to the Auguries of Maddunani of Arzawa; and Uḫḫamuwa, the author of a ritual against an epidemic in the land (CTH 410), also came from Arzawa. The land of Ḫapalla, which belongs to the lands of Arzawa, is the homeland of Ašḫella, the author of another plague ritual (CTH 394).[18]

The various ritual groups are not distinguished solely by their method of magical execution but in addition by more formal aspects. Such, for instance, is the case of the ritual directives of the AZU-priests which are invariably rendered in the third person singular form, while those of the ŠU.GI-magicians often appear in the first person singular or plural forms.

A close study of the ritual literature reveals that it apparently relied on a long tradition. This tradition is indicated by the accuracy and extent of the compositions and their polished style, their rigorous and logical structure, the matching sequence of specific ritual acts, as well as a recurrent cognate usage of the *materia magica*. The same also applies for the employment of ritual jargon which consists of subject-related terminology as well as syntactic particularities.

---

[15] KUB 35.148 rev. iv 25'–27'.

[16] KUB 24.14 rev. iv 31 *a-ni-ia-an-ma-at* URU*ḫa-at-te-li*.

[17] KUB 5.6+KUB 18.54 rev. iii 36.

[18] O.R. Gurney 1977, 51 sq.

Other rituals from Arzawa: CTH 402 Rituel de Malli, contre la sorcellerie". CTH 406 "Rituel de Paskuwatti, contre l'impuissance sexuelle". Bo 3483 is the ritual of Addā Lú URUArzawa. KUB 34.74 is the ritual of [Tapalzu]nawili LÚ URUArzawa. 516/z is the ritual of [Tarḫun]tapaddu Lú URUArzawa, cf. H. Otten 1973a, 81 sq. In KBo 31.6 14'–15' the ritual of the woman MUNUSNÍG.GA.GUŠKIN URUArzawa (also involved in ritual practices in the mantic text KUB 5.6+KUB 18.54 Rs. III 21, 32) is mentioned.

As for the duration of the tradition, there is noteworthy evidence of a close similarity between Luvian (Southeast-Anatolian) rituals and Old Hittite (Central Anatolian-Hattian)[19] and Palaic or Luvian-Palaic[20] rituals. This would argue for a strong and very early link between the two cultural spheres,[21] which is only explained it Central Anatolia and probably even the Pontic coast under intense Luvian influence from the earliest stage of Hittite history,[22] supposition which is supported by the Old Hittite legend of the queen of Kaniš.

The Hittite royal court collected rituals with an apparently insatiable appetite. According to the colophons, ritual experts were summoned to the court from all parts of Asia Minor such as Turmitta[23] in the north of Central Anatolia, Ḫurma[24] in the east, Kizzuwatna[25] in the south-east, Arzawa[26] in the south-west, and Alalaḫ[27] in Northern Syria. The ritual experts explained the rituals to the royal scribes, who then wrote them down and edited them while adding the names and the origins of the experts.

This collecting activity was not only restricted to regions of Asia Minor and Syria. Great interest was also directed towards cathartic and magical rituals, medical texts, and mantic collections from

[19] In this connection, we must above all mention the incantions of the cultic media pertaining to the difficulties of procuring the *materia magica* necessary for the performance of the ritual. These relations are also indicated by the occurrence of Hattian deities in Luvian rituals, as in Šulinkatte (KBo 14.114 4, 7; KBo 14.108.9; KBo 29.3) and Telipinu (cf. V. Haas and G. Wilhelm 1974, 26–28), or place names like Ankuwa (e.g. KBo 29.30 rev. iv 8').

[20] Cf. F. Starke 1985, 37–71.

[21] As for instance in the case of the incantation of Zuwi from Angulla-Turmitta in written Luvian language (KUB 35.148 rev. iv 11'–13'), or the dialogues characteristic for Luvian as well as Hattian incantations, cf. also V. Haas and G. Wilhelm 1974, 26–28.

[22] This would support the view of an immigration of Hittite and Luvian tribes via the the Pontic coast as already held by H. Otten 1973, 64 in reference to the Zalpa document, which states that the Indo-Europeans who arrived at Kaniš had started out from Zalpa.

[23] CTH 412 "Rituel de Zuwi: magie et mythe".

[24] CTH 395 "Rituel de Hantitassu": "Si les années d'un homme sont gâtées".

[25] See for instance the riuals of the AZU-priest Ammiḫatna, also the ŠU.GI-magician Tunnawi, Maštigga (CTH 404 "Rituels de Mastigga, contre les dissensions familiales") etc.

[26] Cf. note 18.

[27] The rituals of Allaituraḫi, the "woman from Mukiš" against withcraft, ChS I/5, no. 1—no. 39, the ritual of Giziya from Alalaḫ (ChS I/2 no. 40).

Babylonia.[28] They were either left in the Babylonian language, as disclosed by an Akkadian healing ritual treated by G. Meier,[29] or else translated into the local language, as disclosed the Hittite translation of an Akkadian *šigû*-ritual.[30] Sometimes they were shown by altered, as in the Hittite medical texts from Boğazköy[31] or the Lamaštu ritual,[32] which also had an Old Assyrian edition next to the Old Babylonian versions.[33] A Hittite recipe for the treatment of an illness from an assault by the demon Lamaštu furthermore quotes a drug described as the "bristle of a white pig,"[34] known from the later Babylonian series.

Since the ritual for the substitute king, which was translated into Hittite,[35] functioned toward off unfavourable omens, its appropriation from Babylonia must have taken place approximately at the same time as the acquisition of the respective omen collections.[36]

Comparing magical techniques—which basically consist of different forms of analogy, and rites of contact and transfer, identification and substitution, attraction and repulsion[37]—as well as the *materia magica* and its application, with those of Babylonian witchcraft, often leads to the discovery of detailed equivalences. A division between an explicitly Mesopotamian and Anatolian witchcraft therefore only seems justified to a certain extent, as the magical repertoire basically stays the same. It hardly seems reasonable to attempt to trace this phenomenon on an historical level, since mutual contact between both regions was well established already long before the Hittite period.

---

[28] Though most of these unknown texts were written during the first half of the first millennium B.C., many were originally compiled some time during the first half of the second millennium B.C.

[29] KUB 29.58+, discussed by G. Meier 1939.

[30] K. van der Toorn 1985, 124–33; see CTH 801.

[31] Edition: C. Burde 1974.

[32] I have elsewhere discussed the Sammeltafel KUB 43.55(+)KUB 59.63 (V. Haas 1990, 549) obv. III 10—rev. IV 16 in OrAnt. 27, 1988, 86–104. The linking element of the rituals gathered on this tablet is the *materia magica* ⁽ᴾᴱ́Š⁾*gapirta*, a rodent. According to W. Farber, 1980–1983, 440, the contents of the fragments KUB 37.66 and 70 are closely linked to the Lamaštu ritual.

[33] Cf. A. Falkenstein 1939, 8–41, 19 sq.: 1–13 and W. Farber 1980–1983, 439–46.

[34] KBo 21.20 obv. I 16'–19'; the text was discussed by C. Burde 1974, 42–46, see also V. Haas 1988, 95 sq. esp. note 36.

[35] Edition: H. M. Kümmel 1967.

[36] Cf. V. Haas 1994, 206–14.

[37] Cf. V. Haas 1980–1983, 244–51.

A comparative, differentiating view of the rituals and ritual techniques within the two cultural spheres is therefore more appropriate.

The influence of Babylonian literature and thus ritual technique on Hittite witchcraft is already evidenced for the Old Hittite Period.[38] The practice of transfering misfortune to human substitutes, as already described in Old Hittite rituals, is sometimes precisely reflected in Babylonian texts, as in the case of a Babylonian ritual preserved in a Hittite copy,[39] and an Old Hittite ritual of the ŠU.GI-magician Zuwi of Turmitta and Angulla,[40] both relating to the supply of a substitute and provisions.

In the 14th and 13th centuries B.C. Hittite incantations designated as *šiptu*, "incantation", began to be written down. Library catalogues were compiled, listing rituals and medical works which frequently contained identical indications to ones in Akkadian texts of the first millennium B.C.

Texts containing the Akkadian term *šiptu* are usually preserved on *Sammeltafeln*. Many are also listed in library catalogues. In addition to the indications, the number of exact equivalences to passages from Babylonian ritual literature is so large, that they manifestly appear to be nothing else but translations from the Akkadian language.[41] Accordingly, a library catalogue[42] cites maladies of the head, throat and eyes, as well as coughs. The indication *mān antuḫšan su'ālu epzi* "if a cough seizes a man" (obv. II 15) is matched by the Akkadian medical text compilation *šumma amīlu su'ālu iṣbassu*.[43] The indication *ma-a-an an-tu-uḫ-ša-an tar-mi-iš*, "if a peg hits a man" (rev. III 11) is akin to the Akkadian *šumma sinništu* ^{GIŠ}*kakka maḫṣat* "if a woman was hit with the peg".[44] The Hittite birth aid ritual on a collective tablet

---

[38] Cf. e.g. CTH 313, An Old Hittite-Babylonian bilingual copy of a hymn dedicated to Adad, editied by A. Archi 1983.

[39] KUB 29.58+, see note 30.

[40] KBo 12.106+ obv. i 11–12; cf. as well KUB 44.4+, F. Starke 1985, 234:12.

[41] Cf. G. Wilhelm 1994, 1.

[42] KUB 8.36; edition: E. Laroche CTH, 188 ff.; last edited by C. Burde 1974, 38–42.

[43] BAM VI 548 I 17, cf. F. Köcher BAM VI, XXVI–XXXI as referred to by G. Wilhelm 1994, 1.

[44] BAM 235:4, 10 sqq. In the parallel text BAM 236 col. ii this paragraph is broken off. In KUB 8.36, rev. III 1–4 follows "from the cart" . . ., which apparently seems to refer to a malady as well.

CAD M/1 74 s.v. *maḫāṣu* 1.a 2' "if a woman is menstruating (lit. wounded by the weapon)"; AHw II 422 s.v. *kakku* II 2.e "to smite with the weapon, to make

ŠI-PÁT hu-wa-an-da-aš ma-a-an-za ha-a-ši na-aš ⌜*Ú*⌝-[*UL*][45] *ḫu-un-ta-ri-ia-it-ta na-an kiš-an hu-u*[*k-mi*] "incantation of the wind: if (a woman) gives birth and is not able to release flatulence"[46] corresponds with the Akkadian indication "if a woman is pregnant and inflated with wind"—*Šumms* MUNUS *'i-ri-it-ma u* IM *ud-du-pat.*[47] To liberate the woman from her flatulence, the Babylonian text only prescribes a drug, whereas the Hittite healer prefers to recite a long incantation of 21 lines in Hattian language. The Hittite ritual term *duddu ḫalzai* "he shall cry for mercy", which appears in some rituals, seems to be the equivalent of the Akkadian expression *šigû išassi* of the so-called *šigû*-rituals.[48] One of these healing rituals connects the body of the patient with the landscape; from that results the equations: mountain = nose, dales = ears, wave = hair, throat = snake and so on.[49] In an old Babylonian incantation against the sickness *merḫu* the physiognomy of the patient is compared with the landscape: "The eyes are sisters; above them (eye-brows) there is a ridge (*kiṣirtu*), beneath them (cheek-bones) there is a wall."[50]

Orientation toward the Babylonian ritual formula is also evident in the well documented Hittite ritual introductions *mān antuhšan alwanzaḫḫantan* and *mān antuhšan nasma* MUNUS-*an alwanzaḫḫantan*,[51] which conforms with the Akkadian series specification *šumma amīlu kašip* "if a person is bewitched". The Hittite solution rituals *lauwaš* SISKUR are formally akin to the Akkadian series specification *ana pišerti kišpi* "for the solution of witchcraft". In this respect, reference should also be made to malady specifications as in Hittite *appatar*, an abstraction of the verb *ep*(*p*-), "to seize, to grab" and dating back to the Akkadian malady specification *ṣibtu*.[52] A good example for the

ill", following the context, probably indicating irregular menstruations, to judge by the incantation signature in BAM 235 14.

45 E. Neu 1968, 60 proposes the reading ^{U}[^{ZU}*ar-ra-* (though hardly likely in view of the Babylonian evidence). As it is known that a woman in the process of giving birth is liable to undergo severe suffering from flatulence, the reading proposed by G. M. Beckman 1983, 86 ⌜*Ú*⌝-[*UL*] agrees with the traces from the signs as well as with the general context.

46 KUB 17.28 obv. ii 7–8.

47 BAM 240 obv. 28'.

48 See K. van der Toorn 1985, 125.

49 KBo 3.8 Rs. III 1–35 und KUB 7.1 iii 1; H. Kronasser 1961, 156ff.

50 AMT 10,1 III 26, siehe B. Landsberger, 1958, 58.

51 808/w as quoted by H. Otten 1973a, 82 note 6.

52 H. M. Kümmel 1967, 14 and G. Wilhlem 1994, 43.

use of Babylonian medical texts by the compilation of a Hittite ritual shows the ritual of Ḫutuši, in which the following prescription appears: "One vessel of water with *laḫni-* mixed in, *alanza(n)*-wood, *ḫatalkišna*-wood (and) *galaktar* he put in the vessel; and she gives it daily (to the person for whom the ritual is performed) to drink.[53]

Examples of ritual details: The utilisation of differently coloured wool types and woollen threads in rituals highlights the symbolic value of colour in Babylonian and Hittite magic. In this sense, colours relate to certain conditions of the bewitched, like the type of spell or illness that had fallen upon him. The different colours therefore probably also reflect the actual tints of the bewitched himself, thus not only referring to the involved types of impurities or demons, but even more so to the categories of fevers. The following example serves as an illustration: "(The spell) with which the king was made blood red (*ešḫarwaḫḫešk-*), [was made yellow] (*ḫaḫlanešk-*), was made black (*danduwaḫḫešk-*), [was made white] (*ḫarganušk-*), that must go back to the land of the enemy."[54] The ŠU.GI-magician "removes the black and the yellow" from the patient "whom the word of impurity had turned black and yellow".[55] In the ritual of the ŠU.GI-magician Alli from Arzawa[56] six differently coloured threads (*gapina-*) as well as a black woollen fleece (^{SÍG}*ešri-*) are needed to counteract seven kinds of spells "if someone is bewitched." Here as well, each colour matches with a specific type of bewitchment. The magician places the threads and the woollen fleece one by one on the knees and the head of the ritual master and entwines after each act specially made images of the threads in order to transfer the respective witchcraft or malady from the patient to the defixion figures. In a fragmented ritual tablet[57] red, blue and yellow wool is used for transferring the disorders of redness and blackness to the red and the blue wool.

In the Babylonian poetry work *ludlul bēl nēmeqi*[58] a sick person describes his condition as being the following: "My eyes let (others)

[53] KUB 28.102 Rs. IV 11'–17', cf. CHD L-N 12. To the formulation *akuwanna pai-/pešk-* "to give to drink" see G. Burde 1974, text B 18'–19', text C 4', text G 21'.

[54] KBo 15.1(= ChS I/5 no. 46), edited by H.M. Kümmel 1967, 111–25, obv. i 27–29.

[55] KUB 7.53+, edition: A. Goetze 1938, obv. ii 46–48.

[56] KUB 24.9+, edition: L. Jakob-Rost 1972.

[57] VBoT 111.

[58] W. G. Lambert 1960, 21–62.

see, that I constantly cry. From washing(?) with tears my cheeks have turned red like fire; my face repeatedly turned black—darkness of my heart. Fear and panic repeatedly turned my skin yellow."[59]

The Babylonian equivalences with the iterative Hittite verbs *ešharwaḫḫešk-* "to make red", *haḫlaḫešk-* "to make yellow" (yellow fever?), and *dankuwaḫḫešk-* "to make black" are the D-stems of the verbs *ṣurrupu* "to hurt intensively, to turn red like fire", *ṣalāmu* in the Dt-stem *ṣutallumu* "to darken, to blacken" and *warāqu* in the Dt(?)-stem "to make yellowish green, to make pale".

An example for the preparation of a drug: beer, wort, and "yeast" are used for the making of drugs from medical plants. Babylonian therapeutical texts name medical plants such as the *kukru*-plant, juniper, black cumin, chick-peas, peas, wheat meal, *ab(b)ukkatu*-resin and *kasû*-meal,[60] which mixed together with "beer deposits" *ina šuršummi šikari*, are processed (*rabāku*) to a decoction. A similar drug is prepared by the Hittite magician Ayatarša in her ritual:[61] She crushes white and black cumin, seeds of the *ānkisa*-plant and other ingredients before mixing the obtained paste with fermented yeast.[62] In some cases Hittite rituals describe pharmaceutic procedures which are not found in the corresponding Babylonian literature, for example the description of the specific materials for production of fumigations and "holy water" (*šeḫelliyaš watar*, akkadian *eggubû*) in the Hurrian-Hittite *itgaḫi* and *itkalzi* rituals,[63] the cooking and infusing of healing plants[64] or various proceedings of drawing out the aromata of plants.[65] An exact instruction for maceration is given by an Hittite-Luwian ritual.[66]

---

[59] [*ina bi*]*takkî šubrā īnājā mi-siš dimāti ṣurrupā usukkāja uṣṣallim pānīja adirat libbīja maškīja utarriqū pirittu u ḫattu*, Tablet I 109–12.

[60] BAM IV 409, edition: F. Köcher 1995.

[61] KUB 7.1 obv. i 1–42, edition: H. Kronasser, 1961, 142–148.

[62] A recipe listing the ingredients yeast and black cumin (against crocodile- and dog bites) also occurs in Plinius, Naturalis Historiae XXIII, 67.

[63] Fumigation: IBoT 2.39 (= ChS I/1 Nr. 3) rev. 20–23; KUB 47.26+ (= ChS I/1 Nr. 46) rev. iii 17'–19' and the ritual of the AZU-priest KUB 41.13 obv. ii 20–23. "holy water": KBo 27.85+ (= ChS I/1 Nr. 2) obv. 23'–26'.

[64] See the ritual of Telipinu from Maşat, edition: H. G. Güterbock 1986.

[65] KUB 28.102 rev. iv 11'–17'; KUB 29.7+ obv. 58, rev. 1.

[66] KUB 9.6+ (= StBoT 30, 1985, 111–113) obv. i 1–21.

I give a detailed statement of such a proceeding in my work, *Materia Magica of Medica Hethitica*, (Berlin, 2003).

The Hittite *materia magica* comprises hundreds of different drugs prepared from plants and plant by-products (seeds, leaves, roots, fruits etc.), minerals, animals and animal products, and bodily secretions, as well as a large array of different figures and tools. To illustrate the cognate use of the *materia magica* in both Babylonia and Anatolia, I would like to present some examples.

As *materia magica* in both Babylonian[67] and Hittite[68] medical science, dog's excrement plays to some extent a significant role. Thus the ŠU.GI-magician Ḫebattarakki adds excrement—UR.GI$_7$-*aš šal-pa-an*—to the barley dog, which she then rubs into the skin of the bewitched (KUB 24.14 obv. I 1–17). In the same ritual she braises parts of a dog: *ŠA* UR.GI|-*ma-at-ta wa-ar-šu-la-an a-wa-an ar-ḫa pár-ḫu-un ŠA* UR.GI$_7$-*ma šal-pa-aš* ^{UZU}UR.GI|^{UZU}GÌR.PAD.DU UR.GI$_7$|-*i̯a ši-mi-ši-i̯a-nu-un* "I have chased away from you the canine *waršula*; I braised dog's excrements, a bone of a dog and a dog".[69] The reason for this action is apparently to chase away the disease germs (*agalmati*—and *anamluli-*) with the ensuing stench.

Another example of *materia magica* consists of garlic, or rather onion. An onion is referred to in a Hittite cathartic ritual[70] for the royal couple to neutralise "all curses" in the following analogic counter-spell: "Afterwards they carry the onion to him (the priest), whereupon he speaks to it in the following way: 'If anyone [speak]s in front of the deity like that: 'In the same way as this onion is wrapped by peelings, and each (peeling) [does not] let go of the other, so shall evil, oath, curse and impurity in front of the temple be wrapped like an onion'. 'See, I have now peeled this onion and have only kept one thin core. In the same manner shall evil gossip, oath, curse (and) impurity in front of the deity be peeled. The deity and the ritual master shall be unsullied from this affair'". Garlic (*šūmū*) assumes more or less the same function in the incantation series Šurpu and

---

[67] CAD K, 71, cf. as well *zē* šaḫ "boar dung," CAD Š$_1$, p. 104.

[68] F. Köcher (1995) was able to demonstrate that such drugs were given secret labels in Babylonian medicine.

[69] KUB 24.14 obv. I 1–17 and 22–24. KUB 24.14 obv. I 1–17 and 22–24. Possibly there are secret labels in the Hittite texts too, but more likely the author of the text understood the drug "dog's exrement" liberally.

[70] The ritual tablet KUB 29.7+KBo 21.41 is considered to be a Late Hittite copy of a Middle Hittite original, E. Neu 1985, 149 sq. and CHD Volume L-N, 235f., 239f., 251, 350, 255; cf. also A. Kammenhuber 1968, 101 fq. note 311.

Maqlû: "By pronouncing the charm of Ea the oath may be peeled off like (this) onion"—*ma-mit ina* MIN-*e šà* ^{d}*é-a* sum.sar.gin$_8$ hé.en.zil,[71] or "May their spells be . . . peeled away like garlic", *kis-pu-sa liq-qal-pu kima šumi.*[72]

One Luvian salt incantation[73] is comparable to an incantation from Maqlû (IX:118–20): "You are the salt which was formed on a pure location . . ." the "pure location" indicating sea and salt lick is designated as the origin for the salt—M]UN-*ša-pa a-a-la-a-ti u-wa-a-*[*ni-ia-ti*] *ú-pa-am-ma-an.*

Many examples of similar ritual practices can be given by the various kinds of manipulation with magic figures. Images of wax are used for burning, and clay figures are used for dilution in water. The crushing of a figure placed on the ground face down word, is illustrated in Maqlû IV:36, as well as in a Hittite and a Luwian ritual.[74] In Hittite rituals we thus also observe the Babylonian habit of spelling out the name on the figure depicting the person undergoing bewitchment.[75]

It is not always clear where such charms come from. Breaking of pottery in the curses of Kumarbi and Teššup, or the well known charm with the pin and the distaff to strengthen weak soldiers or impotent men seem to be of Anatolian origin, since we find this charm in an original historical text of Hattušili I[76] and later in ritual contexts.[77]

The following two instances illustrate the adoption of Akkadian terminology. The first is the Akkadian ritual term *biātu, bâtu,* "to leave for the night". In this instance we are normally confronted with a liquid *materia magica,* which was best left to stand on the roof

[71] Šurpu V–VI 51–52, edition: E. Reiner 1958; cf. also A. Goetze 1947, 318 and V. Haas 1986, 177.

[72] Maqlû V:57, edition: G. Meier 1937.

[73] KUB 35.54 rev. 12–21, cf. F. Starke 1985, 55–71.

[74] KBo 6.34+, edition: N. Oettinger 1976, rev. iii 24–29.

[75] Two defixion figures appear in the ritual of the magician Nikkalzuzzi—one from clay and the other from cedar wood. The first has an inscription giving the name of PU-Šarrum(m)a and the second "the name of the land of the enemy"; see also J. Klinger, *Untersuchungen zur Rekonstruktion der hattischen Kultschicht,* StBoT 37, 1996, 454, note 1. A magician called Manna-DUGUD bewitches three individuals by aid of substitution figures, among whom Šarri-Kušuḫ is probably identical with the son of Šuppiluliuma I, KUB 40.83, edition: R. Werner 1967, 64–67.

[76] KBo 1.11, edition: H. G. Güterbock 1934, 113–130, rev. 16–17.

[77] Examples are listed in I. Wegner 1981, 59–62.

overnight after having been placed there in the evening.[78] The Akkadian expression for this action is given by *ina kakkabi tušbat* "under the star you leave overnight" and equated in Hittite rituals of the AZU-priest with *ANA ŠAPAL* MUL *šeš-*: "Then they go to the waters of purity and bring the waters of purity into the new temple and place them on the roof. Then they (the waters) remain under the stars (*nu ú-i-da-a-ar A-NA ŠA-PAL* MUL^HI.A^ *še-eš-zi*). And they do no (more) on that day.[79] The second example is the Hittite phrase MUL *watkuzi* "a star shimmered" which seems to correspond with the Akkadian expression *kakkabu išḫiṭ*.[80]

The Old-Hittite and Luvian ritual traditions: the two most ancient rituals composed in Hittite language known to us today go back to the time of Ḫattušili I. The first is a rite referred to in the account of the siege of the city of Uršu. The rite was carried out with a whorl and a number of arrows in order to strengthen the Hittite military commander's striking power: "The sons of Lariya (and) Lariya sang with subdued voice the song of Zababa. 'We sprinkled the threshing floor with a flask, a hound . . . a mighty bull they lead away from the threshing floor . . . they removed; a whorl they brought, arrows they removed; a make-up brush they brought, a sankullu-mace they removed.'".[81] In the first paragraph of the so called chronicle of Puḫanu[82] reference is apparently made to a ritual. At the beginning of the text (§ 1) allusion is made to someone—probably a substitute for the king(?) dressing up in "coloured garments", an action normally carried out only in connection with a ritual: "He dresses in coloured clothes; a basket is placed on his head; he holds his bow and he cries out for help—'but what have I done'". The following lines reveal that the basket is filled with ice, apparently symbolising the misfortune that had come over the land of Ḫatti. A ritual act with wine for strengthening the power of the army we find in KBo 3.13, a fictitious inscription of Naram-Sîn in the Hittite language.[83]

---

[78] AHw 124b and CAD B 172b; cf. D. Goltz 1974, 51 sq. and E. Reiner 1995, 48ff. and 52ff.

[79] KUB 29.4, edition: H. Kronasser, 1963, rev. IV 10–14; see also KUB 29.4 obv. ii 46–47 and rev. IV 13; KBo 5.2 obv. ii 28; see also V. Haas 1971, 426.

[80] Cf. G. M. Beckman 1983, 110 with note 283.

[81] KBo 1.11, edition: H.G. Güterbock, 1938, 113–45, rev. 14–18.

[82] Edition: O. Soysal 1987.

[83] Edition: H. G. Güterbock, 1938, 66–80, obv. 17'–18'.

So where are the origins of this oldest Anatolian ritual stratum to be found? The Hittite tradition of festival rituals and associated myths developed entirely independently from Syro-Mesopotamian influences. Whereas Old-Hittite festival rituals are preserved in relatively large numbers, the range of known Old-Hittite original tablets with incantation or cathartic rituals is comparatively limited. Among them is the so called "Old-Hittite ritual for the royal couple" which was written in the first person singular form, therefore rendering the words of a ŠU.GI-magician whose dangerous operations in the court are lamented already by Hattušili I. The intention behind this ritual which lasts for several days is to repel from the royal couple "evil," "common gossip", the *irma*-"illness", *ešḫar*—"blood (deeds)" and *ḫatuga*- "abomination". The structural similarity of this ritual with the festival ritual leads to the assumption that a ritual tradition originating in the festival rituals actually did exist.[84] Some of the magical performances also seem to be of pure Anatolian origin. The magical texts relate to the action of spitting at substitute images and substitute cattle by the royal couple, who for this purpose are holding an iron tongue in their mouths. After this, "mouth washing" is carried out. Also of safe Anatolian tradition is the habit of waving an eagle over a substitute army battalion of clay.

Luvian rituals also tend to be exclusively of Anatolian origin, especially as regards incantation tablets used in the rituals and dialogues rendered in direct speech during ritual performances, as well as fairy-tale-like stories that sometimes allude to mythology. This is the case in the introduction to a recitation referring to "when a man came from the sea".[85] The context of these rituals invariably relates to the healing of a diseased person, be it regarding the arrival or departure of benign deities at the scene where the rituals are carried out, the acquisition of ritual paraphernalia from foreign regions,[86] or the persecution of demonic forces. The function of such dialogues within

[84] This becomes evident from the shift of the site of ritual performance between Ḫattuša, Arinna and Katapa, as well as from the reference to pages, the use of two lances as the requisite of the ruler in the AN.TAḪ.ŠUM^{SAR}- and *nuntarriyašḫa*-festival rituals.

[85] KUB 35.102(+)103 rev. iii 11, see F. Starke 1985, 205.

[86] As in the case of the *tarpatarpa* plant in the birth aid ritual KBo 12.112 (edition: G. M. Beckman 1983, 68ff.) or in the ritual of Zuwi KBo 12.63+KUB 36.70 rev. 1–6.

the ritual context is sometimes not fully understood, as seen in a case of an untenable order from the temple to a group of "abnormal people", the LÚ.MEŠ *ḫurkilaš*, "to make long ways short, and short ways long, to flatten the high mountains and to heighten the low, to catch the wolf with their bare hands, and the lion with their knees, and to halt the flow of the water in the river."[87] Yet such utterances have a tension-heightening effect, thus intensifying the power of the ritual act. They often pertain to the acquisition of highly uncommon and exceptional ritual paraphernalia. By aid of these stories therefore, the ritual tools gain magical value compared to the ones associated with the house, garden or pen.

The incantation tablets: A collection of Luvian pregnancy and birth aid incantations—*hukmaiš armauwaš*—have been preserved, and are designated as the incantations of the house- and hearth-goddess Kamrušepa, as it is she who recites them herself (in the form of her priestess). At the centre are Kamrušepa, the sun-god and their son the tutelary deity of Taurisa. The Kamrušepa myth is one of the incantation motifs which has been preserved in the Luvian, Hattian, and Hittite languages: Kamrušepa is looking down at the earth from her heavenly window, where she notices the calamity challenged by the ritual. She approaches hastly, and with her cathartic rites she begins to take remedial measures.[88]

Sometimes there are short ritual indications relating to the type of occasion on which the incantation may be recited.[89] Occasionally the incantation is introduced by an opening verse such as: "One must go to bring the bodily mother of this child", and then ends in closing phrase: "this child must be lifted in the air with the head hanging down. Then it must be placed at the breast of its mother. May she now be the way she used to be."

Apparently, the recital of the myth accompanies the ritual performance, as seen from the following passage: "One called for the midwife. She lifted the child up. She, Kamrušepa, takes the 9 combs (with the words): 'following maladies shall be combed away: the maladies of the head, the maladies of the eyes, the maladies of the

---

[87] KUB 12.63+KUB 36.70 obv. 18'–27'; cf. J. Puhvel 1986. These tasks are reminiscent of a threat of a series of dreadful apparitions before the magician, KUB 35.145, edition: F. Starke 1985, 231f.:7'–17'.
[88] V. Haas 1994, 439–40.
[89] Edition: F. Starke 1985, 202ff.

ears, the maladies of the mouth, the maladies of the throat, the maladies of the hands.' "[90]

Thus whereas many Hittite ritual performances were imported from Babylonia, the Hittite, Hattian, and Luvian incantations which were integrated into the rituals were themselves flawlessly Anatolian. Such incantations without any ritual context date back to as early as the middle of the third millennium B.C.[91] and could apparently be integrated into any ritual context. A similiar incantation and ritual composition is portrayed by the following quotation from the cathartic ritual of the god Telipinu, who according to the myth had disappeared and subsequently was rediscovered: "Says Kamrušepa to the gods: "Go ye gods, see, Ḫapantali has gone out to graze the sheep of the sun-god. Select twelve rams!' " Kamrušepa purifies the twelve parts of the body, each with a ram according to the *similia similibus* principle known from the Babylonian ritual literature: "Its head corresponds with the head. Its forehead corresponds with the forehead. Its snout corresponds with the nose. Its jaws correspond with the mouth. Its throat corresponds with the throat. Its lungs corresponds with the lungs. The genitals correspond with his genitals".[92] The same motif is also found in Hurrian in the Middle Hittite ritual of the ŠU.GI-magician Aštu.[93]

The Middle Hittite rituals: During the middle Hittite period the Anatolian (Hittite and Luvian) rituals were still being transmitted and compiled, although by this time the corpus of healing and cathartic rituals was enlarged through the addition of a large number of Hurrian ritual texts, which had an affect on the Luvian ritual tradition.[94] Though the Hittite rituals retained their traditional structure, the contents changed, especially with regard to the presiding deities. From now on, Kamrušepa no longer harnessed her carriage to hurry alone to the patient. Ištar from Niniveh as well, along with

[90] KUB 35.88, edition: F. Starke 1985, 207ff.

[91] Compiled by M. Krebernik 1984.

[92] KBo 8.73 (restored according to KUB 17.10 rev. iii 3–5); cf. V. Haas 1971, 422–24.

[93] KUB 48.70 (= ChS I/5 no. 62) obv. ii, KBo 33.200+ (= ChS I/5 no. 63), on this matter see also I. Wegner 1995, 125.

[94] The Luvian rituals as well, were coming under increased Hurrian influence from the 15th century onwards, as seen for example in the reference to Niniveh (^{URU}ninuwa) in KUB 35.30(+) (StBoT 30, 1985, 102f.).

her magical equipment and incantations, travelled from as far away as her home town to Hattuša, the location where the ritual was enacted.[95]

Two serial compilations are essential for our understanding of the ritual customs of that time. The first is a ritual of the ŠU.GI-magician Allaituraḫ(ḫ)i to counteract sorcery, the "woman from Mukiš," which was composed in six tablets. During the Middle Hittite period the incantations were written in Hurrian, whereas during the later Neo-Hittite period versions were copied and translated into the Hittite language.[96]

The second series is a cathartic work of the ritual *itkalzi* composed in 10 tablets in the ritual school of the AZU-priests. In the reign of Tutḫaliya III it was brought from the city of Šapinuwa (Ortaköy) to Ḫattuša where it was copied. The ritual is a compendium of "(incantation) words" of cathartic *materia* in Hurrian language, with the respective ritual instructions in Hittite. The preserved parts of the work are the "(incantation) words for water" (2nd tablet), "for water and rain"[97] (3rd and 4th tablet), for the cedar-tree and the tamarisk (5th tablet), for oil and silver (9th tablet) and according to an excerpt tablet "for gold, silver and lapis".[98] This important series constitutes the basis for the rituals of the AZU-priests, as seen in the case of the Kizzuwatna-priest Ammiḫatna and the cathartic rituals compiled in ChS I/2.

The central deity in the rituals of the ŠU.GI-magicians is Ištar, or Hurrian Šawuška of Niniveh. In one of them it is stated that she hurries from Niniveh to the location of the ritual act, supplied with her incantations and waters of purity. The magician recites the incantations in her name, explicitly stating that the incantations are those of Ištar of Niniveh.

The fact that Ištar of Niniveh, together with her circle including the Babylonian demons Alû[99] and Utukku[100] as well as her paraphernalia, play such an important role in these rituals suggests

[95] CTH 446, edition: H. Otten 1961, obv. II 45–48.

[96] This is shown by the tradition of the ritual of the ŠU.GI Allaituraḫ(ḫ)i, cf. V. Haas 1988a, 117–72.

[97] ChS I/1 no. 6 rev. IV 42' read: [*ḫé-u*]-⌜*wa-aš-ša*⌝ *ud-da-a-ar*.

[98] ChS I/1 no. 11.

[99] KUB 24.7 obv. i 23', v. I. Wegner 1981, 51.

[100] KUB 27. 6 (=ChS I/3-1 no. 6) obv. i 15 and KUB 27.1(= ChS I/3-1 no. 1) rev. iii 46 (erg.).

that the Ninevite tradition from the second millennium was able to survive, although the source material does not reveal why and how such traditions were kept alive. For all that, one of the myths integrated in the ritual of Allaituraḫ(ḫ)i seems to refer to Ištar's abode with her sister Allani-Ereškigal in the netherworld.[101] In some rituals Ištar leaves her home town Niniveh to travel to the place where the ritual is performed. In one of the rituals[102] she is accompanied by her falcon who carries the incantation words and the waters of purity. An incantation of a such ritual refers to the well-known *materia magica* of "heated stones" which had fallen down from the mountains near Niniveh, and subsequently gives an account to their mistress Ištar.[103]

In a birth ritual relating to a Hurrian incantation, possibly originating from Allaituraḫ(ḫ)i, there is mention of the maid of the moon-god Sîn, which thus represents the oldest variant of that well known Akkadian myth.[104]

Even during the Hittite Empire in the thirteenth century B.C. old rituals continue to be performed, although Hurrian incantation components by now appear in Hittite.

In this respect, practically every comprehensive Hittite ritual was handed down in a multi-facetted tradition. The present state of affairs hardly allows for a reconstitution, either of the original form of the rituals, or of the different phases of development the rituals had gone through. This task will be left for generations to come.

My present thoughts were intended to illustrate the scope of the Babylonian influence on Hittite ritual literature. On the other hand I also consider it indisputable that Hittite customs found their way, above all, into the Assyrian tradition. This can be demonstrated by the Assyrian compilation Tākultu,[105] certainly with the first-millennium curse lists, and especially the vassal treaties of Esarhaddon,[106] which are reminscent of the military oaths[107] from the time of Šuppiluliuma I.

---

[101] KBo 12.85+ (= ChS I/5 no. 19) obv. ii 19–27, on this matter V. Haas and H. J. Thiel 1978, 189f.
[102] CTH 446, edition: H. Otten, 1961, 114–57.
[103] KBo 19.145 (= ChS I/5 no. 40) 30'–40'.
[104] V. Haas 1988a, 130–34.
[105] Edition: R. Frankena 1954.
[106] Edition: D.J. Wiseman 1958.
[107] Edition: N. Oettinger 1976.

I hope that my exposé was able to demonstrate that the Hittite rituals, on grounds of their susceptibility to the Sumero-Baylonian ritual literature, are more relevant to Assyriology than has been hitherto believed.

References

Archi, A. 1983: "Die Adad-Hymne ins Hethitische übersetzt," *OrNS* 52, 20–30.

Bawanypeck, D. 2005: *Die Rituale der Auguren*, THeth 25.

Beckman, G. M. 1983: "Hittite Birth Rituals," *StBoT* 29.

Burde, C. 1974: "Hethitische medizinische Texte," *StBoT* 19.

Christiansen, B.: *Die Ritualtradition der Ambazzi. Eine philologische Bearbeitung und entstehungsgeschichtliche Analyse der Ritualtexte* CTH 391, CTH 429 *und* CTH 463, StBoT 48, 2006.

Farber, W. 1980–1983: "Lamaštu," in: *RlA* 6. Band, 439–46.

Falkenstein, A. 1939: "Sumerische Beschwörungen aus Boğazköy," *ZA* 45, 8–41.

Frankena, R. 1954: *Tākultu. De Sacrale Maaltijd in het Assyrische Ritueel*, Leiden.

Goetze, A. 1938: "The Hittite Ritual of Tunnawi," *AOS* 14.

Goetze, A. 1947: "Contributions to Hittite Lexicography," *JCS* 1, 307–20.

Goltz, D. 1974: *Studien zur altorientalischen und griechischen Heilkunde. Therapie, Arzneibereitung, Rezeptstruktur*, Wiesbaden.

Gurney O. R. 1977: *Some Aspects of Hittite Religion. The Schweich Lectures 1976*, Oxford.

Güterbock, H. G. 1934: "Die historische Tradition und ihre literarische Gestaltung bei Babyloniern und Hethitern bis 1200" (Erster Teil), *ZA* 42, 1–95.

Güterbock, H. G. 1938: "Die historische Tradition und ihre literarische Gestaltung bei Babyloniern und Hethitern bis 1200," (Zweiter Teil), *ZA* 44, 45–149.

Güterbock, H. G. 1986: "A Religious Text From *Mašat*," *Jahrbuch für kleinasiatische Forschung* 10, 205–14.

Haas, V. 1971: "Ein hethitisches Beschwörungsmotiv aus Kizzuwatna—seine Herkunft und Wanderung," *Orientalia* 40, 410–30.

Haas, V. 1980–1983: "Magie und Zauberei. B. Bei den Hethitern," *RlA* 7. Band, 234–255.

Haas, V. 1986: *Magie und Mythen in Babylonien*, Gifkendorf.

Haas, V. 1988: "Das Ritual gegen den Zugriff der Dämonin ᴰDÌM.NUN.ME und die Sammeltafel KUB XLIII 55," *OrAnt* 27, 85–104.

Haas, V. 1988a: "Die hurritisch-hethitischen Rituale der Beschwörerin Allaituraḫ(ḫ)i und ihr literarhistorischer Hintergrund," *Xenia*, 117–72.

Haas, V. 1990: "Rezension zu KUB 59," in: *OLZ* 85, 546–49.

Haas, V. 1994: *Geschichte der hethitischen Religion*, Leiden.

Haas, V.—Thiel, H. J. 1978: "Die Beschwörungsrituale der Allaituraḫ(ḫ)i und verwandte Texte," *AOAT* 31.

Haas, V.—Wilhelm, G. 1974: "Hurritische und luwische Riten aus Kizzuwatna," *AOATS* 3.

Haas, V. 2003: *Materia Magica et Medica Hethitica*, Berlin-New York.

Haas, V. 2006: *Die hethitische Literatur*, Berlin-New York, 224–244.

Jakob-Rost, L. 1972: "Das Ritual der Malli aus Arzawa gegen Behexung" (KUB XXIV 9+), *THeth*. 2.

Kammenhuber, A. 1968: *Die Arier im Vorderen Orient*, Heidelberg.

Klinger, J. 1996: "Untersuchungen zur Rekonstruktion der hattischen Kultschicht," StBoT 37.

Köcher, F. 1995: "Ein Text medizinischen Inhalts aus dem neubabylonischen Grab 405, in: Boehmer et al.," *Uruk. Die Gräber*, Mainz, 203–16.
Krebernik, M. 1984: *Die Beschwörungen aus Fara und Ebla. Texte und Studien zur Orientalistik*, Hildesheim—Zürich—New York.
Kronasser, H. 1961: "Fünf hethitische Rituale," *Die Sprache* 7, 140–69.
Kronasser, H. 1963: *Die Umsiedelung der Schwarzen Gottheit. Das hethitische Ritual KUB XXIX 4 (des Ulippi)*, Wien.
Kümmel, H. M. 1967: "Ersatzrituale für den hethitischen König," StBoT 3.
Lambert, W. G. 1960: "*Babylonian Wisdom Literature*," Oxford.
Landsberger, B. 1958: Corrections to the Article "An Old Babylonian Charm against *Merḫu*, *JNES* 17, 1958, 56–58.
Laroche, E. 1971: "*Catalogue des Textes Hittites*," Paris.
Meier, G. 1937: "Die assyrische Beschwörungssammlung Maqlû," *AfO* Beihheft 2.
Meier, G. 1939: "Ein akkadisches Heilungsritual aus Boğazköy," *ZA* 45, 195–15.
Michalowski 1998: "Literature as a Source of Lexikcal Inspiration: Some Notes on a Hymn to the Goddess Inana," in: *Written on Clay and Stone. Ancient Near Eastern Studies Presented to Krystyña Szarzynska on the Occasion of Her 80th Birthday*, edited by Jan Braun et al., Warsaw.
Miller, J. M. 2004: *Studies in the Origins, Development and Interpretation of the Kizzuwatna Rituals*, StBoT 46.
Neu, E. 1968: Interpretation der hethitischen mediopassiven Verbalformen, *StBoT* 5.
Neu, E. 1985: Zum Alter der Pleneschreibung *ma-a-aḫ-ḫa-an* in hethitischen Texten, *Hethitica* 6, 139–59.
Oettinger, N. 1976: Die militärischen Eide der Hethiter, *StBoT* 22.
Otten, H. 1961: Eine Beschwörung der Unterirdischen aus Boğazköy, ZA 54, 114–57.
Otten, H. 1973: Eine althethitische Erzählung um die Stadt Zalpa, *StBoT* 17.
Otten, H. 1973a: Das Ritual der Allī aus Arzawa, *ZA* 63, 76–82.
Otten, H. 1980–1983: Kuwatalla, *RLA* 6. Band, 398.
Puhvel, J. 1986: Who were the Hittite *hurkilas pesnes?*, in: *o-o-pe-ro-si. Festschrift für Ernst Risch zum 75. Geburtstag*, hrsg. von A. Etter, Berlin—New York, 151–55.
Reiner, E. 1958: Šurpu. A Collection of Sumerian and Akkadian Incantations, AfO, Beiheft 11.
Reiner, E. 1995: *Astral magic in Babylonia*, Philadelphia.
Soysal, O. 1987: KUB XXXI 4+KBo III 41 und 40 (Die Puḫanu-Chronik). Zum Thronstreit Ḫattušilis I., *Hethitica* 7, 173–53.
Starke, F. 1985: Die keilschrift-luwischen Texte in Umschrift, StBoT 30.
Strauß, R. 2006: *Reinigungsrituale aus Kizzuwatna*, Berlin-New York.
Taracha, P. 2000: *Ersetzen und Entsühnen. Das mittelhethitische Ersatzritual für den Großkönig Tutḫalija* (CTH *448.4), Leiden-Boston-Köln.
van der Toorn 1985: *Sin and Sanction in Israel and Mesopotamia. A comparative study*, Studia Semitica Neerlandica.
Wegner, I. 1981: Gestalt und Kult der Ištar-Šawuška in Kleinasien, *AOAT* 36.
Wegner, I. 1995: Die hurritischen Körperteilbezeichnungen, *ZA* 85, 116–26.
Werner, R. 1967: Hethitische Gerichtsprotokolle, *StBoT* 4.
Wilhelm, G. 1994: Medizinische Omina aus Ḫattuša in akkadischer Sprache, *StBoT* 36.
Wiseman, D. J. 1958: *The Vassal-Treaties of Esarhaddon*, London.

THE HANDS OF THE GODS: DISEASE NAMES, AND DIVINE ANGER[1]

Nils P. Heeßel
Seminar für Assyriologie, Heidelberg

"The god's hand was heavy upon me, I could not bear it".[2] With these words the righteous sufferer tells us about the consequences of divine displeasure. He is suffering and does not know the reason for it or how to improve his predicament. This is exactly the kind of situation that the complex Mesopotamian system of healing the sick person tried to overcome. In this paper I will try to outline some of the ways that were used to achieve this.

It is instantly recognisable to anyone familiar with Mesopotamian medical texts that the words of the righteous sufferer allude to the phrase "*qāt*(ŠU) DN—hand of the god(s)", which occurs sometimes in therapeutic texts and is ubiquitous in diagnostic texts. The diagnostic texts are either referred to as "diagnostic" or "medical" omens as they frequently state a prognosis about the patient's future; mostly "he will die" or "he will recover", alongside a diagnosis of the stated symptoms. This diagnosis is commonly a "hand of a god".

The schema of the diagnostic texts is as follows:

> "If this and that symptom is present, then this and that diagnosis (usually a "hand of a god") and/or a prognosis (like the mentioned "he will recover" or "he will die").[3]

The diagnostic texts were serialized in the 11th century B.C. by the Babylonian scholar Esagil-kīn-apli, who formed a series of 40 tablets with over 3000 entries.[4] This series was known to the Mesopotamians

---

[1] This paper has been submitted for publication in 1997. In the meantime several of the ideas and texts presented here have been elaborated on in the author's dissertation *Babylonisch-assyrische Diagnostik*, Alter Orient und Altes Testament 43 (Münster 2000). It is a pleasure to thank Dr. David Brown for correcting my English.

[2] W. G. Lambert, *Babylonian Wisdom Literature*, (Oxford, 1960) 48/1. The text has "his hand" instead of "god's hand", but the context makes it clear that the righteous sufferer is addressing himself to a god.

[3] See also H. Avalos, *Illness and Health Care in the Ancient Near East*, (Atlanta, 1995) 130.

[4] For the serialization of the series SA.GIG cf. the interesting text of Esagil-

as SA.GIG, Akkadian *sakikkû*, perhaps best translated as "symptoms".[5] In the Diagnostic Handbook we find "the hands" of an astonishing variety of divine beings.[6] Apart from the great gods like Ištar, Marduk, Sîn, Šamaš, Adad etc. we also encounter less important deities like Ningirsu, Baba, Nusku, Uraš or Išḫara. Equally prominent are demons of all kinds like Lamaštu, Šulak, Kubu, Alû lemnu or Mukīl-rēš-lemutti. Sometimes gods described as "roaming" or "fierce" act as "deputies"[7] to great gods like Anu, Šamaš or Nergal. Widely attested is the hand of a ghost, and one even finds cases of hands of stars, of a sanctuary, of the Underworld, or of human beings.

The meaning of the phrase "hand of the gods", however, has been the subject of some disagreement within the field of Assyriology. According to J. V. Kinnier Wilson the expression "hand of the gods" was used to "express the idea of both 'disease' and 'punishment'",[8] whereas Hector Avalos sees it as "describing an adverse condition, an illness in particular, that was somehow of special interest to the god".[9] Karel van der Toorn, on the other hand, stresses that one cannot translate the 'hand of the gods' as 'the disease of DN', but suggests that "the *qāt* DN constructions, then, intend to localize the source of the signs rather than to give a definite answer concerning the nature and cause of the disease."[10] He further adds, "the issue concerning the meaning of *qāt* DN is confused by such designations as ŠU.NAM.ÉRIM.MA, ŠU.DINGIR.RA, ŠU.^{d}INNIN.NA, ŠU.GIDIM.MA and the like, which are clearly used as names of diseases".[11]

It becomes clear that the major problem concerning the phrase "hand of the gods" centres around the question as to whether the phrase should be viewed as denoting a disease, or as indicating the divine being who apparently sent the disease. Although there is strong

kīn-apli edited by I. L. Finkel, "Adad-apla-iddina, Esagil-kīn-apli, and the Series SA.GIG" in: E. Leichty et al. (eds.), *A Scientific Humanist—Studies in Memory of Abraham Sachs*, (Philadelphia, 1988) 143–159.

[5] This translation was first suggested by J. V. Kinnier Wilson, *Iraq* 18 (1956) 140–141.

[6] For the present see the list in R. Labat, *Traité akkadien de diagnostics et pronostics médicaux*, (Paris, 1951) XXII–XXIII.

[7] M. Stol, *JEOL* 32 (1991–1992) 46.

[8] J. V. Kinnier Wilson, "Medicine in the Land and Times of the Old Testament", in: T. Ishida (ed.), *Studies in the Period of David and Solomon*, (Tokyo, 1982) 349.

[9] H. Avalos, *Illness and Health Care in the Ancient Near East*, (Atlanta, 1995) 134.

[10] K. van der Toorn, *Sin and Sanction in Israel and Mesopotamia*, (Assen, 1985) 78.

[11] *Ibid.*, 199, fn. 304.

evidence for both assumptions, one gets the impression that the cases where a disease is meant are more common amongst the therapeutic texts, whereas in the diagnostic texts most often the divine sender is identified. A closer look at these texts, however, reveals an interesting phenomenon.

First one notices that in the therapeutic texts some "hands" are more common than others. These are especially the "hand of the god", the "hand of Ištar/the goddess"[12] and the "hand of a ghost".[13] One will also notice that these "hands" are always written with the same graphemes (ŠU DINGIR.RA, ŠU ^{d}INNIN(.NA), and ŠU GIDIM.MA or ŠU GIDIM$_{7}$.MA respectively). From two long known references (*šu-dingir-ra-ki* and *šu-gidim-ma-ka*)[14] the Akkadian readings *šudingirrakku*, *šuʿinninnakku*, and *šugidimmakku* have been established and translated respectively as the "hand of the god-disease", the "hand of the goddess-disease" and the "hand of a ghost-disease".[15] All attempts to identify these diseases have been unsuccessful.[16]

When seeking out these "hands" in the Diagnostic Handbook it is striking to see the same "hands" constantly written differently (ŠU DINGIR, ŠU ^{d}*Iš-tar*/^{d}*Iš-tár*/^{d}XV, ŠU GIDIM/GÍDIM/GIDIM$_{7}$). More intriguing still, these different forms of writing are found in those cases where one might expect the divine sender to be identified, whereas the writing in the therapeutic texts, with the correct Sumerian genitive forms, corresponds to the instances where one expects a disease-name.

So, for instance, in an interesting and well-known list in which diseases are related to certain parts of the human body, the "hands of the god and the goddess and of a ghost" appear among disease-names.[17] Here they are written ŠU.DINGIR.RA, ŠU.INNIN.NA and ŠU.GIDIM.MA respectively.

[12] For the problem of distinguishing between the "hand of Ištar" and the "hand of the Goddess" see M. Stol, *Epilepsy in Babylonia*, CM 2 (Groningen, 1993) 36f.

[13] Also very common are the "hand of an oath" and the "hand of mankind". The evidence for these "hands" is, however, rather ambigious.

[14] G. Meier, *AfO* 14 (1941–44), 142/35–36.

[15] The correct transliteration of the ideographic writing of *šudingirrakku*, *šuʿinninnakku*, and *šugidimmakku* should be ŠU.DINGIR.RA, ŠU.INNIN.NA and ŠU.GIDIM.MA, with a point connecting all elements.

[16] For *šugidimmakku* see F. Köcher, "Spätbabylonische medizinische Texte aus Uruk", in: Ch. Habrich et al. (eds), *Medizinische Diagnostik in Geschichte und Gegenwart—Festschrift für Heinz Goerke*, (München, 1978) 25–32; and for *šudingirrakku* and *šuʿinninnakku* compare M. Stol, *Epilepsy in Babylonia*, CM 2 (Groningen, 1993) 33–38.

[17] H. Hunger, *Spätbabylonische Texte aus Uruk* I, (Berlin, 1976) no. 43. Compare the copy on p. 139 where much more is readable than the transliteration shows.

In the therapeutic texts concerning the "hand of a ghost" (BAM 216–230, 469–474, AMT 76/1, 94/2, 97/4,5 etc.), where we expect it to refer to a disease, it is commonly written "ŠU.GIDIM.MA". In almost all of the 47 instances in the Diagnostic Handbook, however, the "hand of a ghost" appears as ŠU GIDIM, without MA. This fits in well with the view that in the Diagnostic Handbook the divine sender of a disease is identified. The same can be noticed for the "hand of the goddess". Always written ŠU.^{d}INNIN(.NA) in therapeutic texts, in all of the 73 instances in the Diagnostic Handbook it is written either ŠU ^{d}XV, ŠU ^{d}*Iš-tar* or ŠU ^{d}*Iš*$_{8}$*-tár*. This may be schematized as follows:

	disease-name	divine "sender"
hand of the God	ŠU.DINGIR.RA	ŠU DINGIR
hand of the Goddess/ Ištar	ŠU.INNIN(.NA)	ŠU ^{d}*Iš-tar* ŠU ^{d}*Iš*$_{8}$*-tár* ŠU ^{d}XV
hand of a Ghost	ŠU.GIDIM.MA ŠU.GIDIM$_{7}$.MA	ŠU GIDIM ŠU GIDIM ŠU GIDIM$_{7}$

Admittedly, ŠU.GIDIM.MA and ŠU.^{d}INNIN(.NA) as well as ŠU.DINGIR.RA do appear in the Diagnostic Handbook. However, these instances only serve to illustrate a disease-nature, as they almost always appear in the protases of the entries.[18]

1. SA.GIG 40, lines 26–27, the tablet concerning babies (TDP 220/26–27):

> DIŠ ^{lú}TUR *ki-ma al-du* U$_{4}$ 2–KÁM U$_{4}$ 3–KÁM GIN-*ma* GA *la i-maḫ-ḫar mi-iq-tu ki-ma* ŠU.DINGIR.RA ŠUB.ŠUB-*su* ŠU ^{d}XV *ek-ke-em-tu*$_{4}$ *šum-šu* BA.ÚŠ
>
> "If the baby, two or three days having passed after it is born, does not accept the milk, (and) *miqtu*(-disease) like the "hand of the god-

[18] The only exceptions are to my knowledge SA.GIG 1/49 (TDP 4/38), 15/29' (TDP 234/29), and 22/59 (TDP 184/9). Here ŠU.GIDIM.MA appears in the apodoses of the entries. In the second instance the text needs collation and in the third the "hand of a ghost" is described as the deputy (*šá-*<*né*>*-e*) of the god Ea and it is probable that it denotes not the divine sender but the disease.

disease" is constantly falling upon him, then it is the "hand of Ištar", "the snatcher" is its name—he will die."

2. The "hand of a ghost" and the "hand of the goddess" appear in tablet 28, in the chapter on epilepsy of the Diagnostic Handbook. Here one disease changes into another.

For example SA.GIG 28/11–13 (TDP 194/47–49):

DIŠ ŠU.INNIN.NA *ana* AN.TA.ŠUB.BA GUR-*šú* ŠU ^{d}XXX : ŠU ^{d}XV *ana* KAR-*šú* . . . ŠU.BI.AŠ.ÀM (= AL.TI)

"If the "hand of the goddess"-disease changes into AN.TA.ŠUB.BA-disease (this is a form of epilepsy), then this is due to "hand of Sîn" //(alternatively) "hand of Ištar". In order to save him. . . ." There follows a recipe and a prognosis: he will recover.

Or: SA.GIG 28/1–3 (TDP 192/37–39):

DIŠ *šum*$_4$*-ma* ŠU.GIDIM.MA *ana* AN.TA.ŠUB.BA GUR-*šú* LÚ BI ŠU DINGIR URU-*šú* GIG *ina* ŠU DINGIR URU-*šú* KAR-*šú* . . . . TI.LA

"If the "hand of a ghost"-disease changes into AN.TA.ŠUB.BA, that man is sick due to the "hand of his city-god". In order to rescue him from "the hand of his city-god . . . ." There follows a recipe, and he will recover.

These remarks clearly illustrate the problems of mixing references to the "hands of the god, the goddess, the ghost" without regard to their context and their style of writing. However, is there a connection between, for example, the "hand of a ghost"-disease (ŠU.GIDIM.MA) and the "hand of a ghost"(ŠU GIDIM) as an indicator of the divine sender of this special disease? In a therapeutic text the diagnoses of symptoms manifested by the patient's temple are named *šugidimmakku*, and the same set of symptoms are identified as the "hand of a ghost" in the Diagnostic Handbook.[19] But there is also a reference which could serve as a counter-example. In the just mentioned tablet 28 of SA.GIG in line 4 we read:

DIŠ AN.TA.ŠUB.BA *ana* ŠU.GIDIM.MA GUR-*šú* SAG.ḪUL.ḪA.ZA TUK.TUK-*ši* ŠU ^{d}XV ŠU MAŠKIM

"If AN.TA.ŠUB.BA changes into the "hand of a ghost"-disease, then he constantly gets the "Provider-of-Evil"-demon (*mukil-rēš-lemutti*), due to the "hand of Ištar/the goddess", alternatively due to the "hand of the Lurker-demon (*rābiṣu*)"."

[19] Compare BAM 482 iii 5 to SA.GIG 4/17 (TDP 34/17) and BAM 482 iii 7 to SA.GIG 4/13 (TDP 34/13).

If there really is a connection we would have expected the "hand of a ghost" in the apodosis and not the "hand of Ištar/the goddess". The same omen also contains a reference which could contradict the idea of differentiating the disease and the divine sender by forms of writing. The "hand of Ištar/the goddess" as the divine sender is written in one of the three manuscripts as ŠU.^{d}INNIN (ŠU ^{d}XV, ŠU ^{d}*Iš-tar* in the others). We have to take this to be one of the inevitable exceptions. Nevertheless, it is likely that the expressions "hand of the god, the goddess and the ghost" sometimes denote a disease and sometimes the divine sender of the disease. The different Akkadian readings (e.g. *šugidimmakku* and *qāt eṭemmi*) for the disease and the divine sender were accordingly distinguished, much more often than not, by means of graphemes.

We have now investigated three "hands" that appear in diagnostic as well as therapeutic texts. But what about all the other "hands" of particular gods that appear frequently as the diagnosis in the Diagnostic Handbook and yet are rare in the therapeutic texts? Similar to a modern diagnostic handbook we would expect the name of a disease to be mentioned after the description of the different symptoms, in order to determine the therapy. For the Mesopotamian Diagnostic Handbook, however, it seems to be more important to identify and name a divine being. The "hand of the gods" is only one, albeit the most frequent, phrase used to name the supposed divine involvement. The gods can also "seize"(DAB/*ṣabātu*), "touch"(TAG/*lapātu*), "strike"(SÌG/*maḫāṣu*) or "reach"(KUR/*kašādu*) the human being and these verbs can even be combined with the phrase "hand of the god".[20] It should be remarked that a "touch by the divine" is common to all these expressions and we should not ignore this fact. Here, so it seems, is a trace of how the Babylonians saw the process of falling sick. It apparently required physical contact between the god and the human being.

It has long been suspected that these identified and named gods are those who actually brought about the sickness of the patient. Yet there has been disagreement about whether the divine being is the cause of the disease or simply its "sender" or "controller". This involves the question as to whether the perceived reason for sickening was human sin or whether sickness could strike without any

---

[20] See M. Stol, *JEOL* 32, 46.

inappropriate behaviour on the human side.[21] Without going into details here, it is worth drawing attention to a few cases in the Diagnostic Handbook where some explanations for the "hand of the god" are stated. These are often introduced by the word *aššu* (MU) "because", and followed by a reference to some particular misbehaviour. An example: SA.GIG 17/79 (TDP 166/79):

> DIŠ *ina* GE_6 GIG-*ma ina ka-ṣa-a-ti ba-liṭ* ŠU [d]*Uraš* MU DA[M LÚ]
>
> "If he is sick in the night and healthy in the morning: It is the "hand of Uraš", because of the wife of a man."

This almost certainly refers to adultery. Marten Stol has rightly observed that "the Diagnostic handbook, in the few cases it mentions human sin, has a marked interest in illicit sexual contacts . . . and in not fulfilling vows made to the gods (*ikribū, kaspu*)".[22] The scarcity of cases in the Diagnostic Handbook where a human sin is referred to, about 30 references in all, demonstrates that the editor of the Diagnostic Handbook was not much interested in the cause of a disease, but in identifying the divine being involved in the sickness of the patient. This may mean that the identification and naming of the divine being was essential in order to heal the patient. As R. Biggs[23] and H. Avalos[24] observed, knowing the name of the god involved ensured the possibility of addressing this god in prayer and in reconciling the god with the patient. Therefore, we can outline two ways in which a sick person was healed. One aimed at coping with the signs of a disease—with it symptoms—and developed an elaborate treatment involving salves, bandages, liquid medicine, etc. as well as rituals and incantations to further the effects of the medicine. These rituals involved instructions such as letting the medicine stand overnight under the stars which, in one way or another, enhanced it.[25] The other way tried to identify the divine sender of the disease through an appropriate method designed to discover the god with whom the patient had problems. Afterwards attempts could be made to heal the patient by reconciling him with this god and

[21] See K. van der Toorn, *Sin and Sanction*, 56–93; H. Avalos, *Illness and Health Care*, 132–134 and M. Stol, *JEOL* 32, 46–47.
[22] M. Stol, *JEOL* 32, 46.
[23] R. D. Biggs, *Reallexikon der Assyriologie,* Bd. 7, 624b.
[24] H. Avalos, *Illness and Health Care*, 135f.
[25] See E. Reiner, *Astral Magic in Babylonia*, (Philadelphia, 1995) 48–53.

thereby sealing off the source of the disease. Calling one method, from a modern point of view, "rational" and the other "magical", however, misses the point.[26] Indeed, in the therapeutic texts incantations are quite common, and in the diagnostic texts prescriptions and recipes do sometimes appear.

It is most regrettable that we do not know which texts were actually used to appease divine anger and reconcile the sick person with the god. These texts were not, as has been proposed,[27] namburbi-rituals, since they coped with problems that an omen had posed long before the effects of that omen—for example a disease—could be felt. K. van der Toorn has argued that the dingir-šà-dib-ba incantations represented the therapeutic counterpart to the diagnostic texts.[28] Yet, as W. G. Lambert[29] noticed, the dingir-šà-dib-ba incantations are addressed to the personal god and goddess, and one would assume that since so much care was taken to identify the gods involved in the Diagnostic Handbook this should lead to therapeutic texts which addressed a greater variety of deities. Here texts like the Akkadian *Šu-ilas* or the eršaḫunga-prayers could be mentioned. Neither should we exclude the possibility that a combination of texts was used. The nam-erim-búr-ru-da texts could have been used against the "hand of the curse" (ŠU NAM.ÉRIM), as could text series like sag-ba,[30] asag-gig, or udug-ḫul. It is very possible that the exorcist had no fixed series of texts which he used to reconcile the divine being with the patient, but decided what action to take according to the situation and the diagnosis he had gained. For example, if the diagnosis were the "hand of a ghost" (*qāt eṭemmi*) he could have used one of the many rituals to expel a spirit.

Thus, were the therapeutic and diagnostic texts separate methods to cope with the same problem of healing a sick person? I think it unlikely that these methods were used independently. Only by

[26] For a rejection of this simple differentiation and a more thorough view of "magic" see T. Abusch, *Babylonian Witchcraft Literature* (Atlanta, 1987) 5.

[27] H. Avalos, *Illness and Health Care*, 136.

[28] K. van der Toorn, *Sin and Sanction*, 123. van der Toorn starts with the incorrect assumption that BAM 315 and 316, as well as *Semitica* 3, 1950, 10 are "diagnostic texts". One could follow van der Toorn much more easily had he drawn parallels to the diagnostic series SA.GIG.

[29] W. G. Lambert, *JNES* 33 (1974) 267–322.

[30] See W. Ph. Römer, in: H. Behrens et al. (eds.), *DUMU-E$_2$-DUB-BA-A, Studies in Honor of Ake W. Sjöberg*, (Philadelphia, 1989) 465–479.

combining various ways of healing would a sick person be treated by all available means. But if these methods are really to be viewed as two parts of the same healing process to be used together, one would like to see some sort of connection between them, as has been discussed at length ever since the publication of Labat's edition of TDP. J. V. Kinnier Wilson was the first to suggest that there was a therapeutic "companion series" to the Diagnostic Handbook,[31] while Karel van der Toorn, as stated above, argued that the dingir-šà-dib-ba prayers incantations served as a counterpart to the therapeutic texts.[32] Most recently Marten Stol, investigating this problem, came to the conclusion that "the Diagnostic handbook was available to the compiler of the therapeutic texts."[33]

A few years ago, the missing link between the therapeutic and diagnostic texts was found. This is tablet 33 of the series SA.GIG, published by Egbert von Weiher in SpTU IV/152.[34] This tablet gives as the diagnosis of the stated symptoms not a "hand of a god" but the disease-name. The structure of this text is similar to the texts we call "*šammu šikinšu*" (the nature of the plant) or "*abnu šikinšu*" (the nature of the stone) and von Weiher named it accordingly "*murṣu šikinšu*" (the nature of the disease)[35] although a reading "*simmu šikinšu*" (the nature of the affected area) following Franz Köcher[36] might be equally appropriate according to the context. The text has the following scheme: "If the nature of the disease/affected area (DIŠ GIG/SIM$_x$ GAR-*šú/šumma murṣu/simmu šikinšu*)—here follow the symptoms—then x is its (the diseases) name (x MU.NI/ x *šumšu*)". This shows that the phrase "If the nature of the disease/affected area is this and that, then x is its name", which sometimes occurs in the therapeutic texts,[37] does not belong to the phrasing of the *asû* as has been proposed,[38] but clearly to that of the *āšipu* since the series SA.GIG forms part of *āšipūtu*.

---

[31] J. V. Kinnier Wilson, *Iraq* 19 (1957) 44–46.

[32] K. van der Toorn, *Sin and Sanction*, 123.

[33] M. Stol, *JEOL* 32, 49.

[34] E. von Weiher, *Spätbabylonische Texte aus Uruk* IV, AUWE 12, (Berlin, 1993) no. 152.

[35] *Ibid.*, 81.

[36] See F. Köcher, "Ein Text medizinischen Inhalts aus dem neubabylonischen Grab 405", in: R. M. Boehmer et al., *Uruk—Die Gräber*, AUWE 10, (Berlin, 1995) 209/21'.

[37] References have been collected by M. Stol, *JEOL* 32, 64.

[38] *Ibid.*, 64.

Furthermore, at the end of this tablet after a ruling, the text assigns the disease-names to certain "hands of the gods". It is most interesting to note that certain "hands" are equated to more than one disease. The "hand of the sungod Šamaš" is equated to nine diseases (the maximum) and the "hand of the Gula (the goddess of healing)" equated to seven diseases. This section cross-indexes disease-names with the "hands of the gods" and is therefore the first clear link between the therapeutic texts and the Diagnostic Handbook.

This elaborate and well-thought-out system aimed at using all available means to further the recovery of the sick person. The symptoms of the disease were viewed as containing vital information about the divine anger that led to the sickness. By using this information to determine the name of the god involved, the exorcist gained the means by which to reconcile the patient with the angered god and thereby eliminate the source of the disease. The patient, who could be sure that the immediate source of his disease was thus eliminated, no doubt looked forward with almost absolute certainty to the end of his suffering. The power of the placebo effect is well-known to modern physicians. On the other hand the pharmacological-therapeutic treatment ensured the recovery from the actual disease and its symptoms. Although we do not know exactly how effective these recipes were, since we have only started to identify the plants and drugs involved, I think we can safely assume that this treatment yielded at least partially positive results.[39] We might surely call this system holistic.

Only now can we fully understand the dismay, the utter wretchedness, of the righteous sufferer quoted at the beginning of this article. In his case this system had failed, leaving him no hope of recovery:

> "My symptoms eluded the exorcist and my omens confounded the diviner, the exorcist has not diagnosed the nature of my symptoms, nor has the diviner put a time limit on my illness."[40]

It becomes clear that this poor wretch had indeed nothing to look forward to, but endless suffering.

---

[39] Compare J. A. Scurlock, *AfO* 42/43 (1995–1996) 252–253.

[40] W. G. Lambert, *BWL*, 44: 108–111 with slight alterations.

List of Cited Literature

Abusch, T., *Babylonian Witchcraft Literature*, Brown Judaic Studies 132 (Atlanta, 1987).
Avalos, H., *Illness and Health Care in the Ancient Near East*, Harvard Semitic Monographs 54 (Atlanta, 1995).
Biggs, R. D., "Medizin. A. In Mesopotamien", in: *Reallexikon der Assyriologie*, Bd. 7 (1987–90) 627–627.
Finkel, I. L., "Adad-apla-iddina, Esagil-kīn-apli, and the Series SA.GIG" in: E. Leichty et al. (eds.), *A Scientific Humanist—Studies in Memory of Abraham Sachs*, (Philadelphia, 1988) 143–159.
Hunger, H., *Spätbabylonische Texte aus Uruk* I, (Berlin, 1976).
Kinnier Wilson, J. V., "Two Medical Texts from Nimrud", *Iraq* 18 (1956) 130–146.
——, "Two Medical Texts from Nimrud (Continued)", *Iraq* 19 (1957) 40–49.
——, "Medicine in the Land and Times of the Old Testament", in: T. Ishida (ed.), *Studies in the Period of David and Solomon*, (Tokyo, 1982) 349.
Köcher, F., *Die babylonisch-assyrische Medizin in Texten und Untersuchungen* I–VI, (Berlin, 1963–1980).
Köcher, F., "Spätbabylonische medizinische Texte aus Uruk", in: Ch. Habrich et al. (eds.), *Medizinische Diagnostik in Geschichte und Gegenwart—Festschrift für Heinz Goerke*, (München, 1978) 17–39.
Köcher, F., "Ein Text medizinischen Inhalts aus dem neubabylonischen Grab 405", in: R. M. Boehmer et al., *Uruk—Die Gräber*, AUWE 10, (Berlin, 1995).
Labat, R., *Traité akkadien de diagnostics et pronostics médicaux*, (Paris, 1951).
Lambert, W. G., *Babylonian Wisdom Literature*, (Oxford, 1960).
—— "Dingir.šà.dib.ba Incantations", *Journal of Near Eastern Studies* 33 (1974) 267–322.
Meier, G., "Die zweite Tafel der Serie bīt mēseri", *Archiv für Orientforschung* 14 (1941–44) 139–152.
Reiner, E., *Astral Magic in Babylonia*, Transactions of the American Philosophical Society 85, (Philadelphia, 1995).
Römer, W. Ph., "Eine Beschwörung gegen den 'Bann'", in: H. Behrens et al. (eds.), *DUMU-E$_2$-DUB-BA-A, Studies in Honor of Ake W. Sjöberg*, (Philadelphia, 1989) 465–479.
Scurlock, J., Review of M. Stol, *Epilepsy in Babylonia*, Cuneiform Monographs 2 (1993)", *Archiv für Orientforschung* 42/43, (1995–1996) 252–253.
Stol, M., "Diagnosis and Therapy in Babylonian Medicine", in: *Jaarbericht van het vooraziatisch-egyptisch Genootschap "Ex oriente lux"* 32 (1991–1992) 42–65.
Stol, M., *Epilepsy in Babylonia*, Cuneiform Monographs 2, (Groningen, 1993).
van der Toorn, K., *Sin and Sanction in Israel and Mesopotamia*, (Assen, 1985).
von Weiher, E., *Spätbabylonische Texte aus Uruk* IV, AUWE 12, (Berlin, 1993).

EPILEPSY IN MESOPOTAMIA RECONSIDERED

Hector Avalos
Iowa State University

Identifying diseases in ancient Mesopotamia has always encountered philological difficulties.[1] Such difficulties are complicated further by the fact that the modern classification of some diseases is still variable, and this includes controversy about whether certain symptoms (e.g., involuntary muscle movements) should be classified as epilepsy. It is in this light that Marten Stol's *Epilepsy in Babylonia* provides a fresh opportunity to review some of the problems involved in the study of Babylonian and Near Eastern medicine in general.[2]

We should first note that the condition identified by Marten Stol as "epilepsy" previously had received little attention from Assyriologists. As Stol notes, Erich Ebeling provided a very brief discussion in the *Reallexicon der Assyriologie* (1938) that did not go much beyond what had been written by Karl Sudhoff, a non-Assyriologist, in 1911.[3] To be fair, neither of those scholars had much information available to them.

In *Epilepsy in Babylonia*, Stol profiles some of the basic historical sources (e.g., Hippocrates' *On the Sacred Disease*) for the study of epilepsy, and announces that his principal aim is to "survey how the Babylonians viewed and treated epilepsy."[4] Stol's examination of Babylonian terminology concludes that the Akkadian *bennu* is the general word for epilepsy, and he argues that the Sumerian an.ta.šub.ba is the more technical name given to "the sudden attack" of epilepsy.

Another important term is *miqtu*, which he admits does not always mean epilepsy, but which is remarkably parallelled by the later European notion of epilepsy as "the falling sickness." There are also

[1] For some examples, see P. B. Adamson, "Some Anatomical and Pathological Terms in Akkadian," *RA* 84 (1990) 27–32.
[2] Marten Stol, *Epilepsy in Babylonia* (Cuneiform Monographs 2. Groningen: Styx Publications, 1993).
[3] *Epilepsy*, 3.
[4] *Epilepsy*, Preface.

demonic entities associated with epilepsy, and these include the enigmatic "spawn of šulpaea," Lugal-urra ("Lord of the roof"), Lugal-nam-en-na, and Lugal-amašpae. He also discusses epilepsy in relation to related afflictions (e.g., "melancholy," "Hand of the God") and demons such as Alû, Incubus, and Succubus.

Stol provides an edition and translation of the extant portions of the Diagnostic Handbook (SA.GIG) (Tablets XXVI, XXVII–XXVIII, XXIX, and XXX) focusing on epilepsy. This work supersedes the old edition of René Labat's *TDP* in some of those sections, and includes tablets (e.g., XXVI) not known to Labat. In addition, Stol provides a new edition of a second diagnostic text, known after its incipit ("If you approach a sick man"). This edition is based on a text (STT 1 89) published by O. R. Gurney. Stol regards it as an older version of the Diagnostic Handbook, and he suggests that the editor of the Diagnostic Handbook composed his version in reaction to it.

Stol's discussion of therapeutics centres on the use of, *inter alia*, stag's horn, blood, fumigation, amulets, and "jasper," a stone often associated with the moon. Indeed, here and in the following three chapters, he outlines the links among epilepsy, calendrics, and the moon, links which have continued into modern times in many cultures.

In his treatment of the sociology of epilepsy, Stol discusses the societal reactions to children struck with epilepsy, as well as some of the legal aspects of epilepsy. He includes discussion of epilepsy in the Code of Hammurabi, Neo-Assyrian contracts, and Greek law. Finally, he delves into the occurrence of epilepsy in animals.

In order to assess the problems involved in identifying "epilepsy" in ancient Mesopotamia one must consider briefly what is in modern medicine meant by "epilepsy," the definition of which can be quite complex and varied. According to one authority: "Epilepsy can be defined as the repeated occurrence of seizures in the absence of an acute precipitating systemic or brain insult."[5] Ernst Niedermeyer's authoritative manual includes an entire chapter on "Differential Diagnosis: Epileptic vs. Non-Epileptic Attacks," and he would classify

[5] W. Allan Hauser, John F. Annegers, and V. Elving Anderson, "Epidemiology and the Genetics of Epilepsy," in Arthur A. Ward, Jr., J. Kiffin Penry and Dominick Purpura, eds., *Epilepsy* (New York: Raven Press, 1983) 269.

as "non-epileptic" those convulsions resulting from hypoglycemia, liver disease, galactosemia, and other conditions.[6] There have also been a number of attempts to impose an international classification of epilepsies which would distinguish convulsive symptoms resulting from conditions outside of a chronic brain lesion associated with "true" epilepsy.[7]

As Owsei Temkin's classic history illustrates, the terms for "epilepsy" could vary from one practitioner to another within the same city.[8] Thus, for Galen (2nd c. CE), the true epileptic fit was marked by the participation of the whole body and loss of consciousness.[9] Yet, in other ancient traditions, an epileptic fit need not involve the loss of consciousness.

In light of this complexity and the problems relating to the modern and ancient definition of epilepsy, it may be said that Stol's approach is only partially successful. He does not provide an adequate discussion of what he means by "epilepsy," and at times he appears to define any type of convulsive activity as "epilepsy." At the very least, one would expect the selection of one modern definition of epilepsy that would have provided a reference point for comparison.

Stol does show that an.ta.šub.ba and its related terms are often associated with what may be involuntary muscle movements. His so-called Second Diagnostic Text (lines 141–166), for example, includes, as symptoms of the disease, the flow of saliva (*ru'tu*([ÙḪ]) *ina pîšu*(KA-*šú*) *illak*(GIN-*ak*) lack of self-awarenes (*ramanšu*(NI-šu) *la*(NU) *idê*(ZU)), and "kicking" (*i*(!)-*nap-pa-aṣ*), though it is not clear that this latter behavior is involuntary or simply reflects the great agony of the patient.[10]

On the other hand, Stol sometimes seems to accept uncritically the definitions of epilepsy derived from other authorities. Thus, in Tablet XXVI: rev. 4–6, Stol adopts J. V. Kinnier Wilson and E. H. Reynolds' identification of certain symptoms (e.g., opening and closing

---

[6] Ernst Niedermeyer, *Compendium of the Epilepsies* (Springfield, Illinois: Charles C. Thomas, 1974).

[7] See Niedermeyer, *Compendium*, 24ff.

[8] Owsei Temkin, *The Falling Sickness* (2nd ed. Baltimore: The Johns Hopkins University Press, 1971).

[9] Temkin, *Falling Sickness*, 49.

[10] *Epilepsy*, 94.

of eyes, loss of speech, and abdominal pain) as indicative of "temporal lobe epilepsy."[11] Yet there is no discussion about other conditions that might also result in such symptoms. Niedermeyer, for example, has cautioned specifically against using abdominal pain as an indicator of temporal lobe epilepsy, and adds that to assign an epileptic basis to abdominal pain is as inappropriate "as ascribing an epileptic basis to habit spasm, merely because the movements resemble myoclonic jerks and the motor cortex is presumably involved in both phenomena."[12]

If we accept the definition of Hauser *et al.*, the best that can be shown is that there were Babylonian terms that may have included what we know as "epilepsy," but which may also have been used for a variety of non-epileptic convulsive seizures. A case in point may be the comparison between *bennu* and an.ta.šub.ba. As stated above, Stol has argued that *bennu* is the name given to recurrent epilepsy in general, while an.ta.šub.ba is the name for the sudden attack. Yet Tablet XXVI: rev. 1–3, indicates that an.ta.šub.ba can be recurrent (*la*(NU) *innassaḫ*(ZI-*aḫ*)/"it will not be eradicated").[13] Tablet XXVI indicates that an.ta.šub.ba may occur at a particular time every year (l. 7: MU.1.KAM *imaqqutaššumma* (DUB-*šú-ma*; var. B. RI-ma) *ana ittišuma* (IGI.DUB-*šú-ma*) *ihiṭṭaššu* (LÁ-*šú*)), something that would not be expected of epilepsy.[14] Stol notes that *bennu* is found after various fevers, yet he concludes that this does "not necessarily mean that *bennu* is feverish."[15] However, this association of *bennu* with fever may indicate that the Babylonian author was using *bennu* for convulsions that might not be true epilepsy, according to some modern classifications.

More problematic are cases where the Spawn of Šulpaea, which Stol identifies as "a severe and almost hopeless form of epilepsy,"[16] turns into "curable an.ta.šub.ba." Yet, in another passage, the Spawn of Šulpaea is described as absolutely hopeless (lines 180–186: "it will

[11] *Epilepsy*, 68; J. V. Kinnier Wilson and E. H. Reynolds, "Translation and analysis of a cuneiform text forming part of a Babylonian treatise on epilepsy," *Medical History*, 34 (1990) 185–198.
[12] Niedermeyer, *Compendium*, 166.
[13] *Epilepsy*, 67.
[14] *Epilepsy*, 58.
[15] *Epilepsy*, 7.
[16] *Epilepsy*, 85.

not go away; you shall burn him with fire in his illness").[17] Likewise, there are many cases in which the "Hand of Ishtar" turns into an.ta.šub.ba, something that indicates not a sudden attack, but a condition, which may have precursors (and perhaps initial signals, sometimes known as the "aura," of an epileptic attack). It is possible that the patient described in these cases was also suffering from more than one condition, that would not have been detected in the symptom lists. In any event, these cases show the fluidity of the diagnosis and terminology of Babylonian medicine.

Stol's view of the role of the *āšipu* and *asû* also needs refinement. He seems to follow Edith Ritter, who defined the former as some sort of "conjurer," because he supposedly focuses on magical therapy, but the latter as a "doctor," because this profession supposedly uses more empirical methods.[18] Such a distinction apparently leads Stol to state that "epilepsy would have required a "conjurer' (*āšipu*) not a doctor (*asû*)."[19] As I have argued elsewhere, such translations for these professions are misleading, and it is best to retain the native Babylonian terms for these consultants.[20] The selection of the *āšipu, asû* and other consultants could depend on economics, the status of the patient, and other factors that are not always reflected in diagnostic manuals or texts which only mention one profession.

In the present writer's view, Stol is assuming too much homogeneity for ancient Babylonian medical practice and terminology. Stol's study shows that *bennu*, an.ta.šub.ba, and the other related terms may describe a variety of conditions marked by involuntary muscle movements. These terms may often, but not always, refer to what most modern physicians classify as epilepsy. Regional and historical variation may have played a far greater role than might be reflected in the main diagnostic texts. Various modern studies of ethnomedicine suggest that inconsistency and variation are a normal part

[17] *Epilepsy*, 96.

[18] *Epilepsy*, 11 *et passim*. Edith Ritter, "Magical Expert = (*āšipu*) and Physician (= *Asû*): Notes on Complementary Professions in Babylonian Medicine," 299–321 in H. G. Güterbock and T. Jacobsen, eds., *Studies in Honor of Benno Landsberger on his 75th Birthday, April 21, 1965* (Chicago, 1965).

[19] *Epilepsy*, 11.

[20] Hector Avalos, *Illness and Health Care in the Ancient Near East: The Role of the Temple in Greece, Mesopotamia, and Israel* (Harvard Semitic Monographs 54; Atlanta: Scholars Press, 1995) 142–167.

of the medical terminology in many cultures.[21] In addition, we should also note that the Akkadian diagnostic manuals published by Stol reflect the work of perhaps a minority of the consultants available in Mesopotamia. Such consultants were élite and literate, as opposed to the majority of consultants in Mesopotamia who may have been folk healers who did not document their diagnoses, terminology, or therapeutic practices.

Such problems have implications for the study of medicine in the ancient Near East. While we should not abandon our efforts to identify diseases as specifically as possible in terms of modern medical classifications, our efforts might be best focused on the social aspects of illnesses in the ancient Near East. For example, Stol's editions of diagnostic texts focusing on a limited illness or group of illnesses might help us explore the extent to which diagnostic manuals could be used to set work priorities within a health-care system. Diagnostic manuals can define work priorities by identifying patients who are not expected to recover, and so perhaps not worthy of further efforts by consultants.

The variety of terms and treatments pertaining to illnesses that have convulsions as a symptom might help us explore how such variety can complicate a patient's therapeutic strategy as well as provide hope for patients who may not be satisfied with previous options. In sum, even if we cannot identify a disease as specifically as we might desire, we still may be able to study how the ancient Mesopotamian peoples described their experiences and what the implications of those experiences were for the broader religious, social, and economic aspects of their culture.

---

[21] For some examples of terminological diversity and inconsistency, see Frederick L. Dunn, "Traditional Asian Medicine and Cosmopolitan Medicine as Adaptive Systems," 133–158 in Charles Leslie, ed., *Asian Medical Systems: A Comparative Study* (Berkeley: University of California Press, 1976); Giles Bibeau, "The Circular Semantic Network in Nbgandi Disease Nosology," *Social Science and Medicine* 15B (1981) 295–307. "After submission of this article, a number of works have been published addressing methodological problems in diagnosis of Mesopotamian diseases. One notable item is: Nils P. Heessel, "Reading and Interpreting Medical Cuneiform Texts: Methods and Problems," Le Journal des médecines cunéiformes 1, no. 3 (2004) 2–9.

LAMAŠTU—AGENT OF A SPECIFIC DISEASE OR A GENERIC DESTROYER OF HEALTH?

Walter Farber
Oriental Institute, Chicago

There are many diseases—or, more cautiously: many states of illness some of which ultimately may lead to death[1]—in ancient Mesopotamia for which the pertinent texts give us a simple rationale: they are said to have been caused by the grip, Akkadian *ṣibtu*, of a certain demon. While for a Babylonian this might be sufficient to explain a person's misfortune in losing her or his health or life, such a seemingly simple aetiology leads the modern scholar to a number of much less simple questions.

First of all, we would like to know in every instance whether the demon is acting on his or her own mischievous behalf, thus afflicting people in an unpredictable or haphazard way, or whether the grip of the demon is ultimately ordered by some higher authority, be it for a general purpose like population control,[2] or because of an individual's sin or other fault.[3] It also has to be asked whether the actions of a specific demon lead directly to a definable disease which can then become the object of diagnosis and subsequent healing practices, or whether the grip of the demon is irreversible once it has occurred, in which case any useful action against it would have to precede the affliction and thus be prophylactic and apotropaic.

If the result of such demonic action is a definable and potentially treatable disease, we can try to find out how the ancient medical practitioner arrived at the diagnosis "grip of demon so-and-so," and how he defined the set of symptoms typical for that particular illness. Looking from a slightly different angle, we could re-phrase this

---

[1] For a useful definition of "Illness" vs. "Disease," see Taber's *Cyclopedic Medical Dictionary*[13] (ed. C. L. Thomas, 1977), D 47f., as quoted by R. D. Biggs, Medizin. A. (RlA 7/7–8, 1990) 626a.

[2] See, most conveniently, M. Stol, *Zwangerschap en Geboorte bij de Babyloniërs en in de Bijbel* (Leiden 1982), 91f.

[3] For a general discussion of 'illness' as a result of 'sin,' see K. van der Toorn, *Sin and Sanction in Israel and Mesopotamia* (Assen 1985), esp. 67ff.

and ask: is the particular demon exclusively responsible for one or more definable diseases, or do his or her activities lead to an array of otherwise non-interrelated symptoms and breakdowns in an individual's health? In the first case, a subsequent question arises, namely whether the demon is actually an independent mythological figure, or rather a secondary personification of that particular disease? As an example for such a personification from a strictly non-Mesopotamian background, but employing imagery very similar to the Akkadian *ṣibit DN*, let me quote a famous couplet of Christian Morgenstern:[4] "Ein Schnupfen hockt auf der Terrasse, auf dass er sich ein Opfer fasse." In general, one would expect in such a case that, just as in Morgenstern's line, the personified (or demonised) disease would have as its name a generic noun or descriptive term directly related to the illness or its symptoms. The Akkadian "Fire" incantations[5] which are addressed to a personified female "demon" *išātu* (literally "fire," then "fever") provide a good example for this principle.

The question of prophylaxis versus treatment also needs some more refinement. While prophylaxis for diseases of natural cause would in most cases seem anachronistic in the ancient Near East, its prominent role in combating demon-induced illness is hardly disputable. One could even speak of a dichotomy in Mesopotamian medicine between cause-oriented treatment, which largely consists of apotropaic and prophylactic measures against demon-induced illness in the widest sense, and symptom-oriented treatment, which would seem to be the normal procedure for dealing with diseases of "natural" causes. Such symptom-oriented treatment is by necessity based on a belief that these symptoms are part and parcel of a particular disease which under positive circumstances can be eradicated by the alleviation or removal of just these symptoms. On the other hand, curing of symptoms would not have any lasting effect in demon-induced diseases since only the physical separation of perpetrator and victim could guarantee long-term healing of such ailments. Reversing the argument, one could say that the more apotropaic or prophylactic elements can be found in a Babylonian prescription or medical ritual, the more likely it will be that we are not looking at a definable disease of natural causes but rather at a general state of

[4] Ch. Morgenstern, *Gingganz* (1919): 'Der Schnupfen' ll. 1–2.
[5] See W. G. Lambert, *AfO* 23 (1970) 39ff.

ill-health brought about by the destructive force of an evil demon. Such a state could, in modern terms, sometimes be described as a "syndrome," or even a "psychosomatic condition," rather than as an individual disease.

Let us now turn to the Lamaštu incantations and rituals, to see how they stand up to some of the tests mentioned above. Texts dealing with Lamaštu have been known for a very long time, with sizeable pieces published as early as 1875[6] and first edited, although in a somewhat strange and unfruitful way, by J. Halévy in 1882.[7] Interest in the texts received a major boost when, in 1902, D. Myhrman published his dissertation "Die Labartu-Texte,"[8] a masterly edition of all the pertinent material that was known at the time. Although he had only texts from Kuyunjik at his disposal, he could already reconstruct major portions of what has since been known as the "Lamaštu Series." In the preface to this edition, Myhrman summarized the evidence gleaned from those texts and described Labartu, as her name was read at that time, first simply as a "Krankheitsdämonin," a demon of disease, and a bit later more specifically as a fever demon.[9] Never since have Assyriologists questioned that the Lamaštu rituals and incantations belong to the realm of medicine (or, more specifically, to the magico-medical corpus). At the same time, the search was on for a more specific definition of the disease or diseases caused by our demon.

A significant step in this direction was to further narrow down Myhrman's description, and to define Lamaštu specifically as a demon of "Kindbettfieber," or puerperal fever. This view, championed by D. O. Edzard,[10] has since been reiterated many times in the Assyriological literature.[11] I myself have also used the term "Dämonin des Kindbettfiebers,"[12] although adding that this definition was "somewhat

---

[6] G. Smith, IV R[1] nos. 62, 63 and 65.

[7] J. Halévy, *Documents religieux de l'Assyrie et de la Babylonie* (Paris 1882), where the texts were 'transliterated' into Hebrew characters; the promised translation never appeared.—For a discussion of the scholarly background of this attempt, cf. J. Cooper, *AuOr* 9 (Fs. M. Civil, 1991) 47ff.

[8] ZA 16 (1902), 141–200; also published separately (with an added vita, and pages numbered 1–60) as *Inaugural-Dissertation*, Strassburg 1902.

[9] Ibid. 145 and 147 (= p. 5 and 7).

[10] *Wörterbuch der Mythologie*, ed. H. W. Haussig, Stuttgart 1961, 48.

[11] See, for instance, V. Haas, *Magie und Mythen in Babylonien* (Gifkendorf 1986) 139ff: "Lamaštu, die Kindbettdämonin."

[12] RlA 6/V–VI (1983) 444b.

simplifying." Especially after being endorsed prominently by W. von Soden,[13] the "Kindbettfieber" theory has also gained acceptance beyond the narrow field of Assyriology.[14]

A different line of argument was proposed by J. V. Kinnier Wilson who, based on a phrase in an Old Babylonian Lamaštu spell, connected Lamaštu with intestinal typhoid infections.[15] This view was further expanded recently by J. Scurlock.[16]

A third approach, first brought to the fore by F. Köcher in 1978,[17] tries to identify Lamaštu as the cause of, or at least a major contributor to diseases of the liver and gallbladder. This argument draws its main evidence from outside the Lamaštu corpus and connects this with a line from the Standard Babylonian series. It was most recently developed in detail by F. Wiggermann.[18]

At the same time, a number of scholars resisted the temptation to connect Lamaštu with any particular disease.[19] The most poignant statement to this effect, predating his theory about liver and gallbladder disease by three decades, comes again from F. Köcher: "Lamaštu kann weder als ausgesprochene Fieberdämonin, noch als blutsaugender Vampir, noch als Erzfeindin der Frauen und Kinder speziell begriffen und verstanden werden. In ihr manifestiert sich vielmehr das Prinzip des Bösen schlechthin."[20] Somewhat similar but with a feminist twist are the conclusions of G. Remler, who contends that Lamaštu's destructive forces are not aimed at producing any specific illness but represent the demonization of the "otherness" of femininity and female sexuality in a male-dominated society. In her opinion, Lamaštu is the completely unpredictable manifestation

---

[13] *Akkadisches Handwörterbuch I* (Wiesbaden 1965) 533a; id., *Einführung in die Altorientalistik* (Darmstadt 1985) 190.

[14] See, for instance, W. Eilers, *Die Āl, ein persisches Kindbettgespenst* (Bayerische Akademie der Wissenschaften, Sitzungsberichte 1979/7, München 1979) 3–5, who sees the 'Kindbettgespenst' Lamaštu as the prototype of several such demons of later times in the Near East.

[15] *JNES* 27 (1968) 245.

[16] *Incognita* 2 (1991) 157f.

[17] In: *Medizinische Diagnostik in Geschichte und Gegenwart* (Fs. for H. Goerke), ed. Ch. Habrich *et al.* (München 1978), 35f, fn. 59. Cf. also the independent remarks by Eilers, *Die Āl* (see above, fn. 14) 4.

[18] In: M. Stol, *Zwangerschap* (see above, fn. 2) 104f.

[19] See, for example, the brief but lucid entry "Lamaštu" in J. Black/A. Green, Gods, *Demons and Symbols of Ancient Mesopotamia* (Austin 1992) 115f.

[20] *Beschwörungen gegen die Dämonin Lamaštu* (Inaugural-Dissertation, Universität zu Berlin 1948; unpublished) 4.

of the basic fear ("Urangst") of anything different and threatening to this male-oriented view of the universe.[21]

The textual material relating to Lamaštu having significantly increased over the last few years,[22] it seems appropriate to revisit the evidence offered by the incantations and rituals. It becomes readily apparent that, thirty years after Köcher's statement quoted above, there is still not the slightest indication in the corpus to suggest that Lamaštu ever had an interest in attacking pregnant women or women in labor. Yes, she is shown watching them, counting their days, and trying to be on the spot at the very moment of birth.[23] But the target of this is always the child, never the mother. It is also significant that there is no evidence that she ever was responsible for stillbirth: only after it is born does the child become of interest to her. Then, however, she makes every possible effort and uses every conceivable trick to snatch, kill and devour the baby. Her attack on the babies is thus aimed at instant death, and not at inflicting a potentially curable disease. The twisted limbs and faces of her victims are vividly described in some incantations, but hardly ever any symptoms usable for a diagnosis. Indeed, a comparison of her activities with SIDS, or Sudden Infant Death Syndrome, a scenario in which any help comes too late, seems admissible.[24] In a way, she thus produces a social *fait-accompli* rather than a curable medical problem, which is underlined by the fact that she even prevents the dead children from getting a normal burial.[25] She is out to deprive the family and/or

[21] G. Remler, *Dämonisierung des Weiblichen: Gestaltung einer Urangst* (unpubl. M.A. thesis, Graz 1991).

[22] See my forthcoming edition of the Lamaštu series and related texts.

[23] Cf., for instance, Lam. I 117–19, where she "counts the pregnant women daily, always follows behind the ones about to give birth, counts their months, marks their days on the wall."

[24] One has to keep in mind, however, that the recognition and medical definition of this syndrome is closely related to a generally low infant mortality in modern societies and an expectation that the average baby will survive early infancy, and that the comparison thus cannot adequately reflect the experience of an ancient mother or physician who had to cope with many more life-threatening dangers for the baby.

[25] This attitude is most clearly expressed in Lam. I 155–60: "(Although) not being death, she cut his (the child's) throat, not being a *gallû*-demon, she twisted his neck, strangled the boy in the wetnurse's lap. (Then,) she did not allow him to be buried in the house, (saying): 'They should place the boy in a red leather bag, as if storing provisions. They should lift him up and take him to the wilderness where they should leave him.'"

society of members of the next generation, and even of any memory of them. No healing rituals for Lamaštu-afflicted babies are known, only prophylaxis and up-to-the-minute apoptropaic measures are called for. In the few cases where the baby is called "the patient," and a prognosis "he will survive" is given, the prescription is also prophylactic and thus obviously meant for the possible but by no means certain event of her attack. I thus can see no evidence from the Lamaštu corpus proper, that she was ever held responsible for any curable medical condition or "disease," even less for puerperal fever, an affliction of the mother and not the baby.

It is true that our view of all this may be somewhat blurred by the fact that symptoms of illness are very hard to define with babies and children still too young to communicate their pain or discomfort. Of overt symptoms discernible to an examining physician, only "heat and cold", i.e. fever and chills of the baby are occasionally mentioned in the Lamaštu texts. I think it is no coincidence that these are at the same time the two most nondescript items in any diagnostic description. We cannot assume that a concept of fever in the modern sense of "consistently and measurably increased body temperature" was on the mind of an ancient patient or doctor. "Heat and cold" is rather, I assume, in most cases a subjective description of discomfort which can also occur for purely emotional reasons. The fact that a Lamaštu incantation could also be used to pacify a crying youngster[26] might thus be interpreted to mean that both the crying and the "chills" were overt signs of the immediate presence of the invisible demon attacking the child at that very moment.[27] It should also be remembered that, according to our texts, Lamaštu is "clad in heat, fever, cold, frost and ice" as part of her destructive aura.[28] This would explain why even those incantations mentioning fever are accompanied by purely apotropaic and prophylactic rituals. I am therefore hesitant to see these passages as an indication that Lamaštu was per se a "demon of fever."

The evidence for Kinnier Wilson's theory that Lamaštu is directly responsible for abdominal typhoid rashes, a symptom which actually

---

[26] W. Farber, *Schlaf, Kindchen, schlaf!* (Winona Lake, 1989) 102ff., l. 18 text l.

[27] For other points of contact between the genre LÚ.TUR.ḪUN.GÁ "to pacify a child," and Lamaštu texts, see W. Farber, ibid. 116f.

[28] Lam. I 62.

can be visually diagnosed even in small children, is also slim. First of all, it should be noted that the one line from an Old Babylonian incantation which is most crucial for this interpretation must actually be emended to yield the reading "She grabbed the baby seven times at his abdomen."[29] This emendation is minor and seems quite plausible, while the unemended text makes no grammatical sense. It is, however, indisputable that the alleged rash itself is not mentioned in the line. Its existence is only inferred from the reference to Lamaštu's grip, and this interpretation is made still less probable by the following line which says: "Pull out your claws, loosen your grip!" This command to the demon emphasizes once more the well-known motif of her deadly grip but at the same time fails to provide any allusion to scars or a rash left behind. The auxiliary evidence brought forth by Kinnier Wilson and Scurlock[30] is in itself inconclusive, and in view of the shakiness of the one pillar on which everything depends, I think we should abandon the idea of Lamaštu as a direct cause of typhoid fever. It may be noted here in passing that by taking a single line out of its context, one could postulate many more Lamaštu diseases. As an example, the line "she has strangled the boy in the wetnurse's lap," quoted in fn. 23, could have led to an interpretation of Lamaštu as an asthma demon, and so on. Fortunately, nobody has made this or other similar claims yet.

The third theory mentioned above, namely that Lamaštu is responsible for gallbladder and liver diseases, does not even need a detailed rebuttal. With the exception of the phrase "you (Lamaštu) make faces yellowish-green,"[31] no evidence connecting her to liver trouble is to be found in the Lamaštu corpus. The argument is thus only based on texts which use other names for the demonic force behind the affliction, specifically *pāšittu* "the Eliminator." Although this name is also occasionally used to describe Lamaštu, there is no proof that all texts mentioning the term are actually speaking of her. Accepting the risk of circular argument, I prefer to adhere to the rather consistent picture of the demon, as it emerges from the corpus of texts directly related to her activities, and to reject any attempt to see her

---

[29] BIN 2, 72, 9; a pronominal suffix *-šu* has to be added, to yield the Akkadian line *ina imšišu adi 7<-šu> iṣbassu.*

[30] See above, notes 15 and 16.

[31] Lam. I 74.

as the cause of definable disease unless this is mentioned in just these texts. This does not detract from the attractiveness of the philological argument about *mārtu pāšittu* and liver or gall disease, which uses sophisticated plays on words and the like,[32] but it prevents me from relating it directly to our demon and her activities.

I thus cannot find any clear evidence from the Lamaštu corpus to connect her activities to any symptoms which unambiguously point to a specific and definable disease afflicting babies and small children. The same can be said about references to Lamaštu from the diagnostic omen series and related texts. Again, the symptoms mentioned there are so non-specific, like shivering, weeping a lot, or being thirsty, that it seems not only impractical but probably simply wrong to interpret them as signs of a definable disease.[33] All the actions taken in the Lamaštu rituals are prophylactic and apotropaic, not therapeutic. At best, we thus can liken Lamaštu's grip on babies to the equally unspecific and untreatable condition we call SIDS and which for a believer might also be seen as preventable only by magico-religious means. Within the ancient Mesopotamian view of human life, I doubt whether such an affliction would even have qualified as a medical case.

The picture of Lamaštu emerging is thus, much in the vein of Köcher's 1948 statement, that of a plainly destructive force which is not out to cause disease but to kill and annihilate. This is further bolstered by the many passages which refer to her attacks on adolescents and adults,[34] on animals,[35] even plants and inanimate features of nature.[36] Again, not a single one of these descriptions brings to the fore any symptoms which unequivocally connect her to any specific disease. Like her assaults on babies, these attacks are simply destructive and not disease-producing. The texts also occasionally

[32] Wiggermann in: Stol, *Zwangerschap* 104.

[33] Cf. Wiggermann, ibid. 106 with very similar conclusions.

[34] See, for instance, Lam. I 67–68: "If she attacks an old man, they call her 'the Annihilator.' If she attacks a young man, they call her 'the Scorcher.'"

[35] E.g., Lam. II 123: "She holds back the ox as it moves around, blocks the donkey as it runs."

[36] E.g., Lam. I 181–86: "By crossing a river, she makes its water murky; by travelling a road, she makes it impassable; by leaning against a wall, she smears it with mud; by leaning against a tamarisk, she scatters its twigs; by leaning against a date palm, she strips it of fresh dates; by leaning against an oak or terebinth, she causes it to shrivel."

make the point that her murderous attempts are unpredictable and unselective.[37] Even though her misdeeds were directed against mankind as a result of a deliberate act by her divine parents,[38] it seems safe to say that her actions are ultimately performed by her own volition, and without any aspect of divine wrath or revenge for sin and disobedience by the afflicted individual. On the contrary, her murderous actions even evoke spontaneous reactions by the gods, to save mankind from her attacks.[39]

There is no doubt that Lamaštu is a primary demon and not a secondary personification of a disease; as a matter of fact, as a daughter of Anu she has family connections right into the center of the pantheon. Neither her name, nor her features as described in the texts or depicted on amulets give any indication that a particular disease is her ultimate *raison d'être*. She is not of the same lowly stature as the personified "Cold-in-the-Head" who is sitting on the back porch waiting for a victim of its very narrow destructive interests. On the contrary, Lamaštu ranks much higher, and is much more dangerous. She is a paramount evil force whose actions can (and regularly do) lead to loss of health and subsequent or immediate death. To call her just another illness-causing demon could be an insulting understatement. To avoid the risk to incur her wrath, the search for a specific Lamaštu disease should be called off.

---

[37] Cf., for instance, Lam. I 125–26: "She spatters venom no matter where, she spatters venom no matter when."

[38] Lam. I 111–13: "Anu, her father, and Antu, her mother, made her descend from heaven in view of her unseemly deeds, and (also) denied her a place of worship on earth."

[39] See, for instance, Lam. II 141–44, where—on hearing her demands for attackable babies—"Anu wept, and the tears of Aruru were flowing: 'Why should we destroy what we have created, and why should the wind carry away what we have produced?'" Manuscript finished September 1997.

WITCHCRAFT, IMPOTENCE, AND INDIGESTION

Tzvi Abusch
Brandas University

In this essay, I shall take up the relationship between witchcraft and disease. Such a treatment is not an *ad hoc* concoction but is surely appropriate, for, as is well-known, "witchcraft is an almost, if not completely, culturally universal explanation for illness, injury, and slow recovery."[1] Mesopotamian anti-witchcraft materials allow us to explore this topic in various ways, but here I can do no more than note a few points of intersection.

Witchcraft may be described as human behavior, demeanor, or speech intended to harm wrongfully another human being by magical means. Envy and hostility characterize the world of witchcraft. In Mesopotamia, witchcraft was held responsible for an assortment of misfortunes. For purposes of this volume on Mesopotamian medicine, I shall ignore the witch as a cause of, *inter alia*, economic breakdown, the break-up of marriage, or the loss of social esteem, and concentrate instead upon illness. However, instead of examining some examples of general physical and psychological deterioration believed to have been brought on by witchcraft and to have led to the victim's death, I will direct my remarks to some specific syndromes or sets of symptoms for which witchcraft, perhaps more than any other cause, was held responsible and which became, therefore, characteristic of the experience of being a victim of witchcraft; I leave the theme of witchcraft as a cause of death for a later occasion.[2]

---

[1] A. F. C. Wallace, *Religion: An Anthropological View* (New York, 1966), 114. In this paper, I have cited Wallace frequently on witchcraft and illness not because I am unfamiliar with the more recent anthropological literature on witchcraft, but because I have generally found Wallace's approach to religion to be illuminating and useful. Particularly helpful have been his treatments of the goals and functions of therapeutic and anti-therapeutic rituals as regards witchcraft and of the psychological dimensions of witchcraft and illness (pp. 113–116, 177–187). It is unfortunate, I think, that this book was pushed to the periphery of the anthropological study of religion by other intellectual currents and did not take the central place that it deserved.

[2] In addition to the sections presented here, the conference paper also included a section on the subjective experience of death and suffering as portrayed in an

I

As I observed many years ago, "the medical texts frequently associate symptom syndromes centering on the stomach, lungs and mouth with witchcraft diagnoses."[3] These problems relate especially to the digestive tract.[4]

In some of these passages, the patient is simply described as having been bewitched (*awīlu šū kašip*)[5] or as having been seized by witchcraft (*awīlu šū kišpū ṣabtūšu*).[6] Other passages are more specific: the victim is said to have eaten or to have drunk witchcraft (*awīlu šū* (*ḫašê maruṣ*) *kišpī šūkul u šaqi*).[7] Still others go so far as to state that the witchcraft was ingested by means of food/bread or beer (*ana piširti kišpī ša ina akali šūkulu* and/or *ana piširti kišpī ša ina šikāri šaqû*) and even to specify that the medium was such foods as cress or garlic (*ana piširti kišpī ša <ina> saḫlê šūkulu; ana piširti kišpī ša ina šūmi šūkulu*).[8]

---

unusual witchcraft text, which has now appeared as "The Internationalization of Suffering and Illness in Mesopotamia: A Development in Mesopotamian Withcraft Literature," in *Magic in the Ancient Near East* = *Studi epigraphici e linguistici sul Vicino Oriente antico* 15 (Verona, 1998), 49–58. (The section of the conference paper that dealt with *zikurrudû*-witchcraft will appear elsewhere.)

[3] See my *Babylonian Witchcraft Literature: Case Studies* (Brown Judaic Studies 132; Atlanta, 1987), 128, n. 89.

[4] For problems relating to salivation, see, e.g., E. Ebeling and E. Unger, "Keilschrifttexte aus Konstantinopel. 1. Ein medizinischer Text aus Kujundjik," *AfO* 1 (1923), 24, obv. 1–2; K 2417 (*AMT* 31/4), obv. 14' and 16'. For problems relating to the 15' lungs but especially the digestive tract, see, e.g., K 249 + (*BAM* 434), i, 13'–15' and variant duplicate K 2614 (*AMT* 48/4), rev. 8'–9'; *STT* 102, obv.1–3; 249 + (*BAM* 434), iii, 10–12 // *BAM* 90: 9'–10'; *BAM* 90: 12'–13'.

[5] See, e.g., *AfO* 1 (1923), 24, obv. 2; K 249 + (*BAM* 434), iii, 12; K 2417 (*AMT* 31/4), obv. 14' and 16'.

[6] See, e.g., K 2478 (*AMT* 50/3): 11'; K 9013 (*AMT* 55/2): 5'; *BAM* 90: 13'; *BAM* 193, i, 10'–11'.

[7] For *awīlu šū kišpī šūkul u šaqi*, see, e.g., *BAM* 190: 23–24 // *STT* 102, obv. 8–9 // *BAM* 193, ii, 4' and partial duplicate K 8469 (*AMT* 48/2): 3 (all these passages are quoted below); *LKA* 154, obv. 6' // *LKA* 157, 157, i, 15–16; *BAM* 232, i, 20' // K 3648 + K 6169 (*AMT* 21/2) + Sm 1280, obv. 21 // *STT* 328, obv. 3'. The last citation is part of a Marduk prayer and ritual (see *Babylonian Witchcraft Literature*, 95, n. 21); a more up-to-date list representing the progress made by the mid-1970's is the following: K 1853 + K 6262 + K 6789 + K 13358 + K 13813 (+) K 7201 + K 10819 (+) K 6996 (+) K 9216 (+) K 431 + K 11260, rev. // K 2493 + K 7102 + K 9081 + K 10352 (+) K 10353 + K 11159 // K 3000 rev. // K 3648 + K 6169 + Sm 1280 // K 5088 + K 6918 + K 11307 // K 8965 // *BAM* 232 // *STT* 129 + 262 (+) 130 (+) 134 (+) 135 (+) 328. For passages which include *ḫašê maruṣ*, see, e.g., K 249 + (*BAM* 434), i, 14'–15' and variant duplicate K 2614 (*AMT* 48/4), rev. 9'; *STT* 102, obv. 2–3.

[8] For examples, see, e.g., *BAM* 161, ii, 11': *saḫlê*, and several occurrences in KUB

This theme already appears as a major focus of the first large group of witchcraft texts, notably those found in Boghazkoi.[9] Note, also, that we now have some nice examples of the use of plants/herbs for witchcraft purposes from Old Babylonian Mari—notably, in AÉM 1/2, no. 314 (p. 76), where the princess Shimatu is accused of trying to use *šammī ša kišpī* against her father Zimri-lim, and in AÉM 1/1, no. 253 (p. 532), where we are informed of a mother's death in an ordeal when she swore that her daughter had not made use of plants of witchcraft when preparing or setting out the materials for the food of a young boy.

II

To illustrate the type of therapeutic treatment undertaken to treat digestive problems caused by witchcraft, let me cite two related but variant prescriptions that exemplify both the therapeutic as well as the textual variations that we frequently encounter in this type of literature, namely (1) *BAM* 190: 22–26 // *STT* 102, obv. 7–11 // *BAM* 193, ii, 2'–7' and (2) K 8469 (*AMT* 48/2): 1–4.

Both prescriptions were intended to be used against witchcraft, and both contain the same symptomology and diagnosis (*BAM* 190: 22–24a // *STT* 102, obv. 7–9a // *BAM* 193, ii, 2'–4' // K 8469 [*AMT* 48/2]: 1–3a). The symptoms are largely of a digestive nature, and the diagnosis stipulates that the patient had eaten and drunk "witchcraft." The two prescriptions thus open in the same way, but they then diverge and prescribe different therapies. The first prescribes (*BAM* 190: 24b–26 // *STT* 102, obv. 9b–11 // *BAM* 193, ii, 5'–7') that, in order to release the witchcraft, various plants are to be crushed together, placed in beer, and left out overnight under the stars. In the morning, on an empty stomach, the patient is to ingest the potion; he will then vomit and get well. Presumably, the purpose of the treatment is to induce vomiting in order to clear the ingested

37, 43 // *KUB* 37, 44 (+) 45 (+) 46 (+) 47 (+) 48 (+) 49 (+) 49(+)50?, 50?; *KUB* 37, 44 (+), i, 13' (= 44, obv, 13'): *šikāri*; *KUB* 37, 43, i, 7' // *KUB* 37, 44 (+), i, 21' (= 44, obv, 21'): *šūmi*; *KUB* 37, 44 (+), iii, 1 (= 45, r. col., 1): *ša*-[; *KUB* 37, 43, iii, 6' // *KUB* 37, 44 (+), iii, 11 (= 45, r. col., 11): *akali*.

[9] These texts are published in *KBo* 8, *KBo* 9, *KBo* 36, *KUB* 4, and, especially, *KUB* 37.

"witchcraft" out of his system. The second prescription, K 8469 (*AMT* 48/2), contains a different therapy: after the shared symptomology and diagnosis, this text prescribes (K 8469 [*AMT* 48/2]: 3b–4) that, in order to release the witchcraft, a plant is to be pounded and the patient is to ingest it with wine; then, possibly subsequent to an enema, he will have a bowel movement and get well. (This is then followed by a second prescription resulting in defecation.)

The aforementioned texts read as follows:

(a) Symptoms and diagnosis:

BAM 190	22	DIŠ NA SAG ŠÀ-*šú ru-púl-ta* TUK-*ši*	SAG ŠÀ-*bi-šú*	
STT 102	7	DIŠ NA SAG ŠÀ-*šú ru-púl-*⸢*ta*⸣ TUK.MEŠ-*ši*	SAG ŠÀ-*šú*	
BAM 193 ii	2'–3'	[	]-*ši*/SA[G]	→
K 8469	1	[N]A SAG ŠÀ-*šú ru-púl-ta* TUK.MEŠ-*ši*	SAG ŠÀ-*šú*	→
BAM 190	23	*ú-ṣa-rap-šú*	NINDA *u* KAŠ	→
STT 102	8	*ú-*⸢*ṣar*⸣*-rap-šú*	NINDA *u* A	→
BAM 193 ii	3'–4'	[	]	→
K 8469	1–2	*ú-ṣa-rap-šú/ur-ra u* GI$_6$ *la i-ṣal-lal*	NINDA *u* A	→
BAM 190	23	LAL UZU.MEŠ-*šú tab-ku*	NA BI [ ]	
STT 102	8–9a	LAL ⸢UZU⸣.MEŠ-*šú* ⸢*tab*!⸣-⸢*ku*!⸣[10]	⸢NA⸣ BI / UŠ$_{11}$.ZU	→
BAM 193 ii	3'–4'	[ ].MEŠ-*šú/ tab-k*[*u*	]	→
K 8469	2–3a	LAL UZU.MEŠ!-*šú tab-ku/*	NA BI *kiš-pi*	→
BAM 190	24a	⸢KÚ⸣ *u* NAG		
STT 102	9a	KÚ NAG		
BAM 193 ii	4'	[ ] ⸢*ù*⸣ NAG		
K 8469	3a	KÚ *u* NAG		

(b) Therapy:

Prescription One

BAM 190	24b	*ana šup-šu-ri* Ú.*ḫa-šu-u* Ú.⸢*tu*⸣*-lal*
STT 102	9b–10	*ana šup-šu-ri-šú* Ú.*ḫa-šu-u* / Ú.⸢*tu*⸣*-lal* →
BAM 193 ii	5'	*ana šup-šú-r*[*i*] Ú.*tu-lal*
BAM 190	25	[.S]IKIL 1-*niš* SÚD *ina* KAŠ ŠUB *ina* UL *tuš-*⸢*bat*⸣
STT 102	10–11	Ú.SIKIL 1-*niš* SÚD *ina* KAŠ ŠUB/*ina* UL ⸢*tuš*⸣*-bat* →
BAM 193 ii	6'	Ú.SIKIL 1-*niš* ⸢SÚD⸣ *ina* ⸢KAŠ⸣ ŠUB *ina* UL *tuš-bat*
BAM 190	26	[*še*]-*rì* NU *pa-tan* NAG ḪAL-*ma* ⸢TI⸣
STT 102	11	*ina še-rì ba-lu pa-tan* NAG-*šú* ḪAL-*ma* TI
BAM 193 ii	7'	*ina še-rì ba-lu pa-tan* NAG-*šú* ḪAL-*ma* TI

---

[10] Copy: ⸢*ta*⸣.

Prescription Two:

K 8469 3b *a-na šup-šu-ri* Ú.*a-ri-ḫa* SÚD
K 8469 4 ⸢*ina*⸣ GEŠTIN.ŠUR.RA NAG-*šu ina* DÚR-*šú* SI.SÁ-*ma* TI

(K 8469 5 DIŠ KIMIN Ú *mat-qu* SÚD *ina* GEŠTIN.ŠUR.RA NAG-*šu ina* DÚR-*šú* SI.SÁ-*ma* TI)

The two prescriptions are partial duplicates. (1) *BAM* 190: 22–26 // *STT* 102, obv. 7–11 // *BAM* 193, ii, 2'–7' and (2) K 8469 (*AMT* 48/2): 1–4 contain identical symptomology and diagnosis; each text then builds upon that same symptomology and attaches related prescriptions which will lead to the expulsion of the witchcraft substance, either by means of defecation or vomiting. *BAM* 190 // *STT* 102 // *BAM* 193 provide one prescription resulting in vomiting; K 8469 (*AMT* 48/2), instead, provides two prescriptions resulting in defecation. (In this context, it is of interest to note that one of our texts, *BAM* 193, ii, 2'–iii, 5, contains a related series of six prescriptions based upon the symptomology and diagnosis of *BAM* 193, ii, 2'–4'; the first, *BAM* 193, ii, 5'–7', is identical with our 'Prescription One', while the fifth, *BAM* 193, iii, 4, is similar to that found in our 'Prescription Two'.) Actually, both K 8469 (*AMT* 48/2) and *BAM* 193 seem to be collections of prescriptions for digestive problems caused by witchcraft; more specifically, witchcraft that had been incorporated through ingestion.[11]

III

An important portion of those anti-witchcraft texts that are characterized by a specific medical concern do, in fact, describe and deal with digestive illnesses. Note the appropriateness of ascribing illnesses associated with ingestion and with the oral cavity to the eating or drinking of "witchcraft," since object intrusion in many cultures is one of the standard causes of illness, and witchcraft regularly makes use of a form of object intrusion in which a foreign poison is magically introduced into the body. But certainly, the fact that digestive

[11] For a similar tablet, see *BAM* 90, a collection of prescriptions for digestive problems caused by witchcraft. (This characterization may also be true for *BAM* 190, but if so, that tablet follows a different organizing principle.)

illnesses often possess a pronounced psychosomatic component might agree with their ascription to (or their association with) witchcraft. In this context, it should be recalled that concern about the hostility of others may often be no more than a projection of repressed hostility in oneself, and, more specifically, that "the intensity of the belief in witchcraft as a cause of illness . . . is definitely related to severity of socialization anxiety."[12]

Another set of physical problems characteristically ascribed to witchcraft belongs to the realm of sexual performance and dysfunction. Here we draw our evidence from the corpus of anti-witchcraft texts but mainly from a corpus of incantations, rituals, and prescriptions designated by the term Šà.zi.ga by the ancient Mesopotamians. The purpose of this latter corpus was to enable a man to attain and to maintain an erection, and, more specifically, perhaps, to deal with the problem of premature ejaculation. Only occasionally do the texts explain the cause of sexual dysfunction. Yet, while several of the Šà.zi.ga texts ascribe sexual dysfunction to the anger of the gods,[13] the most frequently cited cause is the witch and witchcraft.[14]

Witchcraft is responsible for other illnesses and symptoms, but in fact, the two areas that I have singled out account for a disproportionately large portion of witchcraft texts and are among the most significant medical manifestations of witchcraft. Why, particularly, was witchcraft blamed for harming men in the ways that we have described?

I have already provided a partial answer to this question by noting the relationship of witchcraft to psychosomatic illness, to socialization anxiety, and to hostility. Here I shall elaborate this argument. From a male's point of view, food, drink, and sex are closely associated

---

[12] Wallace, *Religion: An Anthropological View*, 185–186.

[13] See, for example, *STT* 280, ii, 1–9 and 25–32 (edition: R. D. Biggs, *ŠÀ.ZI.GA: Ancient Mesopotamian Potency Incantations*, TCS 2, 67) for the anger of Marduk and Ishtar.

[14] See Biggs, *ŠÀ.ZI.GA*, 3 and references there. Additional references: limiting myself to texts edited by Biggs in *ŠÀ.ZI.GA* and without citing further duplicates or additional texts, I note in addition also *LKA* 94, obv. i, 10–11 (p. 12), ii, 18 (p. 13 and notes to this line, p. 16; cf. p. 22 on *AMT* 88/3, 11), iii, 6–7 (p. 14 and notes to these lines, p. 16); *AMT* 88/3, 11–18 (text no. 4, pp. 20–21); *KAR* 236, obv. 18—rev. 23 (and dupls.) (text nos. 11–12, pp. 27–31); *AMT* 88/3, 9–10 (p. 52); *STT* 280, i, 1–27 and presumably 28–59 (pp. 66–67); 81–7–27, 73, obv. 9–15 (p. 69).

with women members of the family, and in these areas, males may sometimes feel themselves to be in a position of dependence and/or vulnerability.[15] Certainly, the experiences of food and drink are associated with a mother. This latter point is significant, since witchcraft accusations have been associated with the intensity of the socialization anxiety experienced in childhood. And in the present context, it is particularly appropriate and useful to recall the theory that

> [t]he process by which illness is acquired . . . may be related to the nature of childhood discipline, and most particularly to the realm of experience . . . in which most anxiety is felt. Thus, for instance, a great deal of anxiety about oral experience in infancy might be associated with beliefs that illness is acquired by eating or drinking something containing magically poisonous substances.[16]

It would agree with some social theories of witchcraft, then, if the source of danger and witchcraft were in the family. But while the ascription of blame for witchcraft activity to members of the immediate family can, in general terms, be documented in our sources,[17] usually the witch is treated as an outsider or marginal member of the social group.[18] Perhaps, women family members were suspect, and there was greater fear and hostility in the Mesopotamian family

---

[15] For an interesting example of male ambivalence towards food because of its association with women, see, for example, the use of "love magic" among the Black Caribs of Belize in S. S. Sered, *Priestess, Mother, Sacred Sister: Religions Dominated by Women* (New York/Oxford, 1994), 134–135:

. . . Black Carib men and women have opposite financial agendas: she wants him to give her money for the household and children; he wants to spend money on alchohol, other women, and gambling. Therefore, women use ritual means to ensure a man's continuing presence in and economic contributions to the home. A woman's "love magic" involves secretly putting some of her bodily secretions into his food. Knowing that women can and do perform such rituals creates an ambivalent attitude toward food. Men love to eat and are dependent on women for food (women control food preparation and distribution), but they are scared of what women have put into the food. Highlighting the ways in which these food rituals enhance interpersonal relationships, Bullard emphasizes that "love magic" encourages men to follow through with co-residence and financial support after a casual sexual relationship.

[16] Wallace, *Religion: An Anthropological View*, 186.

[17] Cf., e.g., Meier, *Maqlû* IV 77–78.

[18] Cf., e.g., Meier, *Maqlû* IV 106–107, 119–128. But, in the present context of bewitchment by food, it should not be forgotten that people, on occasion, may have thought that they had been poisoned by neighbors in village disputes, and that this may have then been attributed to witchcraft (cf. R. Briggs, *Witches and Neighbors: The Social and Cultural Context of European Witchcraft* [New York, 1996], 119, 146–163).

than we have thus far realized. But if this is the case, such feelings about close family members were regarded, not unnaturally, as dangerous and the blame safely projected onto outside women.[19] In any case, bewitching by giving food and drink might be the (real or alleged) deeds of a neighbor who was thought to be a witch;[20] such behavior is normal in a village or small town culture characterized by the close contact of neighbors and by limited resources, competition, and envy.

IV

Yet, while instructive and perhaps even true, the above considerations may not yet explain fully why in the Mesopotamian corpus eating and drinking witchcraft was an important cause of digestive and related illnesses. Another source of information that we should investigate is the description in a number of incantations of the witch giving bewitched food and drink to her victim, while also washing and salving the victim with witchcraft. One example should suffice:

1 ÉN *īpuš kaššaptu kišpīša lemnūti*
2 *ušākilanni ruḫêša lā ṭābūti*
3 *išqânni mašqûtsu ša leqê napišti*
4 *urammekanni rimkīša lu'â ša mītūtiya*
5 *ipšušanni šamanša lemnu ša ḫabāliya*

The witch has performed against me her evil witchcraft,
She has fed me her no-good drugs,
She has given me to drink her life-depriving potion,
She has bathed me in her deadly dirty water,
She has rubbed me with her destructive evil oil.

BRM 4, 18: 1–5 (and dupls.)[21]

---

[19] This seems to be consonant with the fact that in *Enūma Eliš* the maternal opponent in the generational conflict involving Marduk is held at a distance and is associated with a figure who belonged to a much earlier generation and who displayed non-human features (Tiamat) (cf. Th. Jacobsen, *The Treasures of Darkess: A History of Mesopotamian Religion* [New Haven/London, 1976], 186–187).

[20] Cf., e.g., R. Briggs, *Witches and Neighbors*, 113–114, 119.

[21] BRM 4, 18 // Sm 302 (*AMT* 92/1), ii, 11'–14' // K 15177 + Rm 491, obv. 14'–16' and rev. 1'–16' // Rm 2, 314, obv. 13'-rev. 19'. For bibliographical information and an examination of the contexts in which this incantation appears, see my "The Demonic Image of the Witch in Standard Babylonian Literature: The Reworking of Popular Conceptions by Learned Exorcists," in J. Neusner, *et al.*, eds.,

Regarding the actual or original meaning and setting of this commonplace description of bewitching, my student Kathryn Kravitz made what is, I think, a productive observation: the activities of feeding, giving drink, washing, and salving are also the activities of a healer.[22] I find this observation suggestive and appealing, since originally, in my estimation, Mesopotamian witches also performed constructive acts on behalf of clients,[23] and, therefore, the overlap of the activities of a witch and those of a healer in the aforementioned topos suggests that the Mesopotamian witch may also have functioned as a healer. To be sure, the witch is regarded as an evil being in the standard magical and therapeutic texts, but this is a late development (and a distortion). This form of the witch combines several different personages; herein, among others, the roles, activities, and images of several types of lay-persons, especially women who made use of magic and other special techniques, coalesced and were transformed. The original lay witch, it would appear, was both a sorceress and a healer. As a sorceress, she was associated with both constructive and destructive rituals; though, in principle, ethically neutral, these acts were seen by the witch and/or construed by society sometimes as negative deeds, sometimes as positive ones. As a healer or doctor, she, too, could perform destructive acts (including the use of poisons), but, in the main, her intentions were good and her activities were intended to be constructive.

Yet, the healer's transformation into a negative personage is not surprising (nor is it without parallel).[24] Patients often feel ambivalence

Religion, Science, and Magic in Concert and in Conflict (New York/Oxford, 1989), 54, n. 25 and 55–56, n. 29. (I have since identified *SBTU* 2, 22, ii, 37–52 as a duplicate of Sm 302 [*AMT* 92/1], col. i.) For further examples of the topos of giving food, drink, washing, and salving, see, e.g., J. Laesse, *Studies on the Assyrian Ritual and Series bît rimki* (Copenhagen, 1955), 38: 11–15 (and dupls.); W. Mayer, *Untersuchungen sur Formensprache der Babylonischen "Gebetsbeschwörungen"*, Studia Pohl: Series Maior 5 (Rome, 1976), 512: 38–39 (K 72 + and dupls.); *Maqlû* I 103ff; KAR 80, obv. 34–35 (and dupls.). (Most of these examples were already cited by Laesse, *Bît rimki*, 38, n. 86. There are, of course, more examples.)

[22] See, already, Abusch, "Demonic Image of the Witch," 54–55, n. 26.

[23] For textual examples supporting this construction, see *Babylonian Witchcraft Literature,* 131–134, as well as "Ritual and Incantation: Interpretation and Textual History: A Consideration of *Maqlû* VII: 58–105 and IX: 152–59," in M. Fishbane and E. Tov, eds., *"Sha'arei Talmon": Studies in the Bible, Qumran, and the Ancient Near East Presented to Shemaryahu Talmon* (Winona Lake, 1991), 371–375, and "Demonic Image of the Witch," 32–34.

[24] Female healers (but also male ones) are often accused of practicing witchcraft.

vis-à-vis those who try to heal them. This ambivalence is due partly to the patient's feeling of dependence upon the healer. Moreover, a patient who does not recover or perhaps even grows worse might blame the healer for harming him by means of what are normally regarded as standard medical techniques, but are now construed by the self-described victim as forms of witchcraft. Furthermore, those who have the power to help are also thought to have (and also have) the power to harm, and this is true not only of the sorcerer but also of the healer. In any case, in Mesopotamia, the role of the informal female healer is stigmatized by the institutional male magical healers, the *āšipu*, and her activities are designated as destructive and evil.[25]

In support of the claim that the topos derives from the witch's form as healer, I note that the very activities mentioned—giving a person something to eat or something to drink, washing a person, or salving a person—are actually among the most common and typical activities of healing in the medical texts; they are some of the most basic activities of Mesopotamian herbal medicine undertaken by the healer on behalf of his patients.[26]

A further indication that the function of the "witch" as a healer may be the origin of the diagnostic notation that the patient is ill

For early modern Europe and Colonial America, see, e.g., Briggs, *Witches and Neighbors,* 171, 277–279; A. L. Barstow, *Witchcraze: A New History of the European Witch Hunts* (San Francisco, 1994 [1995]), 108–127; R. Godbeer, *The Devil's Dominion: Magic and Religion in Early New England* (Cambridge, 1992), 66–69.

[25] I have discussed this mode of polarization elsewhere, see, especially, "Demonic Image of the Witch," 38–39, and, more recently, "Witchcraft and the Anger of the Personal God," in T. Abusch and K. van der Toorn, eds., *Mesopotamian Magic: Textual, Historical, and Interpretive Perspectives* (Ancient Magic and Divination, vol. 1; Groningen, 1999) as well as the introduction to "Considerations When Killing a Witch: Developments in Exorcistic Attitudes to Witchcraft," in J. Kreinath, *et al.*, eds. *The Dynamics of Changing Rituals: The Transformation of Religious Rituals within Their Social and Cultural Context* (Toronto Studies in Religion 29; New York, 2004), 191–210. Conflict between male medical specialists and female healers has often been cited as an explanation for the treatment of female healers as witches (for references, see, e.g., the works by Briggs and Barstow, cited in the previous note.). Some doubts have recently been raised as to whether this treatment was really a question of gender; cf., e.g., Briggs, *Witches and Neighbors,* 277–278, and J. Sharpe, *Instruments of Darkness: Witchcraft in England 1550–1750* (London, 1996), 174–175.

[26] For these medical activities, cf. E. K. Ritter, "Magical-Expert (= *āšipu*) and Physician (= *asû*): Notes on Two Complementary Professions in Babylonian Medicine," in H. G. Güterbock and Th. Jacobsen, eds., *Studies in Honor of Benno Landsberger* . . . (AS 16; Chicago, 1965), 313–314; D. Goltz, *Studien zur altorientalischen und griechischen Heilkunde: Therapie-Arzneibereitung-Rezeptstruktur* (Wiesbaden, 1974), 56–95, esp. 60–63, 65–70, 91–92; P. Herrero, *La thérapeutique mésopotamienne* (Paris, 1984), 87–113, esp. 88–92, 97–100.

because he has eaten and drunk witchcraft may perhaps be found in the fact that the witchcraft eaten and drunk in these texts is sometimes referred to by the term *šammu*, 'plant' (or 'drug'). This usage is not at all suprising in view of the references to the use of *šammī ša kišpī* (plants/herbs for witchcraft) in the Old Babylonian Mari texts cited earlier in this paper. But more telling is the observation that *šammu*, 'plant' is the very designation used also for medicinal herbs or plants. Perhaps by citing one example of the usage *šammu* = withcraft in the medical texts, we can provide not only evidence of the usage but also a suggestion of how the usage developed.

An example of a text where witchcraft that is eaten and drunk is designated by the term *šammu*, 'plant', is provided by a prescription drawn from a group of therapeutic texts that developed from, or were built upon, inventory lists of therapeutic plants.[27] I have in mind the three parallel prescriptions (1) K 249 + K 2513 + K 2879 + K 8094 + K 9782 + K 10764 + K 12669 + K 12927 + 82–5–22, 996 (*BAM* 434), iv, 3–10 // K 3201 + K 6261 (*BAM* 435), iv, 11–16; (2) *BAM* 190: 27–33; and (3) K 8469 (*AMT* 48/2): 6–10. In K 249 + (*BAM* 434), iv, 3–10 // K 3201 + (*BAM* 435), iv, 11–16 and its parallel *BAM* 190: 27–33, a number of plants to release witchcraft are listed and their total given (22 Ú UŠ_{11}.BÚR.RU.DA [K 249 + (*BAM* 434), iv, 9 // K 3201 + (*BAM* 435), iv, 15]; 23 Ú UŠ_{11}.BÚR.RU.DA [*BAM* 190: 32]). These plants for the release of witchcraft are then stated to be efficacious for the treatment of a man to whom plants, *šammu*, had been given to eat or drink: *ana* NA Ú-*ma* KÚ NAG SIG TÉŠ.BI SÚD *ina* KAŠ NAG (K 249 +

[27] For examples of this class of texts, see, e.g., the prescriptions in K 249 + K 2513 + K 2879 + K 8094 + K 9782 + K 10764 + K 12669 + K 12927 + 82–5–22, 996 (*BAM* 434), iii, 46*–iv, 60 and duplicates: K 249 +, iii, *46'–54' // *BAM* 190: 1–8 // *BAM* 59: 13–20 // *BAM* 161, iii, 1'–7' // K 9684 + K 9999 + Sm 341 + Rm 328 (*BAM* 431), v, 50'-vi, 5' // K 4164 + K 11691 + Rm 352 (+) K 4176 (*BAM* 430), vi, 8–18 // BM 42272, obv. 3–7 (I have not seen this text; for the identification, see Köcher, *BAM*, vol. 5, p. xi, sub. no. 430, vi', 8–18); K 249 +, iii, 55'–70' // K 3201 + K 6261 (*BAM* 435), iii, 1'–11'; K 249 +, iii, 71'–79' // K 3201 +, iii, 12'—iv, 5; K 249 +, iii, 80'—iv, 2 // K 3201 +, iv, 6–10; K 249 +, iv, 3–10 // K 3201 +, iv, 11–16: parallels: *BAM* 190: 27–33 and K 8469 (*AMT* 48/2): 6–10; K 249 +, iv, 11–18 // K 3201 +, iv, 17ff; K 249 +, iv, 19–24; K 249 +, iv, 25–41; K 249 +, iv, 42–50; K 249 +, iv, 51–60. Following a list of plants, the scribe provides a sum total of the plants along with the purpose that these plants serve: e.g., 51 Ú UŠ_{11}.BÚR.RU.DA (K 249 +, iii, 70' // K 3201 +, iii, 11'). Some prescriptions end here; others add a line indicating the mode of ingestion.

(*BAM* 434), iv, 10 // K 3201 + (*BAM* 435), iv, 16); [*ana* N]A Ú-*ma* KÚ *u* NAG SIG *ina* KAŠ SAG NAG-*šú-ma* TI (*BAM* 190: 33). Note that the parallel K 8469 (*AMT* 48/2): 9 renders the meaning of these latter plants explicit, for it designates the therapeutic plants as plants for releasing witchcraft: [ ] Ú.ḪI.A ŠEŠ *ša* NÍG.AG.A BÚR, and thus designates the plants that had been eaten by the patient as witchcraft.

Thus, *šammu* in K 249 + (*BAM* 434), iv, 10 // K 3201 + (*BAM* 435), iv, 16 and *BAM* 190: 33 almost certainly refers to witchcraft. The very use of this word is significant. It demonstrates that the witch was knowledgeable in the use of plants. Some of these plants may even have been poisonous. But plants produce both medicine and poison, healing and witchcraft, and the same plant may even produce both. One may speculate that in a village society without much specialization, the one conversant with the use of plants for healing may have also been conversant with their use for poisoning (and vice versa). Thus, while it is possible that the witch may have used plants for poisons, she may also have used them for healing purposes.

The usage of *šammu*, then, would hearken back to the origin of the topos: the preparation of drugs mainly from plants. Later, at least in the traditional literary sources, the plants were used by the witch exclusively for poisoning and witchcraft. As for the change of *šammu* to *upšašû* in K 8469 (*AMT* 48/2): 9, perhaps it reflects only the specification of poison (plants) as witchcraft (plants) (and, thus, attests as well to the addition of a demonic or magical dimension to the use). But it may also reflect the transmutation of neutral or even healing plants into plants of witchcraft and of acts of healing into acts of witchcraft.[28]

In any case, I suppose that the woman who gave the patient medication and potions made from plants eventually became the woman who used plants exclusively for destructive purposes. Hence, the various activities of the earlier lay healer became the source of, or model

[28] For the correspondence *šammū*: witchcraft, note the usage *šammū zērūti* in *BAM* 237, iv, 29 (DIŠ SAL Ú.ḪI.A *ze-ru-te šu-ku-ul*), and compare *kišpū zērūti* in the opening line of the incantation Rm 545 (*AMT* 67/3): 8'ff. (and dupls.); for occurrences of this incantation and its incipit, see F. Köcher, "Die Ritualtafel der magisch-medizinischen Tafelserie 'Einreibung'," *AfO* 21 (1966), 16: 13, references there, p. 19 ad line 13, and *BAM* 197: 25.

for, the activities of the malevolent witch. This construction is consonant with and may be the consequence of competition between *āšipu* and lay healer. This competition may have been a result of increasing centralization and stratification of state, temple, and economy, and of the domination of all sectors of society by its center. As part of these developments, 'exorcism', especially as a healing profession, as practiced by the increasingly important *āšipu*s expanded its role at the expense of other cultic and healing specialties.

A parallel to this sort of development is actually provided, I would suggest, by the treatments for sexual dysfunction discussed earlier and documented in the Šà.zi.ga texts. The woman partner was originally the active participant and likely functioned in a therapeutic role. This role is overshadowed and taken over by the *āšipu*,[29] and this woman may then have been transmuted into the perverted prototype for, and point of origin of, the witch who is blamed for the male's sexual dysfunction.

We may recall the observation regarding European witchcraft that, "certain women were suspected of witchcraft not because they were powerless but precisely because they were seen to have a great deal of power."[30] Similarly, it may be suggested for Mesopotamia that sex therapist and woman healer were demonized and made into witches.

V

But I would be remiss if I ended on this note and did not touch on one final question, the treatment of which is crucial to an understanding of the relationship of witchcraft and illness; to wit, how is the experience of an illness that is understood as having been caused by witchcraft different from an experience of a like illness that is brought on by a different cause? I cannot provide a full answer; but a partial answer may be suggested if we contrast the mood and behavior of one who ascribes his illness to witchcraft and one who ascribes it to divine wrath occasioned by his own sins.

As I have argued in a study of witchcraft and its relationship to the anger of the personal god, sin and witchcraft are part of two

[29] See Abusch, "Demonic Image of the Witch," 35.
[30] Barstow, *Witchcraze*, 110.

distinct mentalities, the one focussing on forces internal to the individual, the other on forces external to him; the one emphasizing power and guilt, the other powerlessness and innocence. When the individual sins, he is powerful, responsible, and guilty, for sin implies guilt and guilt implies the power to do wrong and to affect another as well as the ability to obtain a pardon. This attitude is rooted in a subjective, personal relationship between human and god and in a sense of personal strength and effectiveness. But when the cause of suffering is externalized, and the sufferer sees himself as affected by witchcraft, he bears neither responsibility nor guilt. He emphasizes his innocence, but also his powerlessness. He becomes a victim; and, as such, he has both the need and the right to go to the god. He is powerless and dependent.

The sinner alienated from his god seeks reconciliation, for the cause of illness, the personal god, is basically good, and one wishes to recreate a positive relationship. The victim of witchcraft, on the other hand, seeks retribution and destruction, for the cause, the witch, is fundamentally evil and must be destroyed so that the sufferer may appease his aggressive/hostile feelings.[33]

If these characterizations are correct, it is reasonable to suppose that these different moods would color or define the experience of illness, as in the following situation: When, for example, a sexual illness, such as was treated in the Šà.zi.ga corpus, was thought to be a consequence of divine anger aroused by sin, I imagine that the illness was experienced as a punishment, that is, as chastisement and/or abandonment. But when the very same illness was thought to have been caused by witchcraft, I imagine that it would have been experienced as assault, that is, as debilitation and emasculation.

The fear of witchcraft grew in importance in Mesopotamia. The growing emphasis on an external human cause as an explanation for failure and suffering took place in an increasingly complex urban world in which the individual was losing some of his traditional supports and was confronted by more extended, impersonal, and hostile social forces. His reaction was to blame witches for his illness and impotence.[34]

---

[33] See my "Witchcraft and the Anger of the Personal God," 92–94.

[34] I wish to thank M. Tolpin and C. Wyckoff for reading the final draft of this paper and suggesting several improvements.

THE DEMON OF THE ROOF

T. Kwasman

Epilepsy illustrates probably more than any other illness a dual tradition of interpretation in the history of medicine.[1] On the one hand, epilepsy has been explained as being caused by demonic powers or the supernatural, and on the other hand by natural or physiological processes. One of the reasons for this is the dramatic way in which epilepsy expresses itself, showing both mental and physical symptoms. However this is not the only reason, since Christianity with its belief in miracle healing played a key role in maintaining the view of epilepsy as a demonic disease, and therefore, supposedly, contributed to the confrontation between irrational and rational medicine, i.e. the dichotomy between magic and science.[2]

The term epilepsy historically designates a wide range of illnesses, since its exact nature can not be adequately determined. Actually, one should speak of "epilepsies". In antiquity, it definitely coincided with, and was related to, various maladies including skin diseases, paralysis, and lunacy.[3] Epilepsy has been the subject of many scholarly treatments. The standard work for the subject was written by Oswei Temkin in 1945. The book was revised in 1971 and contains a bibliography of 1120 articles, books, and monographs. As the title implies, it deals with the history of the illness in the occident.[4] For the Ancient Near East a good part of the research concerned itself with biblical and talmudic sources.[5] Recently, the cuneiform sources

---

[1] The most comprehensive study of the illness is O. Temkin, *The Falling Sickness. A History of Epilepsy from the Greeks to the Beginnings of Modern Neurology* (Baltimore, 1971), 3ff.

[2] Cf. F. J. Dölger, "Der Einfluss des Origines auf die Beurteilung der Epilepsie und Mondsucht im christlichen Altertum", *Antike und Christentum* 4 (1934) 95–109; O. Temkin, *The Falling Sickness*, 91–2; also O. Temkin, *Hippocrates in a World of Pagans and Christians* (Baltimore, 1991), 94–105.

[3] See in general Temkin, *The Falling Sickness*, ix.

[4] O. Temkin, *The Falling Sickness*.

[5] The standard work for the Bible and Talmud is J. Preuss, *Biblical and Talmudic Medicine* (Northvale, 1998). See also W. Ebstein, *Die Medizin im Neuen Testament und*

have been treated comprehensively in a monograph by M. Stol.[6] This study provides a description and treatment of the disease in its oldest forms, and traces the demonological interpretation of the disease through centuries of tradition.

Two texts concerning ancient epilepsy were published in 1994 in an edition of Genizah texts.[7] These documents are now part of the Taylor Schechter Collection in Cambridge. The first text, T.-S. K 1.56, T.-S. K 1.56 (A), is part of a handbook composed of three sections.[8] The first section is a sample text of an amulet. The remaining sections are instructions for various magical purposes, and a theoretical treatise on Sotah (the adulteress). The sample text concerns 'epilepsy', and its contents is largely identical to the second text, T.-S. K 1.147 (B), which is a genuine amulet.[9] This amulet was written for Karam, daughter of Joseph and Tamharun, married to YTR.[10] The editors have dated this text and also T.-S. K 1.56 on paleographical grounds to the 11th century C.E. Originally, the amulet, T.-S. K 1.147, was folded.[11] On the outside of the amulet one sees a caption together with a cartouche which was overlooked by the editors.[12] The caption is almost illegible.

Both versions contain in the first section (1a) an apotropaic incantation intended to protect the client from epilepsy. T.-S. K 1.147 begins with an invocation and continues with a 'pronouncement' of divine names. The incantation ends in 1.11 with the divine and angel names and then continues at the end of 1.21:

> I bound and sealed your bodies by these holy and wonderful names, all demons and all spirits and *mzyq*-demons and *kyyb*-demons and *lilu*-demons and evil *HMHM*-demons and evil *mr*ʿ-demons and evil *lṭb*-

im Talmud (Stuttgart, 1903). A more recent treatment of epilepsy in Jewish sources was made by S. Kottek, "From the history of medicine: Epilepsy in Jewish Sources", *Israel Journal of Psychiatry and Related Sciences* 25 (1988), 3–11.

[6] M. Stol, *Epilepsy in Babylonia.* Cuneiform Monographs 2 (Groningen, 1993).

[7] P. Schäfer & S. Shaked, *Magische Texte aus der Kairoer Geniza* (Tübingen, 1994) vol. I.

[8] P. Schäfer & S. Shaked, ibid. 30.

[9] P. Schäfer & S. Shaked, ibid. 219ff.

[10] The personal name YTR is difficult to interpret.

[11] In the description of the amulet, the editors claim that on the lower edge of the obverse and reverse there are traces of another text. Obviously, these supposed traces are impressions from the ink of the text itself after the amulet was folded.

[12] See plate p. 302 where the caption can be faintly seen. The cartouche has an X, and in each part of the X the Digrammaton.

> demons; and all evil *pg*ʿ- demons of the day and *pyg*ʿ-demons of the night and all evil machinations, and from all evil diseases and the spirit of *plg*ʾ and the spirit that sits in the heart and the spirit that bores through her hands and her feet and all her body!, that you shall be driven out, removed, and be destroyed from the body of Karam, daughter of Tamharūn and daughter of Joseph, wife of YTR,[13] and from the 248 limbs that are in her body and all that dwells with her and that stands with her and sits with her and lies with her, and evil *kp.yn* and evil *mylyn* and evil *mzyqyn* and evil *śṭnyn* and evil *rwḥyn* and *ptkryn* and *bny ʾygry* and *bny ḥṣby* and *bny mzly* and *bny dyqly*, and that you shall come to her no more and not confuse her mind, neither by day nor by night not by any means ever, and you shall not appear to her anymore, and neither in the image of a man, and nor in the image of an animal, and wild animal and bird, rather you shall be destroyed and removed from her and around her 50 cubits, from now until eternity. With (these) names I have adjured and with these names I sealed. Fire: *And the flame of a consuming fire* (Isaiah 29:6; 30:30). Fire upon the rebellious. Before you I wrote and I sealed: Blessed is the Name of His glorious kingdom for all eternity.[14]

In the first two parts of the incantation, the demons are bound and sealed. The section translated above is the actual exorcism. It names the diseases and the demons involved. In l. 26 (B) רוח פלגא "spirit of plg'" is mentioned. In explaining רוח פלגא, the editors make the following observation: "רוח פלגא. Dieser Begriff wird auch in b Pes 111b in Zusammenhang mit zahlreichen anderen Dämonen und Krankheiten erwähnt. Es handelt sich also vermutlich um einen Geist, der eine bestimmte Krankheit verursacht."[15] This *bestimmte Krankheit* is a well known medical term attested in various Semitic languages including Hebrew. Firstly, the above-mentioned passage concerning רוח פלגא in the Babylonian Talmud (Pesachim 111b) needs to be examined. It reads as follows:

האי מאן דמפני אנידרא דדיקלא אחדא ליה לדידה רוח פלגא
האי מאן דמצלי רישיה אנידרא דדיקלא אחדא לי' רוח צרדא

Venice (ca. 152)

[13] After YTR is a text marker. The ? in the edition is superfluous as there is no letter here.

[14] There are certain grammatical inconsistencies in the text which can not be discussed here. See App. A for the full text.

[15] "This concept is mentioned together with numerous other demons and diseases also in b Pes 111b. It deals apparently with a spirit, that causes a certain disease." cf. P. Schäfer & S. Shaked, *op. cit.* 41 n. 12 רוח פלגא.

> If one defecates on the stump of a palm tree, רוח פלגא seizes him, and if one leans his head on the stump of a palm tree, רוח צרדא/צדדא seizes him.[16]

The Rashi gloss translates פלגא into Old French as פלשד"ן "palsy/paralysis."[17] Jastrow defines the term as: רוח פלגא *the demon Palga*, a disease (paralysis?)".[18] פלגא is attested in other Semitic languages such as Arabic, Syriac Mandaic, and Hebrew. For Syriac, Brockelmann defines the term as "apoplexia" and Payne Smith as "ημιπγηγια, *paralysis morbus*".[19] In Mandaic, Drower and Macuch give two definitions: "1. paralysis, and 2. a kind of (paralysis?) demon".[20] Arabic has the meaning "semiparalysis, hemiplegia" and is well attested in medieval medical texts.[21] The word also occurs in Hebrew with the meaning paralysis.[22] It is documented in the works of Asaf

---

[16] Interesting is an apparent gloss to Pesachim 111a, attested in the Munich codex 95, where פלגא is added to זבונים רוח the "demon of immorality" (So the Soncino translation. Jastrow translates "passion" in the sense of "sensuality", 406a). A few talmudic manuscripts have the same variant, cf. R. Rabbinovicz, *Variae Lectiones in Mischnam et in Talmud Babylonicum* (Munich, 1867), vol. VI p. 338 n. ה. See App. C.

[17] For this gloss see A. Darmesteter, D. S. Blondheim, *Les Glosses Françaises dans les Commentaires talmudiques de Raschi* (Paris, 1929), 105 no. 767. Rashbam has רשיי"ן מוו which according to Catane is corrupt; Cf. Mochè Catane, *Recueil des Glosses* (Jerusalem, 1984), 45 no. 698.

[18] M. Jastrow, *A Dictionary of the Targumim, Talmud Babli and Yerushalmi, and the Midrashic Literature* (Philadelphia, 1903), s.v. פלג II 2) 1176.

[19] C. Brockelmann, *Lexikon Syriacum* (Halle, 1928; reprint: Hildesheim, 1982), 570; R. Payne Smith, *Thesaurus Syriacus* (Oxford, 1901), vol. II 3138b 4).

[20] E. S. Drower, R. Macuch, *A Mandaic Dictionary* (Oxford, 1963), 361 s.v. *palga* 2. See also G. Furlani, "I Nomi delle Classe dei Dèmono Presso i Mandei" in: *Atti della Accademia Nazionale dei Lincei* (Rome, 1954) Vol. IX 424 sub *palga o pilgia*.

[21] R. Dozy, Supplément aux Dictionaires Arabes (Leiden, Paris, 1927), 2nd ed. vol. 2 277a s.v. See H. Kroner, *Zur Terminologie der arabischen Medizin und zu ihrem zeitgenössischen hebräischen Ausdrucke* (Berlin, 1921) 39–40. The Arabic is translated by Ibn Tibbon as פלאריש (variant: פלארי׳) "paralyse"; J. von Sontheimer, "Nachricht von einer arabisch-medisinischen Handschrift vermutlich des Ibn-Dschela", Henschels Janus 2 (1847) 256 where *falidch* is translated "Halbseitige Lähmung. Hemiplegia."

[22] E. Ben Yehuda, *A Complete Dictionary of Ancient and Modern Hebrew* (Jerusalem, New York, 1960) Vol. VI .4936 s.v. פלג. According to the unpublished dissertation of A. Melzer, *Asaph the Physician—The Man and his Book: A Historical-Philological Study of the Medial Treatise, The Book of Drugs (Sefer Refuoth)* (University of Wisconsin, 1972) 339, the word is incorrectly pointed. Ben-Yehuda obviously believed that the word was borrowed from Arabic. Note that Pseudo-Ibn Ezra has בפלאג בפלאג; Cf. J. O. Leibowitz, S. Marcus, *Sefer Hanisyonot. The Book of Medical Experiences attributed to Abraham Ibn Ezra* (Jerusalem, 1984) 132 (132v 27). In Ms. Munich 276 fol. 15a Chap. 13, the אורח חיים of Moshe Narbonni, the term is rendered בפאלג (courtesy G. Bos). The modern dictonaries follow Ben-Yehuda.

HaRofe[23] where it describes both paralysis and epilepsy.[24] Also a ריח פלגא (*sic*) is mentioned in *The Sword of Moses*,[25] which Gaster translates as "paralysis".[26]

Morever, it has been surmised that פלגא is related to the Aramaic root פלג "half".[27] Thus it has been identified with hemiplegy and the migraine.[28] Note that the demon mentioned in the above passage of the Talmud with פלגא, צרדא/צדרא, is described by Rashi as "an ache of half the head".[29] This again relates to the notion of migraine, which originates from the Greek word ημικρανια "pain on the one side of the head or face".[30] In contrast, פלגא is quite clearly derived from Greek πληγη "blow, stroke" which has the meaning "paralysis" in such English words as "paraplegia" and "hemiplegia".[31] The two terms fell together on account of the identical spelling. It is worth noting that πληγη is basic to the ancient understanding of paralysis and epilepsy. The underlying concept of epilepsy or paralysis

---

[23] See A. Melzer, *op. cit.* 339, according to which the use of the word in the sense of hemiplegy is supposedly Asaf's coinage. However, the word is also used by Asaf for Greek פרלסיא. An edition based on the Oxford manuscript was made by S. Müntner, *Korot* 5ff. (1971). The main study of Asaf is still L. Venetianer, *Asaf Judaeus. Der älteste medizinischer Schriftsteller in hebräischer Sprache*, Teil I. Strassburg 1916; Teil II. Strassburg 1917.

[24] L. Venetianer, *ibid.* 95 n. 2 & 3.

[25] M. Gaster, *The Sword of Moses* (London, 1896) vol. III 81 1.5

[26] Ibid. vol. I, 320, No. 14. See below n. 27 for the astral medical context.

[27] E. Ben Yehuda, *op. cit.* vol. VI, 4936 s.v. פלג.

[28] E. Ben Yehuda, *op. cit.* vol. VI, 4936 s.v. פלג n. 2; J. Preuss, *op. cit.* 305–306. The *Aruch* s.v. נרד has: פלגא כאב חצי הראש which is identical to the explanation given by Rashi for the demon צרדא. See next note. I. Davidson, *Sepher Shaashuim. A Book of Mediaeval Lore by Joseph ben Meir Ibn Zabara* (New York, 1914) 10, n. 6. See A. Melzer, *op. cit.*

[29] Bab. Talmud Pesachim 111b 2: "צרדא. כאב חצי הראש"; J. Preuss, *op. cit.* 306 n. 94 asserts: "... The explanation of *Rashi* which is found in our texts by the word *palag* probably belongs to the word *cerada* and vice-versa." This follows the explanation of the Aruch. See previous note and I. Davidson there.

[30] H. G. Liddell-Scott, *A Greek-English Lexicon* (Oxford, 1966) 772b.

[31] Ibid. 1417b. Note that the word has the meaning "stroke" which is basic to the ancient understanding of paralysis and epilepsy. These are diseases that strike, i.e. Akkadian *miqtu* AN.TA.SUB.BA. See M. Stol, *op. cit.* The Greek has also the meaning "plague" which is reminiscent of Hebrew מכה/מכות. Note the relationship of the pest god Nergal to the roof demon; see note 35 below. See J. Preuss, *op. cit.* The Greek is used in the medical works of Alexander Trallianus as "apoplectic stroke". It is possible that Trallianus is the Alexander of a Latin text which has fragments of a Hebrew translation. See M. Steinschneider, *Die hebräischen Übersetzungen des Mittelalters und die Juden als Dolmetcher* (Reprint, Graz, 1956) 778, 838. Both "paraplegia" and "hemiplegia" are cases where half the body is paralysed.

as a "striking disesase" is comparable to Akkadian *miqtu* AN.TA. ŠUB.BA.[32] It is evident that רוח פלנא is a spirit that causes paralysis/hemiplegia and is related to epilepsy.

Epilepsy Demons

In the Genizah texts, additional demons concerning epilepsy are mentioned: בני אינרי "roof-demons", בני הצבי "jug demons", בני מזל "constellation demons", and בני דקל "palm(tree) demons".

1. בני אינרי *"sons of the roof"*[33]

Besides the Akkadian sources, the בני אינרי occur frequently in incantations and related texts of late antiquity such as magic bowls and metal amulets composed in Mandaic, Syriac and various Babylonian Aramaic idioms. For example, Text H 1. 2, a magic bowl written in a Standard Babylonian Aramaic, one finds: ושבעה בני "and seven roof demons".[34] In another bowl, Text A 1.2–3, the roof demons are found in a sequence:

> ... לכל שידא ולבו לנבו לשידי ולבר אינרי ולכל ירורי ליליין ומבכלין סטני
> ופתכרי ולוטתא ושיפורי ושמתתא וחומרי ירוחי וירורי ונאלי ולטבי ובאלבי
> ובני אינרי ... FN 35a

An interesting text in Mandaic, organized like an Akkadian omen series, is entitled: *qwbly' ls'hry' wld'ywy' wlšydy' wlbr 'ng'ry'* "Charms against *shr*-demons and *dews* and *šēdus* and roof demons".[35] In a Mandaic incantation dealing with various diseases and called *š'pt' d̲-š'mbr'* "incantation of the *šambra*-plant" the following is quoted: *wkwl rwh br 'ng'ry'* "and each spirit of the roof demons"[36] In an

---

[32] See M. Stol, *op. cit.*
[33] T.-S. K 1.56 1a:17 has בני אונרא (p. 31 of the edition). They are translated on p. 35 as "Dachgeister". The comments on p. 42 ad 1.17 that אונרא could be a 'Steinhügel' or "Götzenaltar" and that the "Söhnen des Götzenaltars" may be "eine Metapher für Götterbilder" are contradictory and can be safely ignored.
[34] C. H. Gordon, "Aramaic and Mandaic Magical Bowls", *Archiv Orientální* 9 See App. E II. (1937) 85–6. See App. E II.
[35] E. S. Drower, *The Book of the Zodiac (Sfar Malwašia)*, (London, 1949), 77 [120 1.18–19]. See App. E III.
[35a] See App. E I.
[36] E. S. Drower, "A phylactery for Rue" Orientalia NS 15 (1946) 331 1.6.

unpublished Mandaic lead roll in the British Museum, the following demon list is attested:

wlṭbyʾ wpʿgyʾ wpʾlgyʾ wbnyʾ ʿngʾryʾ[37]

In the Babylonian Talmud, these demons are called and Rashi states explicitly that they are demons of the roof.[38] In Pesachim 111b they are mentioned with other demons:

בי פרחי רוחי דבי זרדתא שידי דבי איגרי רישפי

Venice ca. 1520

"Caper tree-demons (בי פרחי) are רורי; sorb-bushes (בי זרדתא) are שידי; demons of the roof (בי איגרי) are רישפי".

The רישפי do not occur in the amulet or parallel text. רשפי are attested otherwise as a a category of the מזיקים (Ber. 5a).[39] The Aruch records a variant reading to the talmudic text: ודבי נגרי רישפי "demons of the smithy are רישפי".[40] This adapts the term to the basic meaning of רשף which is "glow, flame, spark". The רישפי are actually derived from the West Semitic deity Rašap who is identical to the Sumerian Nergal.[41] Nergal is an underworld and pest deity who has a definite connection with the Mesopotamian roof demon.[42]

The common word in Hebrew for epilepsy is נכפה which is not attested before late antiquity. The medieval term is חולי נופל.[43] A clear term for the disease in Biblical Hebrew is not attested although attempts have been made to identify epilepsy in the Bible.[44]

The בני איגרי as noted above are very ancient, although in Jewish sources they are first attested in late antiquity. They are well known from magic bowls as well as in Syriac and Mandaic.[45]

---

[37] BM 132947 + 1.40–42. (courtesy Ch. Müller-Kessler).

[38] Rashi (Pesachim 111b): "בי איגרי. שדים המצויים בגנות רשפי שמם".

[39] It also has the meaning "pain" according to the Aruch.

[40] *Ha-Aruch* (Lublin, 1874). s.v. רשף. The phrase is an emendation.

[41] F. Gröndahl, *Die Personennamen der Texte aus Ugarit* (Rome, 1967) 181. In general see E. von Weiher, *Der babylonische Gott Nergal*, AOAT 11 (Neukirchen, 1971).

[42] In the myth "Nergal and Ereškigal" (El-Amarna version) fourteen personified illnesses are named as gatekeepers for the underworld. Gates 9–12 are: 9. d.*bé-e-en-na* 10. d.*ṣi-i-da-na* 11. d.*mi-qí-it* 12. d.*bé-e-el-ú-ri*. These illnesses are all forms of epilepsy or related to it. See E. v. Weiher, ibid. 86.

[43] See S. Kottek, *op. cit.* for references.

[44] J. Preuss, *op. cit.* 299–302.

[45] This demon occurs frequently in magic bowls: cf. C. H. Gordon, "Aramaic and Mandaic Magic Bowls in the Istanbul and Bagdad Museums", *Archiv Orientália* 6 (1934) 319–322; "Aramaic Incantation Bowls" *Orientalia* 10 (1941) 123. In bowls belonging to Mahdukh, daughter of Newandukh, the demon occurs very frequently. There are at least 17 bowls belonging to this client and thus it is possible that we

The origins of the roof demons are clearly to be found in the Mesopotamian demon *bēl-urri*/LUGAL-*urri*/LUGAL-*ugri* "Lord of the roof".[46] Stol was the first to identify this demon with the Syriac *bar ʾeggāra*. There is some confusion, however, concerning the Akkadian word *igāru* which has the meaning "wall," although it means "roof" in other Semitic languages.[47] It is most likely that the distinction was originally not very great and it seems that in some cases roofs and walls were not necessarily separate components of a building.[48]

Brockelmann defines *bar ʾeggāra* as "daemon lunatici" and Payne Smith "lunaticus".[49] A study of this demon in Syriac was made by G.J. Reinik.[50] It occurs in the Peshitta and Cureton version in Matthew 17:14–18 where Jesus heals an *epileptic* child:

---

are dealing here with a medical dossier on epilepsy. Until now only one bowl has been published, cf. S. Shaked, "'Peace Be Upon You, Exalted Angels': on Hekhalot, Liturgy and Incantation Bowls", *JSQ* 2 no. 3 (1995) 197–219. The reason for the large number of bowls may be due the fact that epilepsy is a recurring disease. I wish to express my gratitude to D. Levene for providing me with information on the bowls. For Mandaic references see G. Furlani, *op. cit.* 431–432 sub *br engaria o angaria* where the correspondence to Syriac is discussed. Cf. Drower, Macuch, *op. cit.* 69 s.v. *br ʿ ngaria*. T. Nöldeke, *Mandäische Grammatik* (Reprint, Darmstadt, 1964) 122 §104b.

[46] M. Stol, *Epilepsy in Babylonia* (Cuneiform Monographs 2, Groningen, 1993).

[47] AHw 366a s.v. *igāru*. S. Kaufman points out that in the Egyptian Aramaic papyri that the word has the meaning "wall" as in Akkadian; S. Kaufman, *The Akkadian Influences on Aramaic* (AS 19, Chicago, 1974) 57. M. Stol, *op. cit.* 17–18; J. Hoftizer & K. Jongeling, *Dictionary of the North-West Semitic Inscriptions* (Leiden, New York, Köln) 1995, 12, s.v.'gr4. See Jastrow, *op. cit.* where "איגר.. [vaulted] roof..., opp. חומה."

[48] Stol discusses this problem and makes the suggestion that in Southern Iraq houses made of rushes were built in such a manner that the wall and roof were indistinguishable; cf. M. Stol, *op. cit.* 17–18. Kaufman makes a similar point (see previous note). Note that such houses are known from Tell Halaf and are called θόλοι <θόλοι (fem.) "round building with conical roof rotunda". Also θολόσ (masc.) means "mud, dirt". See Liddell-Scott, 803a. Kaufman's reference to two Old Babylonian LU fragments (MSL XII 201) is interesting. lú.é.gar8.da.šub.ba = ma-aḫ-ṣa-am be-el ú-ri-im "attacked by the (demon called) Lord of the Roof" (CAD M I 115 s.v. *maḫṣu*), which refers to an epileptic, shows that the distinction between wall and roof was not necessarily maintained. See M. Stol for a detailed discussion *op. cit.* 18–19.

[49] K. Brockelmann, *op. cit.* R. Payne Smith, *op. cit.* vol. I, 580b with references from Bar Bahlulis. For the relationship between lunacy, demons and epilepsy which occurs in late antiquity and the Byzantine period see O. Temkin, *op. cit.* 86. For recent Byzantine literature cf. K. Leven, "Die 'unheilige' Krankheit-*epilepsia*, Mondsucht und Besessenheit in Byzanz", *Würzburger Medizinhistorische Mitteilungen* Bd. 13 (1995) 17–57, and G. Makris, "Zur Epilepsie in Byzanz", *Byzantinische Zeitschrift* 88/2 (1995) 363–404.

[50] G. J. Reinik, "Der Demon 'Sohn des Daches' in der syrischen exegetischen Literatur", *Studia Patristica* XVI Part II (1985) pp. 105–113.

"And when they rejoined the people a man came to him, knelt down before him and said, 'Lord, have pity on my son, who suffers severely from epilepsy (*bar ʾeggāra*); often falling into fire and as often in water. And I took him to your disciples, but they were unable to heal him. "O faithless and perverse generation!" Jesus exclaimed. "How much longer am I to be with you? How much longer am I to bear with you? Bring him here to me." He then rebuked the lad; the demon came out of him; and that moment he was well.'"[51]

The Greek term for which *bar ʾeggāra* is used is σεληνιαζεσθαι, "to be diseased by the moon".[52] That this word is clearly being employed to describe epilepsy is evident from the parallel text in Mark where the symptoms described are of an epileptic attack. It is thus certain that Matthew uses the word "diseased by the moon" which is translated into Latin as *lunaticus* to describe epilepsy.[53] Insanity, madness, epilepsy, and skin diseases are related and are caused by the phases of the moon. It is this reason that the word "diseased by the moon" can be used for lunatic; insanity, madness, epilepsy and skin disease all being "moon diseases."

Returning to the above passages from the New Testament, we noted that Syriac translates Greek σεληνιαζεσθαι (diseased by the moon) as *bar ʾeggāra* "demon of the roof". The Old Syriac Gospel has in its Sinaitic version an interesting variant to Math. 17:15. The Sinaitic version has *rūḥ pelga*.[54] This is the רוח פלגא mentioned in the Geniza texts and it is quite clear from the Syriac variant that

[51] See G.A. Kiraz, Comparative Edition of Syriac Gospels Aligning the Sinaiticus, Curetonianus, Peshîṭta & Ḥarklien Versions. Vol. I Mathew. Leiden 1996. The translation follows E.V. Rieu, *The Four Gospels* (London, 1961) and the Syriac text. The italics have been added by the present writer.

[52] W. Bauer, *Griechisch-Deutsches Wörterbuch zu den Schriften des Neuen Testaments und der übrigen urchristlischen Literatur* (Berlin-New York, 1971) 1480. In general see A. Lesky, J. H. Waszink, "Epilepsie", *Reallexikon für Antike und Christentum* V (1962) 819–831. An interesting aside is that in alchemist terminology mercury is called *tyānē dbar ʾeggāre* "urine of the *bar ʾeggāra*", see G. J. Reinink, *op. cit.* 105 n. 3, who quotes M. Bertholet – R. Duval, *La Chemie au Moyen Age*, Tom II. *L'Alchemie Syriaque* (Paris, 1893) 46:10. According to D. Goltz, *Studien zur Geschichte der Mineralnamen in Pharmazie, Chemie und Medizin von den Anfängen bis Paracelsus* (Sudhoffs Archiv Beih. 14, Wiesbaden, 1972) 269–271, Semitic languages do not have a word for mercury but use a loan word i.e. Arabic *zībaq* which is Persian in origin.

[53] See M. Stol, *op. cit.* 121–130, and see next note.

[54] T. C. Falla, "Demons and demoniacs in the Peshitta Gospels", *Abr Nahrain* 9 (1970) 60, p. 48. See G. J. Reinink, *op. cit.* 106, n. 3.

פלגא is related to epilepsy. The spirit *Palga* "paralysis" is a disease caused by the epilepsy demon *bar ʾeggāra*.

2. בני חצבי *"vessel demons"*

The amulet lists בני חצבי after the "roof-demons", which is read in the text edition as בני חצבט. The ט which is designated as damaged is a י. This agrees with the endings of the other demons mentioned in the group. The letter ך of the word בשכבך of the adjoining column has been written into the י thus making the י look like a ט. The demons בני חצבי are attested in a magic bowl published by C.H. Gordon.[55] They are most likely to be identified with Mandaic *haṣbia* "jugs, pitchers" and are thus "vessel demons".[56]

3. בני מזל *"constellation demons"*

The next group of demons are the בני מזל "constellation demons". That stars and the zodiac play a role in determining illness and well being is a principle of astro-medicine.[57] In the astronomical work ראשית חכמה of Ibn Ezra such illnesses are among other features caused by the constellations and stars. Hemiplegy חולי הפלג is mentioned as being caused by the zodiac sign Pisces and as והפילוג caused by Saturn.[58] Epilepsy in the form of skin diseases (leprosy) and lunacy is especially associated with celestial bodies and often in association with the moon. In Babylonian sources epilepsy (*bennu*) is caused by the "Star of Marduk" which is Jupiter.[59]

---

[55] *ArOr* 9 (1937) 86, 87; Text H: ויבני חיצבי. In l. 2 the בני אי{ק}נירי are mentioned.

[56] Drower, Macuch, *op. cit.* 125b s.v. *haṣbia* 2. See App. F.

[57] See E. Reiner, *Astral Magic in Babylonia* (Transactions of the American Philosophical Society, vol. 85 Part 4, 1995).

[58] R. Levy, F. Cantera, *The Beginning of Wisdom. An Astrological Treatise of Abraham Ibn Ezra* (Baltimore, 1939) xxxvi, xliv [15v] (Hebrew section). The French version has *la partison* and *jerre le partement*, see p. 73 and n. 28d 2. where the margin has "paralisis," and p. 84 and n. 36c 1, where the variants have "apoplexia, paralisis and separatio." Saturn is considered generally to be an "evil" star that affects the body; see for example: S.A Wertheimer, *Batei Midrashot* (2nd edition, Jerusalem, 1989), Bd. II 35 no. 15 and n. 88. See also F. Klein-Franke, *Iatromathematik im Islam.* Hildesheim (1984) 105; O. Temkin, *op. cit.* 93, 94, 176.

[59] M. Stol, *op. cit.* 15–16; 116–117.

LUGAL-irra the roof demon is also associated with the constellation Gemini.[60]

4. בני דקל *"palm demons"*

The next set of demons are the palm demons: בני דקל. The palm-tree as well as other trees and bushes are mentioned in the tractate Pesachim of the Babylonian Talmud as housing demons.[61] Regarding the palm-tree the following is stated (Pesachim 111a):

> Resh Lakish said: There are four things for which he who does them has his blood on his head and forfeits his life. These are: defecating between a palm tree and a wall; passing between two palm trees; drinking borrowed water, and passing over poured water, even if his wife poured it before him. 'Defecating between a palm tree and the wall': this was only said when there is not four cubits [space], but when there is four cubits we don't care. And even when there is not four cubits [space], it was only said only when there is no other way [to pass]; but if there is another path, we don't care.

The text makes it clear that demons are harmful if a person is in a position where they have no room to pass. In places where demons can freely move they are harmless. This is underlined in the following passages (Pesachim 111a):

> 'And one who passes between two palm-trees'. This was only said where a public domain does not cut across them; but (where) a public domain cuts across them, we don't care.

After discussing the dangers of shadows (palm trees cast shadows), the Talmud makes the following statement mentioned above (Pesachim 111b):

> "If one defecates on the stump of a palm-tree, the demon *Palga* seizes him, and if one leans his head on the stump of a palm-tree, the demon צרדא seizes him".

The Talmud connects the palm tree directly with the demon *Palga* and thus gives us background information on paralytic epilepsy.

---

[60] M. Stol, *op. cit.* 117ff.

[61] For the relationship of trees and demons see still W. Robertson Smith, *Lectures on the Religion of the Semites* (1889) 126, 169ff.

The palm tree is a major item of Near Eastern culture which goes back to hoary antiquity. There does not, however, seem to be a cuneiform source to the Talmudic passages. We may assume that such a source exists, since the palm tree is one of the oldest industries in the Near East. Interesting information, however, is found in another geographical region: Ethiopia and from a text called "The Mirror of Solomon".[62] This document, written in Ge'ez, tells of Solomon's meetings with various demons and how he gained knowledge about demons by asking them about their activities. In one section, he addresses a demon called Daqleš, obviously a demon of the palm tree.[63]

The text states:

> Salomon spoke to the demon called *Daqleš*. . . .: "How do you make man ill?" He answered: "First: I take the hands and feet and drive his spirit out. Second: I blow over his eyes like blood, make him fall backwards and I eradicate his senses. Third: I twist the mouth so that he cannot speak anymore."[64]

The text continues describing the illness point by point. The second part of the same section gives a prescription for medication of the disease, and the third part gives the various names of God and mentions two demons. One of these demons is called *bāryā*, the Ethiopian word for epilepsy.[65]

Conclusion

Roof, seizure, constellation and palm demons are all causes for what may be called "ancient" epilepsy. The sources concerning these demons are scarce. The demons themselves dwell and originate in

[62] O. Löfgrun, "Speigel des Salomo", in *Ex Orbe Religionum Geo Widengren* (1972) vol. I, pp. 220–222.

[63] *daqal* as a palm is not attested in Ge'ez. It has the meaning "mast of a ship". See W. Leslau, *Comparative Dictionary of Ge'ez (Clasical Ethiopic)* (Wiesbaden, 1987) 139b s.v. *daqal.*

[64] The English follows Löfgrun's German translation, cf. note 56.

[65] *bāryā* has the meaning "slave, one in the service of a demon, epilepsy". See W. Leslau, *op. cit.* p. 108b s.v. *bārya.* Leslau also comments that "According to the popular belief, the *bārya* is a spirit that brings on epilepsy." See also S. Strelcyn, *Médecine et plante d'Ethiopie* (Warsaw, 1968) 505, 557. Is this word somehow corrupted from *bar 'egarra?*

high places. The demons are part of a common Near Eastern culture in which the demonological character of an illness was part and parcel of its understanding of disease. The Talmudic era in which our texts seem to be closely associated which had many influences: Greco-Roman, Persian, Egyptian, and Babylonian. The demons in the Geniza texts are much older than the presumed date of the 11th century. These demons survived centuries of tradition. The importance of the Geniza fragments, however, is not only the identification of diseases linked to certain demons, enabling us to classify the type of text, but the role they play in helping us to understand certain passages of the Babylonian Talmud. Thus for example passages mentioned in the tractate Pesachim 111a–112b may now be seen in a different perspective. The Geniza documents show that among the illnesses in Pesachim ancient epilepsy and related diseases such as stroke, mental illness, and skin diseases are being described. There is still much to be studied and investigated. In describing generally the picture we have from the present, we may perhaps call it an inverted system. Thus diseases which are considered to have their causes in physiological and biological processes within the body are described in the demonological tradition externally. The picture which emerges does not necessarily support the observation that ancient epilepsy represents a dual tradition of interpretation of the disease, a demonological and rational, but more a mirror image of the one to the other.

APPENDICES

Appendix A

A T.-S. K. 1.56
B T.-S. K. 1.147

§1 A [9] [אס]רית והתמית נופכון באלו השמות
B [21]... אסרית אנא [22] והתימית [23] נופיכון באילו השמות הקדושות
בי

§2 A כל שדין וכל רוחין [10] וכל [מזי]קין וכייבין
B והמפוארות כל שידין וכל רוחין [24] ומזיקין וכייבין

§3 A והמהמון בישין ומרעין בישין ולטבין ביש...
B ולילין והמהמין בישין ומרעין בישין ולטבין בישין

§4 A [11] [וכל פגעין ביש]ין ופגעאי דממא ופגעאי דליליא וכל עובדין
B [25] וכל פגעין בישין ופינעי דימאמא ופינעי דליליא וכל עובדין

§5 A [12] [בישין ומכל] מ[רעין] בישין ורוח פלגא ורוח דיתבא בלבא ורוח [13] [דנקבא בידיה]
B בישין [26] ומכל מרעין בישין ורוח פלגא ורוח דיתבא בליבא ורוח דנקבא בידיה

§6 A [וב]רגליה ובכל גופיה בשם אל אתיה אסיא [14] [ ] הוה אהה
B [27] וברגליה ובכל גופיה

§7 A שתפקון ותרחקון ותתבטלון מן [15] [גופיה ד...]
B שתיקפון ותיתרחקון ותיתבטלון [28] מן גופיה דכרם בת תמהרון ובת יוסף

§8 A ומן מאתים וארבעים ושמנה אברים שיש בו [16] [וכל דדאיר עמה ודקאים] עמיה
B [29] אשת יתר . ומן רמח איברים שיש [30] בגופה וכל דדאיר עימה ודקאים עימה

§9 A ודיתיב עמה ודשכיב עמיה [17] [. . .]
B [31] ודיתיב עימה ודשכיב עימה [32] וכפ.ין! בישין ומילין

§10 A [. . . ביש]ין ופתכרין בישין ובני אונרי [18] [ ]
B [33] בישין ומזיקין בישין [34] ושטנין בישין ורוחין בישין ופתכרין בישין ובני אינרי ובני הצבי!

§11 A [. . .] . . . [ו]בני דקלי בשם יה יה יה וה צבאות [19] [. . .] . . . יה שלא תבואו אליו
B ובני מזלי ובני דיקלי שלא תבואו אליה

§12 A לא ביום ולא בלילה [20] [בשום פ]נים בעולם ולא
B [35] עוד ולא תבלבלו את דעתה [36] לא ביום ולא בלילה בשום פנים בעולם ולא

§13 A תתראו לו לא בדמות אדם ולא [21] [בדמות]
B [37] תתראו אליה עוד ולא בדמות אדם ולא בדמות

§14 A חיה ולא בדמות בהמה ולא בדמות עוף **אלא** [22]תבטלון ותתרחקון
B [38]בהמה וחיה ועוף **אלא** תתבטלון ותתרחקון ממנה ומסביב לה חמישים אמה.

§15 A מעתה ועד עולם בשמות שהשבעתי **ב** [1]ובאלו השמות חתמתי
B [39]מעתה ועד עולם בשמות הישבעתי ובאילו השמות חתמתי

§16 A נלהביה נראויה **אש** להבה מלפני **אש** [2]אוכלה על המורה ועל הממרה מכם
B [40]**אש** ולהבה **אש** אכלה **אש** מעל המורה מלפני מכם

§17 A כתבתי וחתמתי ברוך [3]שם כבוד מלכותו לעו ועד
B [41]כתבתי וחתמתי ברוך שם כבוד מלכותו לעולם ועד

Appendix B

§§2–6: The demons mentioned here are well attested. An exception are the המהמין, mentioned in §3, which are probably medieval as they are unknown in Late Antiquity. At the end of the list, in §§5–6, three types of רוחין—demons are mentioned: 1. רוח פלנא 2. רוח דיתבא בליבא 3. רוח דנקבא בידיה וברגליה ובכל גופיה.

I. רוח פלנא

רוח פלנא is attested in Babylonian Talmudic Aramaic (BTA), Standard Literary Babylonian Aramaic (SLBA), Syriac and Mandaic sources.[1]

a. *Babylonian Talmud (BTA)*

> האי מאן דמפני אנירדא דדיקלא אחדא ליה לדידה רוח פלנא האי מאן דמצלי רישיה אנירדא דדקלא אחדא לי' רוח צרדא
>
> Venice (ca. 1520)

---

[1] In the commentary on רוח פלנא, the editors of Geniza text make the following observation: "רוח פלנא. Dieser Begriff wird auch in b Pes 111b in Zusammenhang mit zahlreichen anderen Dämonen und Krankheiten erwähnt. Es handelt sich also vermutlich um einen Geist, der eine bestimmte Krankheit verursacht." This remark did not take into consideration the information given in the available literature., see further below and n. 16. For the term Standard Literary Babylonian Aramaic (SLBA), see for the moment C. Müller-Kessler, "The Earliest Evidence for Targum Onqelos from Babylonia and the Question of its Dialect and Origin" JAB 3 (2001) 181–198 and also from the same author "Die Stellung des Koine-Babylonisch-Aramäischen auf Zauberschalen innerhalb des Ostaramäischen" in: N. Nebes (ed.), *Neue Beiträge zur Semitistik*. Wiesbaden (2002) 91–103.

> "If one defecates on the stump of a palm tree, רוח פלגא seizes him. If one leans his head on the stump of a palm tree, רוח צדרא seizes him." Pes 111b

In the above passage the manuscript sources consistently have the reading רוח פלגא. The demon is also attested in Pes 111a in manuscripts: רוח זנונים ופלגא Munich 95 and רוח פלגא Ox.366 (Opp. Add. fol. 23).

b. *Incantation Bowls (SLBA)*

1. [7]..ופנעה וסטנה ונאלה וכל פתיכרין כולהון ופיקדין ואיכרין וחומרין וזידנין *ופלגא ופגאי* מחץ ומחצא [8]וריפסא ופניחא

Gordon H[2]

2. [25]כל שידי ודיוי וליליאתה וכל חילמי סנין *ופגעי ופלג* וסטני ושופטי בישי ומריבין ומבכלאתא

Moriah I[3]

3. [18]..מן שידי ומן דיוי ומן סטני ומן דהלולן ומן מריבין ומן שופטי
[19]בישי ומן סיוטי *ומן פגעי ומן* פלגי ומן {ת}סטני ומן חילמי סנין ומן כל רוחי בישאתה

Geller A[4]

4. [2] *wbʿbdy byšy šydy šbṭy plgy pgʿ yrwdy rwḥy? byšʾ* 11 N 77[5]
5. [2] . . . *lšbqh mn kwlh plgh* TMHC 7 No. 9: 2Pl. 6 l.[6]

c. *Mandaic Sources*

1. [22]. . . *pʾlgyʾ* [23] *zykryʾ wpʾlgyʾ nwqbʾtʾ*—TMHC 7: 41f.: 22–23 (= DC 43Aa; *šʾftʾ d̲-qʾštynʾ*)

---

[2] C. H. Gordon "Aramaic and Mandiac Magical Bowls", Archiv Orientální 9 (1937) 86–90.
[3] C. H. Gordon, "Magic Bowls in the Moriah Collection" Orientalia 53 (1984) 220–221.
[4] M. J. Geller, "Four Incantation Bowls", G. Rendsberg et al. (eds.), The Bible World. Essays in Honor of Cyrus H. Gordon. New York. 49.
[5] S. Kaufman, "Appendix C. Alphabetic Texts" in: M. Gibson, *Excavations at Nippur. Eleventh Season.* OIC 22 1975 151.
[6] C. Müller-Kessler, *Die Zauberschalentexte in der Hilprecht-Sammlung, Jena, und weitere Nippur-Texte anderer Sammlungen.* TMHC vol. 7. Wiesbaden 2005.

2. rydpʾ ḏ-pʾlgʾ ḏ-pʾgrʾ—DC 46:124:14 (ʾlmʾ ryšʿy zwṭʾ)
3. sʾṭnyʾ wsʾrnbw wpʾlgyʾ—DC 47:333:2
   pygʾ ḏ-(ʾw) pʾlgʾ DC 47:332:18
4. wpygyʾ wpʾlgyʾ DC 43 J: 186–187, (šafta ḏ-qʾštynʾ 'incantation of cramps')
   wpygyʾ wpʾlgyʾ ḏ-bnyʾ ʿngʾryʾ DC 43 J: 190 (šafta ḏ-qʾštynʾ 'incantation of cramps')
5. wpygyʾ wpʾlgyʾ wbrngʾryʾ—DC 20:50[7] = DC 43 e:8 (qmʾhʾ ḏ-dʾhlwly)ʾ
6. wlṭbyʾ wpʾgyʾ wpʾlgyʾ wbynʾ ʿngʾryʾ—BM 132947: 40–42 (unpublished lead roll)
7. wlpygyʾ wlpʾlgyʾ—DC 51:688 (pyšrʾ pwgdʾmʾ ḏ-myʾ)
8. pygyʾ wpylgyʾ—Gy 279:5 (and DC 22:274)

רוח פלנא is generally defined as a demon that causes paralysis or apoplexy.[8] פלנא is often associated with the Aramaic root פלג "half".[9] Accordingly, it has been identified with hemiplegy and migrain.[10] Although the association with פלג seems to make sense, it does not completely fit the description of this disease. It is, therefore, more likely that פלנא is derived from Greek πληγή/πλαγά "blow, stroke"

---

[7] B. Burtea, "Ein mandäischer magischer Text aus der Drower Collection" in: Studia Semitica et Semticohamitica. Festschrift für Rainer Voigt anlässlich seines 60. Geburtstages am 17.Januar. 2004. AOAT 317 71–96.

[8] See M. Sokoloff, *Dictionary of Jewish Babylonian Aramaic*. Ramat-Gan 2002 911a s.v. 2# פלנא (DJBA); M. Jastrow, *A Dictionary of the Targumim, Talmud Babli and Yerushalmi, and the Midrashic Literature* (Philadelphia, 1903), s.v. פלג II 2) 1176 (Jastrow). E.S. Drower, R. Macuch, *A Mandaic Dictionary* (Oxford, 1963), 361 s.v. *palga* 2 (MD). See also G. Furlani, "I Nomi delle Classe dei Dèmono Presso i Mandei" in: *Atti della Accademia Nazionale dei Lincei* (Rome 1954) Vol. IX 424 sub *palga o pilgia*; C. Brockelmann, *Lexikon Syriacum* (Halle, 1928; reprint: Hildesheim, 1982), 570 (LS). R. Payne Smith, *Thesaurus Syriacus* (Oxford, 1901), vol. II 3138b 4).

[9] So most dictionaries e.g. DJBA 911a s.v., Jastrow 1176. s.v.

[10] The word has entered Hebrew with this interpretation see E. Ben Yehuda, *A Complete Dictionary of Ancient and Modern Hebrew* (Jerusalem, New York 1960) Vol. VI. 4936 s.v. פלג n. 2; J. Preuss, *op. cit.* 305–306. The *Aruch* s.v. נרד has: פלנא כאב חצי הראש which is identical to the explanation given by Rashi for צדרא (the Rashi text has been exchanged—this is the explanation for פלנא) see, A. Kohut (ed.), *Aruch Completum sive lexicon vocabula et res, quae in libris targumicus, talmidicus et midraschicis* Vienna 1928 vol. 2 p. 355. The explanation has entered the ms. Columbia X893 T141: רוח כאב חצי הראש פלנא. According to A. Melzer the use of the word in the sense of hemiplegy is supposedly Asaf's coinage, see *Asaph the Physician-The Man and his Book: A Historical-Philological Study of the Medial Treatise, The Book of Drugs (Sefer Refuoth)* (University of Wisconsin 1972) 339 (unpublished dissertation). However, the word is also used by Asaf for Greek פרלסיא see, L. Venetianer, *Asaf Judaeus. Der älteste medizinischer Schriftsteller in hebräischer Sprache*. Teil I. Strassburg 1916. Teil II. Strassburg 1917 95 n. 2) & 3).

which fits the definition apoplexy.[11] The idea of "a blow, stroke" is fundamental to the ancient understanding of diseases like paralysis or epilepsy and is the reason for the close association of פלגא with the roof demon. The underlying concept of a malady as a "striking disease" is also found in such words as Akkadian *miqtu* and Hebrew מכות terms that are familiar to us even today when we speak of a stroke or someone stricken with a disease. As the above attestations show, פלגא commonly occurs together with פגעי (*pygy'*).[12] This demon is more general in nature than פלגא and precedes it in the lists. In Mandaic, not only are *pygy'* and *p'lgy'* often attested together but also occur with *br 'gry'* "the roof-demon". In Syriac, *rûḥ pelgâ* occurs in the New Testament in Mathew 17:15 (Sinaitic version) for *bar 'eggārâ* and will be discussed below.

Appendix B1

Ia. רוח צרדא/צדרא

In the above passage from Pes 111b a demon called רוח צרדא/צדרא is mentioned but does not occur in our excerpt. The demon is also attested in Hul 105b:

> ואמ' אביי מריש הוה אמינ' האי דלא שקיל מידי מפתור' כי נקיט איניש כסא למשתי שמא יארע דבר קלקלה בסעודה אמ' לי מר משום דקשי לרוח צרדא
> Soncino 1489

The manuscript sources have variant spellings for the demon name:

> צרדא Vat 120–121, Hamburg 169, Vat 122; צדדה Vat 123; צדרא JTS 1628

In the passage from Pes 111b the manuscript sources have the following spellings:

> צרדא Munich 95, Munich 6, JTS 1608, Vat 109; צרדה Ox 366; צדרא JTS 1623; צדדה Vat 125, Vat 134; צדדא Columbia X893 T141

---

[11] H. G. Liddell, R. Scott, *A Greek English Lexicon*. Oxford 1966 1417b s.v. Both "paraplegia" and "hemiplegia" are cases where half the body is paralysed.

[12] DJBA 887a s.v. פגעא gives a non-descript definition: "a type of demon". See MD 370a s.v. *pygy'*. The demons should be separated from the main entry which has the meaning "deaf-mute, deaf". A relationship to פקע is doubtful. Furlani, *op. cit.* p. 424, suggests the meaning "accidents". C. Müller-Kessler gives the following meaning for the term: "Plage, Schlag, Bedrängnis" see, *op. cit.* p. 186 s.v. *pg'ʿ*.

צדרא is also attested in an incantation bowl:[13]
(...ותיתסי מן [4]רו(ח) צדרא! די נקישא לה (בפת עינה...)[3]

"... and may she be healed from *ṣdrʾ* that strikes her in her eye ball..." M 001

In Mandaic, the expression *bʾynʾ ṣʾrdʾ* is attested in DC 43 e:7 (B) and the parallel text DC 20:16 (A) (*qmʾhʾ d̲-dʾhlwlyʾ*):[14]

A [16]...*yʾ dʾywʾ* [17] *d̲-ʾynyʾ qʾlqʾ bʾynyʾ ṣʾrdʾ*[18] *wʾwyrʾ*
B [7]...*yʾ dʾywʾ dʾnʾt qʾlqʾ bʾynʾ* [8] *ṣʾrdʾ ʿbyrʾ*

The expression also occurs in DC 49:23.[15] In addition, *ṣʾrdyʾ* occurs together with *pygyʾ* in the passage *kwl pygyʾ (w)ṣʾrdyʾ* in DC 44:715 (*zrʾztʾ d̲-hybyl zywʾ*).

There is a graphic confusion in the Talmudic sources between ד and ר. Whereas, Mandaic consistently has the spelling *ṣʾrdʾ*, five of the eight manuscript sources for Pes 111b have צדרא/ה and the remainder צרדא/ה. In the passage from Hul 105b all manuscript sources have צרדא with the exception of Vat 123 which has the reading צדדה. The bowl text M001 has צדרא.[16] The original form of the word is likely צרדא and is related to the Akkadian verb *ṣadāru* "etwa 'schief werden, liegen'".[17] The verb is used in connection with the eye , nose, and mouth.[18] This is a form of paralysis where there is a loss of control over a body part and is used for such conditions as crossed-eyes. DJBA, based on Syriac, defines צדרא as "vertigo".[19] The attestation in the incantation bowl M001 where *ṣdrʾ* strikes the client in the eye ball as well as the Mandaic attestations do not fit the meaning vertigo but rather the meaning crossed-eye, cocked-eye or eye convulsions.[20] The Akkadian term for "dizziness, vertigo" is

---

[13] S. Shaked, "'Peace Be Upon You, Exalted Angels': on Hekhalot, Liturgy and Incantation Bowls", JSQ 2 no. 3 (1995) 197–219.
[14] B. Burtea, *op. cit.* p. 22.
[15] MD 397a s.v. *ṣrd*.
[16] The edition reads צדרא but the facsimile does not support this reading. See also DJBA 953 s.v. 2# צדרא.
[17] See DJBA 953 s.v. 2# צדרא. AHw 1073a s.v. *ṣadāru*. The suggestion of Shaked *op. cit.* p. 209 n. 60 comparing *rwḥ ṣrdʾ* with Hebrew *ʾṣbʿ ṣrdʾ* is incorrect.
[18] CAD Ṣ 229a.
[19] DJBA 953a 2# צדרא with reference to LS 622a s.v. *sdrʾ*.
[20] *ʾynʾ ṣʾrdʾ* has the meaning "slanted eye, cross-eyed or eye convolutions" and is a condition where there is a loss of control over eye movements. The definition given in MD 397a s.v. *ṣrd* as "with a blighting eye" is based on the the meaning of צדרא as torpidity.

ṣidānu "likewise attested as a demon: d.*ṣi-i-da-na* and which might have some influence on the term due to its similarity.[21] צדרא when used with the eye clearly has the meaning crossed-eye, etc. but when the word is used without a body part it has the meaning of being in an inclined, sloping or lopsided state e.g. dizziness or vertigo.

Appendix C

II. רוח דיתבא בליבא and רוח דנקבא בידיה וברגליה ובכל גופיה

In §5, רוח דיתבא בליבא "a demon that dwells on the heart" follows רוח פלנא. This demon belongs to a category of illnesses that are expressed by the construction: *demon* + יתב + -ב/-ל.[22] This is followed by ורוח דנקבא בידיה וברגליה ובכל גרפיה which is not attested in Late Antiquity and is likely a medieval addition. In Babylonian sources from Late Antiquity, demons are only attested until now as existing outside of the body.[23] This is evident in the term *demon* + יתב + -ב/-ל where the demon dwells or sits on a certain body part. Also in §§8–9 the demons are described with the verbs יתיב, קאים, דאיר and שכיב demonstrating that they are outside of the body.

Appendix D

§§9–10: A second and shorter demon list occurs in this section. It also begins with general categories of demons and ends with four specific sets of demons: בני איגרי "roof-demons", בני חיצבי "jug demons", בני מזל "constellation demons", and בני דיקלי "palm(tree) demons".

[21] AHw 1100a s.v. *ṣidānu* 2.

[22] Ch. Müller-Kessler, „Dämon + YTB ʿL- Ein Krankheitsdämon. Eine studie zu aramäischen Beschwörungen medizinischen Inhalts." in: Munuscula Mesopotamica. Festschrift für Johannes Renger. Ed. B. Bock, E. Cancik-Kirschbaum, Thomas Richter. AOAT 267. Münster 1999 341–354.

[23] Possession is unknown in Akkadian sources, see M. Stol, Epilepsy 51–53. This is probably true for all Mandaic and Jewish sources from Late Antiquity originating in Babylonia.

III. בני אינרי "sons of the roof"-epilepsy demon[24]

The roof-demon is one of the main Babylonian 'epilepsy' demons. Its origins are to be found in the Mesopotamian demon *bēl-urri*/ LUGAL-*urri*/ LUGAL-*ugri* "Lord of the roof".[25] Stol connected this demon with Syriac *bar ᵓeggārā* but did not take into consideration other sources.

a. *Babylonian Talmud (BTA)*

In the Babylonian Talmud, בי אינרי are attested in Pesachim 111b with other demons:

בי פרחי ררחי דבי זרדתא שידי דבי אינרי רישפי

Venice ca. 1520

Caper tree-demons (בי פרחי) are רוחי; sorb-bushes-demons (בי זרדתא) are שיד; demons of the roof (בי אינרי) are רישפי.

The third category of demons רישפי is conspicuous. Since the first sets of demons are רוחי and שידי, we would expect the third set also to be a well known demon category such as דיוי. Besides incantation bowls, however, דיוי are not attested in Jewish sources. Otherwise in incantation bowls מזיקיו, חרשי בישין and לילין are attested with רוחין ושדין. The רישפי are mostly considered to be מזיקין based on a passage in Ber 5a: ואין רשף אלא מזיקין. It is unclear, however, why רישפי occur here instead of מזיקין. The Aruch records a variant reading to the Talmudic text: ודבי ננרי רישפי which appears to have the meaning "demons of the smithy are רישפי".[26] This adapts רישפי to the basic meaning of רשף which is "glow, flame, spark". The רישפי are perhaps to be connected with the West Semitic deity *rašap* who is identified with Nergal.[27] Nergal is an underworld and pest deity

---

[24] בני אונרא (p. 31 of the text edition) are translated on p. 35 as "Dachgeister". The comments on p. 42 ad l.17 of the amulet text that state that אונרא could be a 'Steinhhügel' or "Götzenaltar" and that the "Söhnen des Götzenaltars" maybe "eine Metapher für Götterbilder" can be safely ignored.

[25] M. Stol, *Epilepsy in Babylonia* (Cuneiform Monographs 2, Groningen 1993).

[26] Op. cit. s.v. רשף vol. 7 p. 310. It is possible that בי ננרי is somehow conflated from בני אינרי.

[27] F. Grondahl, *Die Personennamen der Texte aus Ugarit* (Rome 1967) 181. In general, see E. von Weiher, *Der babylonische Gott Nergal*. AOAT 11. (Neukirchen 1971).

who has a definite connection with the Mesopotamian roof demon.[28]

The use of בי for expected בני is odd. DJBA has separate entries for דבי אינרי and דבי זרדתא under the lemma דבי (< בי + -ד) "belonging to, associated with".[29] The first set of demons בי פרחי, is listed in DJBA s.v. פרחא and is translated as "among the caper shrubs".[30] It is also given a separate entry as -בי פרחי n. (uncertain) s.v. 1# ביתא.[31] Thus בי is interpreted as deriving from בית and דבי or from the preposition בין although in the case of בי אינרי it is evidently a variant of בני אינרי. More importantly is to note that the construction with בר is well attested for demons and is used to designate a type, species, or an association (even a resident of a place).

b. *Incantation Bowls (SLBA)*

1. ...כל רוחין בישותא דיכרא וניקבתא ושידין ושובטין ירורין ופגעין
דיכרי ופתיכרי ולילין וחלחולין [2]וליתנין
Gordon H [32] ופרגוס ושבעה בני איקנרי וקיריא...

2. [8]...כל סטני בישי וחרשי בישי ומעבדי תקיפי 9 ושידי ודיוי ו ופתכרי לטבי
ובני איגרי מן ביתיה ד

Gordon 5[33]

[10]...אשבעת עליכון את בר איגרי קלילא איסרא טבא דאישתמש בביתיה[11]...
די...

3. [2]...לכל שידא ולבו לנבו לשידי ולבר איגרי ולכל ירורי ליליין ומבכלין
סטני ופתכרי ולוטתא ושיפורי
[3]ושמתתא וחומרי וחוחי וירורי ונאלי ולטבי ובאלבי ובני איגרי.ורוחי טומאה
ולילין דיכרי וניקבתא.....

Gordon A[34]

---

[28] In the myth "Nergal and Ereškigal" (El- Amarna version) fourteen personified illnesses are named as gatekeepers for the underworld. Gates 9–12 are: 9. d.be -e-en-na 10. d.ṣi-i-da-na 11. d.mi-qi -it 12. d.be -e-el-u -ri. These illnesses are forms of epilepsy or related to it. See E. v. Weiher, *ibid.* 86.

[29] DJBA 311a s.v. דבי.

[30] See DJBA 931b. It is also given a separate entry as -בי פרחי n. (u ncertain) s.v. 1# ביתא; DJBA 217a.

[31] DJBA 217a.

[32] C. H. Gordon, "Aramaic and Mandaic Magical Bowls", *Archiv* Orientální 9 (1937) 85–6.

[33] C. H. Gordon, "Aramaic Incantation Bowls", Orientalia (1941) 123: ll. 8, 9, 10.

[34] C. H. Gordon, "An Aramaic Exorcism", Archiv Orientální 6 (1934) 321–322.

The spelling איקנדרי in Gordon H. is exceptional. The following קירייא is translated by Gordon as "towns" but is more likely to be associated with Mandaic *qyry't'* "creatures".[35]

c. *Mandaic*[36]

1. [48]... *wbngry'* ... [50]: *wpygy' wp'lgy' wbrng'ry'* ... DC 20:48, 50[37] = DC 43 e:8 (*qm'h' d̲-d'hlwly*)'
2. [25]... *br* [ʿ] *ng'ry' zykry' wbt* [ʿ] *ngry' nwqb't'* ZST 41f:25 = DC 43 Aa:25 (*šafta d̲-q'štyn'* 'incantation of cramps') followed by *s'rnbw*
3. *wlṭby' wp'gy' wp'lgy' wbyn' ʿng'ry'*.—BM 132947: 40–42 (unpublished lead roll)
4. *wkwl rwh br 'ng'ry' wkwlhyn qyry'th*—DC 47:331[38] (*š'pt' d̲-š'mbr'*)
5. A section of the *sf'r m'lw'šy'* is entitled: *qwbly' ls'hry' wld'ywy' wlšydy' wlbr 'ng'ry'* "Charms against *shr*-demons and *dews* and *šēdus* and roof demons."[39]
6. An unpublished text has amulets against *br ʿng'ry'*—DC 43:GI, GII.
   zyw' ʿtb'ṭ'l 'n't brʿng'ry' mn PN (personal name) l. 30
   'n't ʿnbw bry ʿng'ry' l. 40
   zh' br ʿng'ry' l. 44 often with variants and followed frequently with mn . . .
   zh' 'n't br ʿng'ry' zykry' wbr ʿng'ry' nwqb't' mn PN l. 55
   wpygy' wp'lgy' wkwl bny' 'ng'ry' mn PN ll. 70–72
   h'zyn š'pt' d̲-br ʿng'ry' rb' wzwṭ' end of GII.

In Mandaic, the *br ʿng'ry'* are often grouped according to gender or size. These descriptions also occur for other demons although the designations for size is somewhat rare. Its occurrence with *pygy'* and *p'lgy'* is common. The association with *ʿnbw* and *srnbw* would seem to point to the fact that *br ʿng'ry'* is to be connected with Mercury and not the moon. Mercury is the planet associated with the zodiac

[35] See MD 4121/b s.v. *qyry't'* and see below the Mandaic section.

[36] In general see G. Furlani, *op. cit.* 431–432 sub *br engaria o angaria* where the correspondence to Syriac is discussed. Cf. Drower, Macuch, *op. cit.* 69 s.v. *br ʿngaria* and T. Nöldeke, *Mandäische Grammatik* (Reprint Darmstadt 1964) 122 §104b.

[37] Burtea, *op. cit.* p. 74.

[38] E. S. Drower, "A Phylactery for Rue" Orientalia (1946) 324–326.

[39] E. S. Drower, The Book of the Zodiac (*Sfar Malwašia*). London, 1949 77 [120 ll. 18–19].

signs Gemini and Virgo.[40] This is similar to Akkadian, where *LUGAL-urra* in a Seleucid text is associated with the constellation Gemini.[41]

d. *Syriac*

In Syriac, Brockelman defines *bar ʾeggārâ* as "daemon lunatici" and Payne Smith "lunaticus".[42] A study of this demon was made by G. J. Reinik.[43] It is attested in the Peshitta in Matthew 17:14–18 where Jesus heals an *epileptic* child.

The Greek term for *bar ʾeggārâ* is *selhniazesqai*, "to be diseased by the moon", a verb.[44] Matthew uses the word "diseased by the moon" which is translated into Latin as *lunaticus* to describe a form of epilepsy.[45] Insanity, madness, epilepsy, and skin diseases are illnesses that are caused by the phases of the moon.

Also the Old Syriac Gospel has in its Sinaitic version an interesting variant to Mathew. 17:15. Whereas the Cureton manuscript has *bar ʾeggārâ* the Sinaitic version has *rûḥ pelgâ*.[46]

---

[40] Ibid. 70 [109 ll.].

[41] M. Stol, *op. cit.* 117f. and for Virgo see p. 116.

[42] C. Brockelmann, *op. cit.* R. Payne Smith, *op. cit.* vol. I 580b with references to Bahlulis. For the relationship between lunacy, demons and epilepsy which occur in Late Antiquity and the Byzantine period see O. Temkin, *op. cit.* 86. For recent Byzantine literature cf. K. Leven, "Die 'unheilige' Krankheit-*epilepsia*, Mondsucht und Besessenheit in Byzanz", *Würzburger Medizinhistorische Mitteilungen* Bd. 13 (1995) 17–57 and G. Makris, "Zur Epilepsie in Byzanz", *Byzantinische Zeitschrift* 88/2 (1995) 363–404.

[43] G. J. Reinik, "Der Demon 'Sohn des Daches' in der syrischen exegetischen Literatur", *Studia Patristica* XVI Part II (1985) pp. 105–113.

[44] W. Bauer, *Griechisch-Deutsches Wörterbuch zu den Schriften des Neuen Testaments und der übrigen urchristlischen Literatur* (Berlin New York 1971) 1480 s.v. In general see A. Lesky, J. H. Waszink, "Epilepsie", *Reallexikon für Antike und Christentum* V (1962) 819–831. An interesting aside is that in alchemist terminology mercury is called *tyānē dbar ʾeggāre* "urine of the *bar eggāra*" see G. J. Reinink, *op. cit.* 105 n. 3 who quotes M. Bertholet – R. Duval, *La Chemie au Moyen Age*, Tom II. *L'Alchemie Syriaque* (Paris 1893) 46:10. According to D. Goltz, *Studien zur Geschichte der Mineralnamen in Pharmazie, Chemie und Medizin von den Anfüngen bis Paracelsus* (Sudhoffs Archiv Beih. 14. Wiesbaden 1972) 269–271 Semitic languages do not have a word for mercury but use a loan word i.e. Arabic *zībaq* which is Persian in origin.

[45] See M. Stol, *op. cit.* 121–130 and see next note.

[46] T. C. Falla, "Demons and demoniacs in the Peshitta Gospels", *Abr Nahrain* 9 (1970) 60 p. 48. See G. J. Reinink, *op. cit.* 106 n. 3.

IV. בני חצבי

בני חיצבי has been read in the text edition as בני הצבט.[47] חצבא is in this context a "jug, vessel" (variant: חיצבא).[48] The demons בני חצבי are attested in incantation bowls as בני חיצבי:

ויבני חיצבי Gordon H 1.5[49]
רוח חיצבאי M 001:6[50]

The last attestation is given a separate entry in DJBA s.v. חיצבי and is defined as „a disease" and refers to Mandaic *hyṣby'*, *h'ṣwby'*.[51] *h'ṣwbty'* occur in a Mandaic incantation bowl:

h'ṣwbty' zykry' wh'ṣwbty' nwqb't' TMH 7 41f:29.[52]

It is probable that a distinction was made between רוח חיצבי and בני חיצבי, the former being a disease or spasm demon and the latter the vessel-demons.

V. בני מזלי

The next group of demons in the Geniza texts are the בני מזלי "constellation demons". In incantation bowls מזלי are attested usually together with כוכבי but not as בני מזלי i.e. demons. That stars and the zodiac play a role in determining illness and well being is a principle of astro-medicine.[53] In Babylonian sources epilepsy is also designated as *bennu* and may be caused by the "Star of Marduk" which is Jupiter.[54] *LUGAL-urra*, as mentioned above, is associated with the constellation Gemini.[55] In the astronomical work ראשית חכמה of Ibn

---

[47] The ט which is designated as damaged is a י. The letter ך of the word בשכבך of the adjoining column has been written into the י thus making the י look like a ט.

[48] DJBA 478b s.v. translates "pitcher".

[49] Please provide footnote text.

[50] S. Shaked, *op. cit.* 207f.

[51] DJBA 458b. s.v. and MD 147 s.v. *hyṣby'*, 126 s.v. *h'ṣwby'* 1.

[52] *h'ṣbwty'* have been designated as "Krug-Dämon; Zuckungsdämon", see C. Müller-Kessler, *op. cit.*, index p. 199 s.v.

[53] See E. Reiner, *Astral Magic in Babylonia* (Transactions of the American Philosophical Society, vol. 85 Part 4 1995).

[54] M. Stol, *op. cit.* 15–16; 116–117.

[55] M. Stol, *op. cit.* 117ff.

Ezra illnesses are among other features caused by the constellations and stars. חולי הפלג is mentioned as being caused by the zodiac sign Pisces and as והפילוג caused by Saturn.[56] Epilepsy in the form of skin diseases (leprosy) and lunacy is especially associated with celestial bodies and often with the moon as seen in the New Testament passage above.

VI. בני דיקלי

The next set of demons are the palm demons: בני דיקלי. The palm-tree as well as other trees and bushes are mentioned in the tractate Pes (111a ff.) of the Babylonian Talmud as housing demons. In the passage from Pes 111b quoted above רוח פלגא seizes someone who defecates at the stump of a palm tree. Unfortunately, there are no other references to בני דקלי although a demon *daqleš* is attested in Ge'ez.[57]

Epilepsy or its symptoms are caused by demons that hit or attack from places over or above the victim and thus is clearly associated with height. Heigh places cast shadows or are places where there is dim light and it is the discussion about shadows in which we find 'epilepsy' demons in the Babylonian Talmud (Pesachim 111a–112b). It is the type of light (dim and shadowy) that set the conditions under which 'epilepsy' demons thrive and consequently places that

[56] R. Levy, F. Cantera, *The Beginning of Wisdom. An Astrological Treatise of Abraham Ibn Ezra* (Baltimore 1939) xxxvi, xliv [15v] (Hebrew section). The French version has *la partison* and *jerre le partement* see p. 73 and n. 28d 2. where the margin has "parlisis" and p. 84 and n. 36c 1. where the variants have "apoplexia, paralisis and separatio." Saturn is considered generally to be an "evil" star that affects the body; see for example: S. A. Wertheimer, *Batei Midrashot.* 2nd edition Jerusalem 1989. Bd. II and n. 88. See also F. Klein-Franke, *Iatromathematik im Islam* Hildesheim. 1984. 105; O. Temkin, *op. cit.* 93, 94, 176.

[57] O. Löfgrun, "Speigel des Salomo" in *Ex Orbe Religionum Geo Widengren* 1972 vol. I pp. 220–222. *daqal* as a palm tree is not attested in Ge'ez. It has the meaning "mast of a ship". See W. Leslau, *Comparative Dictionary of Ge'ez (Clasical Ethiopic).* Wiesbaden 1987 139b s.v. *daqal.* The third part of the text mentions two demons one of which is called *bāryā*. *bāryā* has the meaning 'slave, one in the service of a demon, epilepsy'. See W. Leslau, ibid. p. 108b s.v. *bāryā*. Leslau also comments that "According to the popular belief, the bārya µ is a spirit that brings on epilepsy." See also S. Strelcyn, *Medecine et plante d'Ethiopie.* Warsaw 1968 505, 557. Is this word somehow derived from *bar 'egarra*?

are heigh and throw such light are exactly the places where these demons can attack and where epilepsy can be contracted. The above Geniza incantation texts are for warding off epilepsy and are a valuable source for our knowledge of the demonacs behind the disease.

PHLEGM AND BREATH—BABYLONIAN CONTRIBUTIONS TO HIPPOCRATIC MEDICINE

M. J. Geller
University College, London

It is remarkable that nothing of Babylonian medicine and relatively little of early Greek medicine is based upon human dissection. This is in spite of the fact that dissection had been ongoing in Egypt as a consequence of mummification, although little of this knowledge seems to have filtered through to anatomists elsewhere.[1] In Babylonia, most of the knowledge of internal anatomy was based upon the pseudo-science of extispicy—the examination of the entrails of sheep, especially the sheep's liver, although the lungs and kidneys as well—as providing omens for predicting the future. It is only the third-century B.C. Greek physicians Herophilus (practicing in Alexandria) and Erasistratus who appear to have based their knowledge of anatomy on human dissection and vivisection, although in a later age Galen himself studied anatomy from apes and pigs rather than human subjects.[2]

Why did Babylonian physicians not indulge in human dissection? Surely they must have been curious, perhaps inevitably encountering gaping wounds on the battlefield.[3] The medical literature is silent on the subject. Although we assume that Babylonians, like Greeks, had taboos against dissection, there is no direct incontrovertible evidence for such a taboo. The Babylonians had taboos against many other activities, including nose-blowing in public, taking a false oath, urinating into canals, adultery, and so forth, but nothing is mentioned about touching or cutting up dead bodies.[4] Of course no argument

---

[1] H. von Staden, *Herophilus and the Art of Medicine*, (Cambridge, 1989), 29f., that mummification had little influence on medicine.

[2] See *ibid.*, 29–30, and 139–40, 147, suggesting that for a Greek physician in Alexandria, the practice of mummification may have served as justification for a temporary breach of a taboo against human dissection. See also the excellent discussion in J. Jouanna, *Hippocrates*, transl. M. B. DeBevoise (Baltimore, 1999), 310–314.

[3] Cf. George Sarton, *A History of Science*, (New York, 1959), II, 92, in which he speculates that the Babylonians' rudimentary knowledge of human anatomy was based upon dissections of animals and results of warfare.

[4] Cf. W. W. Hallo, Biblical abominations and Sumerian taboos, *JQR* 76 (1985),

from silence is convincing, and fear of ghosts is well-documented in Babylonia, but we are forced to fall back upon a common-sense explanation: dissection was instinctively fell to be potentially dangerous. They had no rubber gloves, and insufficient knowledge of hygiene, and any physician could easily have contracted the disease which the patient made a corpse of in the first place.

An equally simple explanation for the ignorance of anatomy can be derived from comparing Hippocratic methodology with that of Galen, from a much later period. Both Babylonians and early Greek doctors specialised in external examination of the patient, because there was actually little to be learned from studying the internal anatomy of a corpse. Although both groups of doctors knew enough to identify the major organs, a knowledge of morbid anatomy would not have told them much about the course of disease without the use of instruments, such as the microscope, or even a thermometer. Most theory of the inner workings of the body was based upon analogy with the visible world, e.g. a comparison between wind and breath, but there was no clear idea in either system about digestion or the circulation of the blood.[5] It was not until Galen that experimentation was introduced to try to explain the relationship between arteries carrying blood and the transpiration of air in the lungs, i.e. an active attempt was made to find out what happens when the arteries of a dog are ligatured or when a boy was forced to breathe into a bladder for an entire day, or how the pulse is affected by the insertion of a bronze tube into an exposed artery.[6] These experiments represented a radical departure from previous methods of observation, which advanced the study of physiology only minimally.[7] Rather, Galen was intent on actively testing the properties of the circulatory system, to see what would result from interference with normal processes. Although he invariably drew wrong conclusions from his research, such thinking nevertheless represented a radical departure from any type of scientific observation which had previously been carried out.

Mesopotamians could have learned a lot about internal anatomy from sheep. For instance, in cuneiform sources there are many more

21–40, and K. van der Toorn, *Sin and Sanction in Israel and Mesopotamia*, (Groningen, 1985), neither of which refer to any taboo regarding dissection of humans.

[5] See Jouanna, *Hippocrates* 313f. on the 'limits of Hippocratic physiology'.

[6] Furley and Wilkie [full ref. thru 42.], pp. 125, 201, and 179, and see 47–57.

[7] See G. E. R. Lloyd, *Magic, Reason, and Experience* (1979), 200: 'observations were more often deployed to illustrate and support theories than to test them'.

detailed descriptions of the sheep's heart than for the human heart. The Akkadian word for heart, *libbu*, normally refers in medical texts to the stomach or other internal organs:[8] for the sheep, we have words for the 'rear part of the heart' (*warkat libbim*) the 'upper part of the heart' (*elēnu libbim*), the 'joint of the heart' (*kiṣir libbim*), the 'thick part of the heart' (*kubur libbim*), the 'middle of the heart' (*qabliat libbim*), the 'right side of the heart' (*imitti libbim*), the pericardium (*šaman libbim*), the 'fortress of the heart' (*dūr libbim*),[9] and the 'apex of the heart' (*rēš libbim*).[10] For human anatomy, we have merely the word *libbu*, 'heart'.[11] For sheep, we know the word '*tallu*' for 'diaphragm', but no word for the human diaphragm. As for the sheep's intestines, we have terms for the caecum, the ileum, and entrance of the colon, as well as a specialised word for rectum.[12] Other organs featured prominently, governed by the peculiar logic of omens: the spleen was prominent as a dark organ, hence predicting trouble. Great attention was paid to the gall-bladder, identifying its head, middle, and neck, as well as its cystic duct and tip (lit. nose). Three lobes of the lungs were examined, as well as kidneys. The extispicy priests had terms for the portal vein and vena cava, while there is not even a special word for 'vein' or 'artery' in human anatomy. There are even rare specialised terms for the sheep's urethra and perhaps even for the prostate gland.[13] But most of all, the sheep's liver was studied in minute detail, as can be seen in clay tablets in the form of sheep's liver used for training in extispicy, with many characteristics of the physiognomy of the sheep's liver being catalogued.[14]

---

[8] Similarly, Gr. *kardiē* in the Hippocratic corpus usually refers to the stomach, and even in modern anatomy the *cardia* refers to the upper third part of the stomach.

[9] See TDP 126:40 for a reference to BÀD *libbi* in human anatomy, although it is doubtful whether it refers to the diaphragm. U. Jeyes, *Old Babylonian Extispicy*, (Leiden, 1989), 77, suggests that in sheep the *dūr libbi* refers to the 'terno-pericardiac ligaments by which the pericardium is attached to the sternum'.

[10] Jeyes, *Extispicy*, 77. One should include a reference to the *kubuš libbim* 'turban of the heart' in YOS 10 41: 76, although the term *kubšu* commonly refers to the lungs of the sheep; see also *išid libbim* the 'base of the heart' (CAD I 240) and *šer'ānu*, the 'veins of the heart' (YOS 10 42 i 14).

[11] One has the term *takaltu libbi* in BAM 159 I 21, for *takaltu* (lit. pouch), see TDP 78 67; N. Heeßel, *Babylonisch-assyrische Diagnostik* (Münster, 2000), 265 note to 14–15, suggests that this part of the anatomy cannot be successfully identified, but according to MSL 9 35: 66 (Hg. commentary to Hh. XV), *takaltu* refers to the lungs (*hašû*).

[12] Jeyes, *Extispicy*, 80–81, 95.

[13] *Ibid.*, 80, 95.

[14] See von Staden, *Herophilus*, 163, that 'it is striking that the nomenclature they

Although such terms referring to animal anatomy could theoretically be applied to humans, in reality Babylonian terminology for internal organs of the human body is sparse. Physicians only recorded information about the major organs, such as the heart, lungs, kidneys, bladder, liver, intestines, and urethra. As has been pointed out by Marvin Powell, there distinction is made between the urethra and the ureters.[15] There is no obvious word for 'pancreas' or prostrate gland, and no specific term for the esophagus or diaphragm. The brain was a mystery, and the word *muhhu* used to describe it is etymologically related to the word for 'bone marrow'.[16]

The descriptions of the internal organs in early Hippocratic medicine are not much more informative than those of their Babylonian predecessors and colleagues, and similar vagueness applies to descriptions of internal organs, veins, the nerves, and even the brain, although some improvements in knowledge can be noted in Greek science, as one would expect. Nevertheless, the vagueness of Greek terms like 'phleps' for 'blood vessel' is similar to the Akkadian term *šer'ānu*, which can mean 'blood vessels' and 'sinews', really any stringy part of the anatomy.[17]

Important progress in the relationship between Babylonian and Hippocratic medicine has been made by Marten Stol, (although see J. G. Westenholz and M. Sigrist, 'The Brain, the Marrow and the Seat of Cognition in Mesopotamian Tradition, *Le Journal des Médecines* (2006): 1–10. *Cuneiforms*) who argued that 'there is a close relationship between epilepsy and melancholy in Greek and later medicine', and that 'people suffering from an excess of black bile are the melancholics'.[18] Without repeating Stol's argument, it is sufficient for our

[early Hippocratic authors] use for the liver is even simpler and more restricted than that of Greek hepatoscopy'.

[15] M. A. Powell, 'Pharmaceuticals in Mesopotamia', *apud* I. and W. Jacob, *The Healing Past*, (Leiden, 1993), 64.

[16] See Hippocratic treatises offered widely differing explanations for the functions of the brain, while Aristotle considered the brain to be a cooling agent to cool the blood, but the anatomy of the brain is remarkably well-described by Herophilus, see von Staden, *op. cit.* 155ff., and 248.

[17] A. L. Oppenheim, 'On the observation of the pulse in Mesopotamian medicine', *Or. NS* 31 27ff. Another Greek term corresponding to *šer'ānu* is *tonos*, referring to 'nerves', 'strands', and similar stringy anatomical features, cf. Volker Langholf, *Medical Theories in Hippocrates* (Berlin, 1990), 145. There are many other parallels between Akkadian and Greek terms for the anatomy, such as Greek *kholē*, 'gall', which refers both to bile and to the gall bladder (see Langholf, *ibid.*, 40), which applies to Akkadian *martu* equally well.

[18] M. Stol, *Epilepsy in Babylonia*, (Groningen, 1993), 27–32. See Langholf, *Medical*

discussion to point out that the spleen in Babylonian terminology was considered to be the 'black organ', the dark colour being caused by the presence in the spleen of bile. Stol further suggests that the condition in Babylonian medicine described as *hīp libbi*, literally 'heart-ache' could refer to melancholia.[19] It is just possible that even in Babylonia 'melancholy' was conceived as a physical condition caused by the presence or excess in the body of black bile.[20] It must be stressed that there is no clear reference in Akkadian texts to 'black bile' in any special meaning relating to melancholy or epilepsy, although 'black bile' is known as an ordinary disease symptom,[21] as is yellow bile. In fact, bile can come in any of the four diagnostic colours:

> If (the patient) vomits black bile from his mouth [. . .,
> if the patient vomits red bile from his mouth [. . .,
> if the patient vomits yellow bile from his mouth [. . .,
> if the patient vomits white bile from his mouth [. . .[22]

The question is whether Stol's observation associating melancholy and epilepsy in both Babylonian and Greek medicine can be placed within a larger context. The cardinal plank upon which Greek medicine rests is the four humours, characterised by the four colours red, white, yellow, and black, based upon the body fluids blood, phlegm, and yellow and black bile.[23] These humours are not only

---

Theories, 136–7, commenting on the four humours, cites *Epidemics* VI 5.8: 'The tongue indicates the humour: Yellow tongues are *bilious*, and *bile* is from greasy food. Red ones are from *blood*. Black ones are from *black bile* (dry ones from sooty burning and from the uterus). White ones are from *phlegm*.' Langholf then cites *On the Nature of Man*, which has black bile as a 'corrupted product of the blood, or of blood plus bile'. Finally, Langholf, *Medical Theories* 137 refers to the 'black disease' in *Diseases* II 73.

[19] Stol, *Epilepsy*, 28f. The fact that Stol is on the right track here can be seen retrospectively in Islamic medicine, which understood a clear connection between a superfluity of black bile and mental illness; see Michael Dols, 'Insanity in Byzantine and Islamic Medicine', *apud Symposium on Byzantine Medicine*, ed. J. Scarborough, (Dumbarton Oaks Papers 38, Washington, 1984), 138.

[20] Volker Langholf quotes from an undated anonymous treatise *On Foodstuffs*, which he argues is late in its language but early in its content, and contains the line, 'the spleen causes black-biled blood and is harmful', referring to eating the spleen of an animal; see Langholf, *Medical Theories*, 268. Galen certainly saw the connection between black bile and melancholia in his treatise on *Treatment by Venesection*, see P. Brain, *Galen on Bloodletting* (Cambridge, 1986), 83; Robert Parker, *Miasma: Pollution and Purification in Early Greek Religion* (Oxford, 1983), 246, saying that a popular theme in comedy was an excess of black bile as a cause of madness.

[21] *marta ṣalimta.*

[22] *Cf.* TDP 64: 49'–52'.

[23] *On The Nature of Man*, 4, see G. E. R. Lloyd, *Hippocratic Writings*, (London,

associated with the four seasons, but also with the attributes 'hot', 'cold', 'dry', and 'wet', respectively.[24] At first glance, Greek medicine appears in this respect to be fundamentally different from Babylonian medicine. Babylonian medicine often ascribed the ultimate causes of disease to divine punishment, brought on by the agents of demons and ghosts.[25] For this reason, Babylonian medicine—although a distinct discipline—would never quite be divorced from magic. The physician and incantation priest either worked together or in competition with each other, but both shared the same view that disease was brought on by external forces and influences, to be dealt with through magic and rituals on one hand, and through drugs and palliatives on the other. This view of medicine stands in essential contrast to the theory of humours, which saw disease as an internal imbalance within the human body, which had to be corrected through venesection and drugs. The contrast, however, is not as stark as it might seem: Greek still preserved notions of the 'dunameis', the powers or forces which influenced health,[26] just as Babylonians also had ideas of internal disorder or imbalance, as we shall see shortly.

But what about the four humours themselves? As it happens, the Babylonian diagnostic handbook is a very stylized document with a formulaic structure, and each part of the human anatomy is subject to the same general questions. Does the particular organ respond to heat or cold, is it dry or wet, hard or soft, is it on the right or left side? And, of course, what colour is it? There are only four choices: is the organ red, white, yellow, or black? But perhaps this is a coincidence, not related to the four Greek colours of the Greek humours? Consider the following passage from the diagnostic handbook:[27]

35 If his internal organs are red, he will live.
36 If his internal organs are yellow, it is critical.
37 If his internal organs are black, he will die.
38 If his internal organs are black and the internal veins are distended, and he belches wind from his mouth, until the third day he will die.

1983), 262, and see Lloyd's introduction, 26. According to von Staden, *Herophilus*, 243ff., even Herophilus remained wedded to the humoral theory of pathology, despite his many differences with Hippocratic authors.

[24] *Ibid.* 27, and 263ff.

[25] See M. Stol, 'Diagnosis and therapy in Babylonian medicine', *JEOL* 32 (1991–92), 42–65, especially 44–47, (although some disease names are not associated with demons or are personalised).

[26] Lloyd, *Hippocratic Writings*, 29.

[27] Labat, TDP 120.

40 If his internal organs are stretched, it is worrying.
41 If his internal organs are dark, his illness will be prolonged.
42 If his internal organs are thin, he has no attack.
43 If his internal organs are dried out, he will die.
44 If his internal organs are stopped up, it is the Hand of Damu.
45 If his internal organs are swollen, his illness will be prolonged, it is worrying.
46 If his internal organs are swollen, and the internal veins[28] are distended, if the Hand of [. . .].
47 If his internal organs are swollen and his internal veins are distended and he spews forth yellow (bile), . . .
49 If his internal organs are swollen and his internal veins <are distended> and he spews forth yellow (bile), up to day 31 it is the Hand of [. . .].

It would be wrong to suggest that the Babylonians had a theory of 'humours', as had the Greeks.[29] The Babylonians, in fact, were rather poor on theory.[30] In the same way, the Babylonian scribes wrote no treatises explaining medicine (or any other discipline), as the Hippocratics were fond of doing; the closest the Babylonians come to theory

[28] sa šà-*šú*.

[29] See, for instance, Plato's *Timaeus* 81, ascribing the origin of diseases to the four elements which compose the body, namely earth, fire, water, and air. Plato (ibid. 83f.) then proceeds to explain that these elements, compacted into creating flesh, can decompose into the blood, causing disease, and this process can be detected by various colours in the blood. The oldest part of the flesh is thus black and bitter, which can become red when mixed with blood. When further diluted the mixture becomes green, and decomposition through inflammation becomes yellow. Plato labels these mixtures as 'bile'. He then gives further labels to bile, as either 'acid phlegm' and 'white phlegm', the latter of which is formed by a bubbling in the blood which forms a white foam. Although Plato's description is not entirely transparent, nevertheless it clearly represents an attempt to systematise medical theories of his day of the four humours, to explain the relationship between blood, bile and phlegm and the colours that these bodily fluids present to the observer.

[30] They still used a value of 3 for π, although an approximate of 3 1/8 can be found in a text from Susa, see D. J. Struik, *A Concise History of Mathematics*, (New York, 1967), 29, and see also O. Neugebauer, *The Exact Sciences in Antiquity*, (New York, 1969), 47–48, in which he concludes that the Babylonians never progressed beyond the level of pre-scientific thought, until the last few centuries of cuneiform records. Struik argues (*op. cit.* p. 30) there is no evidence that Babylonians relied upon theorems, such as Pythagorus, in solving mathematical problems, but simply prescribed the rule for solving the problem as, 'do such, do so'.

Others would agree. See E. D. Phillips, *Aspects of Greek Medicine*, (New York, 1973), 14, that 'among well-known civilizations by whose medicine the Greek science was influenced, it appears that the Mesopotamian civilizations were not so important for theory in spite of their passion for listing disease, and for numerical lore about disease'.

is a late scholarly list of diseases associated with parts of the body.[31] The Babylonians were fond of lists, and kept extensive records of data, without formulating general observations or treatises. Nevertheless, we must not discount their scholarship or knowledge, nor is it without parallel: the Babylonian diagnostic handbook is actually quite similar to the Hippocratic collections of medical aphorisms, both in form and in content. Greek medical aphorisms, for instance, describing the appearances of urine, are similar to Babylonian symptoms of kidney disease derived from the appearance of a patient's urine. Compare, for example, the following passages from Babylonian and Greek medicine, respectively:

> If his urine is like ass urine, that man suffers from 'discharge' (*mūṣu*) disease.
> If his urine is like beer dregs, that man suffers from 'discharge' disease.
> If his urine is like wine dregs, that man suffers from 'discharge' disease.
> If his urine is like clear paint/glue, that man suffers from venereal 'discharge' disease. . . .
> If his urine is like *kasû*-juice,[32] that man is overcome by 'sun-fever'.
> If his urine is yellow, that man [suffers] from stricture of the groin.
> If his urine is white and thick, that man [suffers] from a dissolving calculus.
> If his urine is like *duhšu*-stone, that man [suffers] from a calculus.
> If his urine is as normal, his loins and epigastrium hurt [him]; that man suffers from stricture of the bladder (var. rectum). = BAM 7 No. 5. 114 1–9.
>
> Those whose urine during a fever is turbid like that of a beast of burden . . . suppuration is avoided if the urine which flows is thick and white. . . . Blood or pus in the urine indicates ulceration of the kidneys or of the bladder. Small fleshy objects, the shape of hairs in the urine which is thick, mean there is a discharge from the kidneys. Thick urine containing bran-like particles indicates inflammation of the bladder. The sudden appearances of blood in the urine indicates that a small renal vessel has burst. A sandy urinary sediment shows that a stone is forming in the bladder.[33]

---

[31] H. Hunger, *Spätbabylonische Texte aus Uruk*, I 43, see F. Köcher, 'Spätbabylonische medizinische Texte aus Uruk', in *Medizinisches Diagnostik in Geschichte und Gegenwart*, (Festschrift H. Goerke, Munich, 1978).

[32] I.e. red, as known from dyeing recipes, see OLZ 95 (2000), 409–412.

[33] Chadwick, J. and Mann, W. N., *Hippocratic Writings*, ed. G. E. R. Lloyd (London, 1983), p. 221. See M. J. Geller and S. L. Cohen, 'Kidney and urinary tract disease in ancient Babylonia, with translations of the cuneiform sources', *Kidney International*, 47 (1995), 1811–1815, see especially 1814.

The Hippocratic corpus, therefore, contains both collections of data as well as explanatory treatises. Here, then, is a pattern which emerges from the evidence: although the theory of four humours was certainly not invented in Babylonia, Greek theories of humours, on the other hand, were ultimately based upon categories and observations of data which resemble important components of the earlier medical corpus of Babylonia.[34]

It would be unfair, however, to imply that Babylonian scholars made no attempt to systematise their knowledge or organise their data into comprehensive groupings. Like the Greeks, they still had to grapple with the problem of trying to diagnose disease without the benefit of any detailed knowledge of human internal anatomy. The result is that the word *libbu* could potentially refer to the heart, stomach, spleen, or bowels, and the plural *libbū* referred to internal organs generally. Perhaps this was intentional: diagnosis was an art, a *technē*, and symptoms referring vaguely to the internal organs of the chest or belly or lower abdomen might be misleading if they were too specific; it was left was to the diagnostician to decide which specific organ was being referred to. Since the symptom lists were organised from head to foot in descending order, the diagnostician would have a good idea about which part of the anatomy was being described, but the practitioner might decide it was stomach rather than bowel which was the diagnostic problem. We must always reckon with the probability that an oral tradition of diagnosis accompanied the written handbooks or reference tablets.

One other factor which is relevant to the comparison between Babylonian and Greek diagnostic data is the fact that Babylonians looked for three colours within their nosology, namely red, yellow (or green) and black, but not white. In Greek humoural theory, the colour white was associated with phlegm, which is synonymous with mucous and was thought to be a primary element like gall, in explaining disease; 'phlegmatic' was a meaningful diagnostic term in Greek medicine. Not only is the colour 'white' mostly absent from Babylonian symptom lists, but the word for phlegm hardly appears in Babylonian diagnostic handbook.[35] It is difficult to distinguish the term since the

---

[34] The situation in Babylonian and Greek astronomy is roughly comparable, for which see D. Pingree, *apud* S. Dalley ed., *The Legacy of Mesopotamia*, Oxford University Press (1998), 125–38.

[35] See TDP 88 18, úh.me-*šú i-š*[*al-l*]*u*, and *ibid.* 180: 30, úh-*su i-šal-lu*, cf. CAD R 435, "he vomits up his phlegm"?

Akkadian word *ru'tu* more commonly refers to spittle or saliva than phlegm,[36] indicating that relatively little significance was attached to this body fluid. Another term for phlegm, *su'ālu*, actually means *coughing* but rarely "phlegm", and is equally rare in medical contexts. Nevertheless, one passage in the Akkadian medical corpus is worth noting, a text against cough: diš na (*šumma amēlu*) ki.min *su-a-lam peṣâ*(babbar) *ittanaddâ*(šub.meš), 'if man (suffers from ditto [= cough]), and continually spits up white phlegm'.[37] Nevertheless, the phlegm here is simply a symptom of disease and is not being treated as a body fluid which can cause other diseases unrelated to cough or respiratory problems.[38]

The evidence, however, is equivocal, since Greek medicine can sometimes be employed to help elucidate Babylonian texts. The Greek concept, for instance, of wind (*pneuma*) circulating in the body as a cause of disease is prominent, and probably has nothing to do with the many references to wind (*šāru*) in Babylonian medicine, which mostly means flatulence.[39] In Greek medicine 'wind' (*pneuma*) or breath (*physa*) was vital in circulating throughout the body, and if any part of the body was cut off from this breath, paralysis resulted.[40] In the case of 'epilepsy', the Hippocratic corpus specifies that phlegm

---

[36] CAD S 340. See also the word *rupuštu*, phlegm or saliva, which occurs occasionally in medical texts, although once referring to the epigastrium (*rēš libbi*), see CAD R 415, BAM 575 ii 45.

[37] AMT 50, 3: 6.

[38] One interesting term in Akkadian medicine is *hīlu*. Stol mentions in the epilepsy diagnoses, for instance, a substance which he translates (rather clumsily) as 'strong water'. The word is probably *hīlu*, 'resin', and the context says that 'if (the demon of epilepsy, Lugalgirra) has seized the epileptic, . . . and if he has 'resin' (in his body) . . . it is critical', and he can expect to die. The word *hīlu* here for 'resin' may possibly be analogous to mucous, understood as a cause of epilepsy.

[39] Flatulence is well known in Greek medical writing as well, although often mentioned in the context of diet and regimen, with texts advocating special diets and regimen for patients suffering from flatulence. See, for example, *Diocles of Carystus*, ed. Philip van der Eijk (Leiden, 2000), 304–307, advocating that flatulent people (*physôdês*) should eat simply and go to bed immediately after dinner, and wake up late.

[40] Cf. Philips, *Aspects*, 53–55. There is a distinction made between 'wind' (*pneuma*) in nature, which is equated with food and drink in terms of bodily nourishment. When *pneuma* is found outside the body, it is called '*aer*', but when circulating within the body (within the vascular system) it is *physa*, or 'breath'. The function of the breath is to cool the body, but if the breath was stopped from moving in any part of the body, that part becomes paralysed. This view of circulating air throughout the body was later systematised, since it became widely accepted after Praxagoras that the arteries circulated *pneuma* while the veins circulated blood throughout the body; see von Staden, *Herophilus*, 173–174.

can interfere with the air flow in the body, resulting in the loss of voice and consciousness, and loss of control of motor movement in the limbs.[41] One treatise in the Hippocratic Corpus, *On Breaths*, argues that all diseases are caused by winds (*pneuma*) in the body.[42]

An interesting but hitherto unnoticed parallel occurs in Babylonia. Although Babylonian medicine does not by any means recognise as comprehensive a role for 'phlegm' as a factor in disease as does Greek medicine,[43] nevertheless the condition described above in the treatise on Sacred Disease may have already been known in Mesopotamia with similar terminology. The Akkadian disease name *zikurrudû* is borrowed from the Sumerian term zi.kur.ru.da, which has been interpreted in various ways and is understood as the disease brought on by black magic and witchcraft. A literal translation

[41] Chadwick & Mann, in Lloyd, *Hippocratic Writings*, 243 (on the Sacred Disease), and von Staden, *Herophilus*, 249, explaining that the Sacred Disease 'attributed aphasia, for example, to the inability of air or *pneuma* to reach the brain when phlegm blocks the vessels which serve as air ducts'.

[42] See J. Jouanna, *Hippocrates*, transl. M. B. DeBevoise (Baltimore, 1999), 282, citing the monist philosophy that air was the sole cause of all disease. See also *ibid.*, 59–60, quoting from the 1st or 2nd cent. A.D. treatise *Anonymous Londinensis*, 'Hippocrates says that breaths [*physai*] are causes of disease, as Aristotle has said in his account of him.' The text goes on to elaborate how breaths in the form of vapours cause disease in the body, either by sudden changes or by being hot or cold.

Galen's treatise *On the use of Breathing* refers to 'psychic pneuma', which he does not define, but he explains that 'since the emptying of the pneuma from the hollows in the brain, when it is wounded, at once makes men both motionless and without feeling, it must surely be that this pneuma is either the very substance or the soul of its primary organ.' (translation D. J. Furley and J. W. Wilkie, *Galen on Respiration and the Arteries* [Princeton, 1984], 121).

[43] See CAD S *su'alu*, which defines this term as referring to both coughing and phlegm, but the word is more likely to refer to phlegm produced by coughing, as does the onomatopoeic word *hahhû*, 'to cough'. The term *ru'tu*, however, is more likely to refer to 'phlegm' as part of human pathology, since it also means 'spittle' or even 'poison' in other contexts. In medicine *ru'tu* is described as either being white, black, red, or yellow/green. It is not, however, associated with 'bile', as in Hippocratic texts, although 'bile' (Akkadian *martu*) does occur frequently as a symptom on its own, which can be vomited or evacuated from the anus (CAD M[1] 298–9); nevertheless, CAD assumes that *martu* can also refer to 'gall-bladder disease', although it is just as likely that the disease is actually 'bile', in line with Hippocratic texts. The main difference between the Akkadian and Greek evidence is that a patient is not described as 'phlegmatic' or 'bilious' in Babylonian texts in the same comprehensive manner as is common in Hippocratic medicine.

for *zikurrudû* is 'breath cut off',[44] and may well correspond to the cutting-off of *pneuma* in Greek medicine. That this understanding of the Sumerian idiom zi.kur.ru.da is correct can be confirmed from an Akkadian incantation, which calls for the driving out of the Namtar (fate)-demon, which 'is present to cut off my breath' (*ša ana nakās napištīya izzazzū*), an obvious reference to the condition known as *zikurrudû*.[45]

Although the disease *zikurrudû* appears in texts associated with witchcraft,[46] the interesting question is whether it attempts to refer to a specific disease, at least within Babylonian disease taxonomy. Within the medical corpus, texts dealing with *zikurrudû* present physical symptoms associated with this condition: (if a man suffers from *zikurrudû*) and 'is constantly disturbed by cramps, his eyes *flicker*,[47] he suffers paralysis in his muscles, all his teeth hurt, and he drinks beer and eats bread but he *was afflicted* . . .'.[48] A second description in the same text describes the symptoms thus: 'If a man suffers pain in the sinews of his right thigh, his muscles are wasted away and his limbs are stiff, he is deranged, he forgets whatever he has done, his 'phlegm' (*ru'tu*) is white. . . ., it is the 'hand' of *zikurrudû*-disease, he will die'.[49] It is certainly worth noting here that the Akkadian symptoms also refer to *ru'tu peṣītu*, 'white phlegm', which is likely to refer to phlegm or sputum in this context rather than spittle.

These symptoms of *zikurrudû* bear comparison with the Hippocratic treatise on *The Sacred Disease*, which explains the cooling function of breath on various internal organs. The text then states, 'If the phlegm

[44] We prefer this translation to the possible alternative translation, 'life cut off', which is not consistent with the characteristic concrete imagery of Babylonian disease names, such as *hīp libbi* or *himiṭ ṣēti*, etc.

[45] W. Mayer, 'Sechs Šu-ila-Gebete', *Or.* 59 (1990), 471, 24.

[46] This is a condition which was thought to be caused by witchcraft, e.g. L. W. King, *Babylonian Magic and Sorcery*, (London, 1896), 12: 1, Maqlû *passim*, and E. Ebeling and F. Köcher, *Literarische Keilschrifttexte aus Assur*, (Berlin, 1953), 144: 30. See Marie-Louise Thomsen, *Zauberdiagnose und schwarze Magie in Mesopotamien*, (Copenhagen, 1987), 40–45, 53.

[47] Agreeing with the translation of Thomsen, *Magie*, 41 ('seine Augen flacken') against CAD A/2, 'his eyes discharge a putrid liquid', since the meaning suggested by CAD is medically less probable. CAD Š/1 295 reserves judgement and cites but does not translate this clause.

[48] Thomsen, *Magie*, 41, and BAM 449 iii 13'–15' and duplicate *ibid.*, 455 iii 4'–5'. Neither CAD nor Thomsen translate the verb *i-le-hi-ib*, but we provisionally suggest that it be considered a IV-stem of *la'abu*, i.e. *illehib* < *illîb*.

[49] Thomsen, *Magie*, 41, and BAM 449 iii 24'–27'.

be cut off from these passages, but makes its descent into the veins . . ., the patient becomes speechless and chokes; froth flows from the mouth; he gnashes his teeth and twists his hands; the eyes roll and intelligence fails, and in some cases excrement is discharged'.[50] The passage goes on to describe a froth on the lips, choking which leads to (uncontrolled) defecation, and kicking movements in the limbs as secondary results of the cutting off of air in the blood.[51]

There is good reason to assume a closer relationship between *zikurrudû* and descriptions of cutting off of the breath in Hippocratic medicine. *Nikis napišti* (see BMS 12: 108), is not only a variant of *zikurrudû*, but it is also a literal translation of the Sumerian term. Furthermore *nikis napišti* is itself a disease name in Mesopotamia, similar in form to other descriptive disease conditions which are associated with natural phenomena, such as fever known as *himiṭ ṣēti* ('sun-heat') and a condition known as *šibiṭ šāri*, 'blast of the wind'. One must bear in mind, however, that there is no Akkadian (or even general Semitic) word for 'air', corresponding to Greek *αηρ*; Akkadian only has *šāru* 'wind' (parallel to Greek *πνευμα*) and *napištu* 'breath' (corresponding to Greek *φυσα*).[52] It is clear, however, that the 'cutting-off of the breath' (zi.kur.ru.da // *nikis napišti*) results in serious difficulties, as does the cutting off of *pneuma* or *physa* in Greek medicine, as a result of the vessels being blocked by phlegm. It is extremely likely that 'cutting off of the breath' was associated with difficulty in breathing and the presence of mucus, since the two phenomena often occur together with breathing difficulties, e.g. asthma, pneumonia, infection, etc. Furthermore, the difficulties in breathing associated with 'cutting off of the breath' were ascribed to other conditions in the body, such as wasting away of his muscles and mental disorientation. It is likely that both systems of medicine were describing similar although not identical conditions.

[50] Hippocrates, Loeb II 159 (trans. W. H. S. Jones). A textual variant adds, 'These symptoms manifest themselves sometimes on the left, sometimes on the right, sometimes on both sides'. An later passage in the same context adds (translation of Chadwick): 'when the blood-vessels are shut off from this supply of air by the accumulation of phlegm and thus cannot afford it passage, the patient loses his voice and his wits. The hands become powerless and move convulsively for the blood can no longer maintain its customary flow. Divergence of eyes takes place . . .'

[51] Stol, *Epilepsy*, 27.

[52] See 'On Breaths' iii 1–6, giving the distinctions between the three types of 'air'.

WOMEN'S MEDICINES IN ANCIENT JEWISH SOURCES: FERTILITY ENHANCERS AND INHIBITERS

John M. Riddle
North Carolina State University

A characteristic of our age is the attention that we pay to gender issues. Historically, it was mostly males, who knew little about the physiology and problems of women, but who were the practitioners of high medicine. The complexities of a woman's uro-genital and reproductive systems are such that specialized knowledge and care are required, or so we believe today. The biases are so great that the state of Louisiana in the 1920s in the United States made it a misdemeanor to provide for the "sale or advertisement of . . . any *secret* drug or nostrum purporting to be *exclusively for the use of females*" (italics supplied).[1]

Considering its importance, all too little is known about medicine in Biblical and Talmudic times and even less about women's medicine. It is true that Julius Preuss (1861–1913) in his *Biblisch-talmudische Medizin* included one short chapter (XIII) on gynaecology and another (XIV) on obstetrics. The latter, incidentally, contained a section on the psychic maternal influences on the foetus.[2] Fred Rosner's *Medicine in the Bible and the Talmud* (1977; revised 1995) discusses Mar Samuel, one of the medical sages of the Talmud, whose specializations included (in his words) obstetrics, gynaecology and foetal development, embryology, and teratology.[3] For the most part the physiology of the body is such that gender as a factor in medical care is only a small part of overall medical procedures. But, where gender is a factor, the medical knowledge needed for women's distinctive problems is critical. Aided by inferences from the surrounding cultures

---

[1] Louisiana 1924, p. 385, Act 95 of 1920 (Dunn, *Dunn's Food*, 2: 923–924).

[2] Julius Preuss, *Biblisch-talmudische Medizin. Beiträge zur Geschichte der Heilkunde und der Kulture überhaupt* (New York: Ktav Publishing House, 1911; new matter, 1971), pp. 453–5 for psychic influences.

[3] Fred Rosner, *Medicine in the Bible and the Talmud*, (Yeshiva University Press, 1995), pp. 216, 223–224.

of Egypt, Mesopotamia, and later the Greeks, we may surmise that most full-time medical practitioners were men, who knew less about women's problems than they did about generic humans or males in particular. Midwives existed but how distinctive they were has been a matter of scholarly discussion that I shall largely pass over. In this paper I shall explore some aspects of medical lore about women and postulate that Jewish women administered among themselves when problems arose and, equally important, when they sought to preserve good health through nutrition, regimen, and hygiene.

In the words of John Noonan, the Hebrews had a "mistrust of sex."[4] There was God's injunction: "increase and multiply; fill the earth" (Gn 1:27–8). The Talmud (*Yevamot* 63b) and Mishnah (*Yevamot* 6:6) amplify the meaning.[5] Many scriptural passages advance pro-natal positions.[6] Sexual intercourse had as its purpose procreation, and sex was not intended for pleasure-seekers to satisfy lusts, although mutual pleasure was an acceptable motive among married couples.[7]

While there is no mention of intentional abortion or contraception in the Old Testament, both occur in the Talmud, Tosefta, and Mishnah. Contraception and abortion were acceptable in some situations according to rabbinic writings.[8] An important Talmudic statement delineated the acceptable circumstances for contraception in the so-called *Baraita* of the Three Women:

> Rabai recited before R. Naḥman: Three [categories of] women may use an absorbent (*mokh*) in their marital intercourse: a minor, a pregnant woman and a nursing woman. The minor, because [otherwise] she might become pregnant and as a result might die. A pregnant woman because [otherwise] she might cause her foetus to become a *sandal* [a flat fish-shaped abortion due to superfetation]. A nursing woman, because [otherwise] she might have to wean her child prematurely [owing to her second conception], and he would die. And what is a minor?: From the age of eleven years and one day. One

[4] John T. Noonan Jr., Contraception. *A History of Its Treatment by the Catholic Theologians and Canonists*, Enlarged ed. (Cambridge, Ma., 1986), p. 33.

[5] *Yebamoth* 62b (Babylonia Talmud, Epstein trans., *Seder Nashim* 1:426–7); *Yebamot* 6:6 (Jerusalem Talmud, vol. 21, Neusner, trans.); see also, Fred Rosner, "Contraception in Jewish Law," in *Jewish Bioethics* (New York, 1979), p. 89.

[6] E.g., Gn 1:22, 15:5, 22:17, 9:1, 26:4, 16:10; Dt 7:13–4, Ru 4:11, Jb 1:2, 42:13.

[7] Noonan, *Contraception*, p. 32; (for mutual pleasure) Rosner, "Contraception in Jewish Law," p. 90.

[8] Rosner, "Contraception in Jewish Law," p. 91ff.; Jakobovits, "Jewish Views on Abortion," pp. 120–122.

> who is under [this age when conception is not possible] or over this age [when pregnancy involves no fatal consequences] must carry on her marital intercourse in the usual manner.[9]

Julius Preuss called this a contraceptive absorbent tampon.[10] The absorbent (*mokh* in Hebrew) was hackled wool or flax used as a pessary, similar, I presume, to those pessaries mentioned in the Egyptian papyri.[11] Rabbinic opinion differed on whether the three examples were exclusive and exhaustive of the conditions for permissible contraception or merely illustrations. In the sixteenth century Rabbi Solomon Luria interpreted the passage as meaning a woman could use a contraceptive pessary if pregnancy would be dangerous.[12]

Illustrating comparative insight into the relationship between magic and medicine is a cuneiform tablet of the Assyrian period that discusses a wool pad as a pessary, not for aborting but for curing sickness that accompanies pregnancy. Drugs of vegetable origin whose names we cannot translate were heated over a fire and mixed with oil and beer, soaked in a woollen pad and inserted into the vagina. This was done twice daily. In case this procedure did not work, various magical devices were used.[13] A cuneiform recipe from Aššur refers to the application of pomegranate to wool which was then placed in the vagina/uterus.[14] Modern animal experiments show that the pomegranate is truly a contraceptive.[15] I suspect that the text

[9] *Yebamoth* 12b (Babylonia Talmud, Epstein, trans., *Seder Nashim* 1:62).

[10] Julius Preuss, *Biblical and Talmudic Medicine*, Fred Rosner, ed. and trans. (New York: Sanhedrin Press, 1978), p. 381.

[11] Although Feldman, *Birth Control in Jewish Law* (p. 170), says wool or cotton.

[12] Rosner, "Contraception in Jewish Law," p. 94.

[13] H. W. F. Saggs, *Might that Was Assyria* (London, 1984), p. 138.

[14] See R. Campbell Thompson, *A Dictionary of Assyrian Botany* (London, 1949), p. 315, 11 (hereinafer *DAB*) and Erich Ebeling, *Keilschrifttexte aus Aššur religiösen Inhalts* (Leipzig, 1919), p. 194, iv, 18 (hereinafter *KAR*). Thompson notes the uncertainty of identification of the part of the pomegranate applied to the wool, although he refers to its use in treating a "woman's disease." For parallel uses of pomegranate in the treatment of disease, see *CAD* N/2, p. 346b and *KAR* 192, r, 17 (application of the "flour of the fruit", ZÍD ***inbi***, to the sick place). It should also be noted that Thompson's identification of the designation **GIŠ.NU.ÚR.MA** $\mathbf{KU_7.KU_7}$ as a "species" of pomegranate is probably incorrect. It appears to identify a sweet taste associated with the pomegranate. For other references to the pomegranate, see Asaph Goor and Max Nurock, *The Fruits of the Holy Land* (Jerusalem: Israel Universities Press, 1968), pp. 70–88.

[15] Eric Heftmann, Shi-Tze Ko, and Raymond D. Bennett, "Identification of Estrone in Pomegranate Seeds," *Phytochemistry* 5 (1960): 1337–9; P. D. G. Dean, D. Exley, and T. W. Goodwin, "Sterpid Oestrogens in Plants: Reestimation of Oestrone in Pomegranate Seeds," *Phytochemistry* 10 (1971): 2215–6; M. L. Gujral,

indicates that it was not to cure a woman's disease, as previously suggested, but for use as a contraceptive pessary. Soranus (fl. 98–138 C.E.) gave five recipes using pomegranate as a contraceptive pessary. One recipe said: "Grind the inside of fresh pomegranate peel with water, and apply [in the vagina]"; another: "Moisten alum, the inside of pomegranate rind, mix with water, and apply with wool."[16] Knowing this circumstantial evidence that other ancient societies employed a contraceptive pomegranate pessary with wool as a pad, one can postulate that the Talmudic pessary was similar in composition and effect.

A more controversial interpretation is made when again, *mokh*, the pessary, was mentioned in another Talmudic passage as preventing pregnancy (*Niddah* 3a–b).[17] In a discussion of the exact beginning of the period of impurity (*i.e.*, onset of menstruation as detected by menstrual blood) the question arose as to what happens if a woman is using a *mokh*, thus absorbing the fluid and thereby delaying by days the perception of impurity. In the context the presumption is that the use of the contraceptive pessary was routine.

Bitter Medicines

The Talmudic passage, however, is different from the abortifacient, oral route, "cup of bitterness" that has a long history contributing as much to our misunderstanding as to our understanding. Numbers 5:11–31 discusses the so-called suspected adulteress; the woman is told:

> [5: 19] be thou free from this water of bitterness that causeth the curse. [20] But if thou hast gone aside, [21] . . . the Lord make thee a curse and an oath among thy people, when the Lord doth make thy thigh to fall away, and thy belly to swell; [22] and this water that causeth the curse shall go into thy bowels, and make thy belly to swell, and thy thigh to fall away." [English translation of Soncino edition of the Bible]

D. R. Varma, and K. N. Sareen, "Oral Contraceptives. Part I: Preliminary Observations on the Antifertiliy Effect of Some Indigenous Drugs," *Indian Journal of Medical Research* 48 (1960): 46–51 at 50.

[16] Soranus, *Gynaecology* 1. 62 (Temkin trans., pp. 64–65; Greek in Ilberg ed., pp. 46–7).

[17] *Niddah* 3a–3b (Epstein, ed. *Tohoroth* 1:10).

The "water of bitterness" can be drunk harmlessly by the faithful wife, but the serious consequences enumerated will affect the *sotah*, or wayward woman. If the woman was faithful, she remains unhurt, presumably, from the cup of roots, and she conceives by seed from her husband. The procedure is comparable to the trial by ordeal familiar to the early Middle Ages. Interestingly, in the first statement the thigh falling away was followed by the swelling of the belly, but in the second the swelling occurs first.

Fred Rosner examined whether the bitter waters might have some rational (i.e., to us, scientific) basis.[18] Preuss considered other opinions on the subject that included the possibility that the cup was "a designated remedy which is harmful to an already initiated pregnancy."[19] Wilhelm Epstein thought that the cup was nothing more than holy water with a little dust from the floor of the suspected woman's home, but the results of her drinking it may have been a secondary expansion of the uterus caused by pregnancy or a form of dropsy (*Wassersucht*) sometimes associated with pregnancy.[20] C. J. Brim translates the phrase *nafla yerecha* ("her thigh shall fall away") to mean "it will fall out of her genital tract," a meaning accepted by the translators of the New English Bible.[21] If she were to be pregnant, not only would she abort but she would have also secondary complications like abdominal swelling and sterility. An innocent woman, that is, non-pregnant, would be unaffected by drinking the bitter water. Brim added medical anthropological accounts of similar parallels in traditional societies, including specifically an ordeal by "bitter water" in which unfaithfulness was tested.

Julius Preuss rejected an interpretation of a medicinal effect from the bitter water on the grounds that not all extra-marital sex ends in pregnancy, hence, the bitter water would be a poor test for adultery. He favoured a psychological meaning whereby a guilty woman would be so afraid that her actions would betray her that she would react violently to the ritual. The guilt and fear would produce the stress-induced physical consequences.[22] In accepting Preuss' viewpoint,

---

[18] Rosner, *Medicine in the Bible*, pp. 239–47.

[19] Preuss, *Bibl. Talm. Medicine*, p. 473.

[20] Wilhelm Epstein, *Die Medizin im Alten Testament* (Stuttgart: Ferdinand Enke, 1901), pp. 136–7.

[21] C. J. Brim, *Medicine in the Bible* (New York: Froben Press, 1936), p. 374.

[22] Preuss, *Bibl. Tal. Med.*, p. 474.

Fred Rosner asserts that no Talmudic opinions require divine intervention or magic, and no abortifacient could be a true test for adultery. It follows that the operation was predicated on stress imposed on a guilty party.[23] The Talmudic *Sotah* (27b; 28a; Num. Rabbah 9:9) says that an adulterous man is likewise tested. The rabbinic interpretation would obviate a rational or pharmaceutical explanation, unless, of course, the woman's knowledge of that man's adultery reduced her stress. Such a reading is truly far-fetched.

The *Gospel According to the Egyptians* (mid-2nd century) has Salome saying: "I will have done better had I never given birth to a child." To her the Lord replied: "Eat of every plant, but do not eat a plant whose content is bitter."[24] This passage establishes a connection between bitter plants and birth control. Let us assume that the "water of bitterness" in Numbers 5:11–31 is a solution, either a tea (concotion) or boiled concentration (decoction), the common, timeless presentations of herbal medicines. The bitter plant of the apocryphal gospel is postulated to be the same "medicine" as in Numbers. There is more inferential evidence in later times, to be presented below. The total testimonial evidence produces a strong possibility that the bitter waters in Numbers 5: 19–22 was a strong abortifacient, perhaps made too strong by a punishing priest.

Root Medicines

The Talmud also has passages that speak of "root medicines" that result in sterility. The Hebrew *ʿqr*, meaning sterility or barrenness, is the equivalent of the Latin, *sterilis* (adjective) or *sterilitas* (noun). In the Babylonian Talmud, a woman inquired as to whether she could take a root poison to prevent having a child. Rabbi Hiyya replied that God's injunction to be fruitful applied to men and, because men were the aggressors in sexual union, the charge did not apply to women.[25] The Tosefta says, "A man is not permitted to drink a cup

---

[23] Rosner, *Medicine in the Bible*, pp. 245–6.

[24] *Gospel of the Egyptians* through Clement of Alexandria, *Stromata*. 3. 66 (John Ferguson trans., 85:297); Wilhelm Schneemelcher, "The Gospel of the Egyptians," in: *New Testament Apocrypha*, 2 vols. Edgard Hennecke and W. Schneemelcher, eds. (Philadelphia: Westminster Press, 1963): 1:166–78, esp. 167.

[25] *Yebamoth* 65b in *The Babylonia Talmud* (Epstein ed., *Seder Nashim*, 1/3:436–437).

of roots (*ikarin*) in order not to beget, and a woman is not permitted to drink a cup of roots (*ikarim*) in order not to give birth."[26]

Not surprisingly, Jewish rabbinic opinion was divided on this issue. Rabbi Joḥana b. Beroḳa asserted that God's injunction applied to both genders.[27] The Mishnah added a different perspective: a man was excused from propagation after "he already has children." One rabbi said that the Mishnah meant two male children, another, a boy and a girl. Maimonides and Caro interpreted the passage to mean that the roots would cause permanent sterility, not temporary; thus a male could not be excused for a lifetime without attempting to propagate the race.[28]

Explicit in these passages is the notion that males could continue sexual unions but that they too could practice birth control. How? The only clear reference is to root drugs for males and females. There was one male contraceptive specified in ancient, classical medical literature: the seeds of a plant called *periklymenon* are drunk by men in order to become sterile, according to Dioscorides.[29] The problem is that we cannot identify the plant. Later, in the Renaissance, Dioscorides' Greek plant name was identified as honeysuckle (*Locerna periclymenun* L.), but there is doubt that honeysuckle is what the ancient Greeks meant by the term.

Ancient Greek women celebrated a festival during which boughs of the chaste tree (*Vitex agnus-castus* L.) were placed beneath their beds so that they could be chaste during the festival.[30] A Galen treatise and another pseudo-Galenic work related that the chaste tree was placed beneath the beds of athletes and that priests ate it presumably because it prevented erections. It was a cure for priapism.[31]

---

[26] *Yebamoth*. 8. 4; on meaning of *ikarin*, see Jastrow, *Dictionary*, 2:1074. I am grateful to Profs. Samuel Levin and to Josef Schatzmiller for assistance in translating this passage. The translation by Noonan (*Contraception*, p. 51) incorrectly says that a woman *is* permitted to take the drug. For a discussion of the Talmudic passage, see Feldman, "Birth Control in Jewish Law," pp. 235–244.

[27] *Yebamoth*. 65b.

[28] Rosner, "Contraception in Jewish Law," p. 93; Feldman, *Birth Control in Jewish Law*, pp. 240–243.

[29] *De materia medica*. 4. 14.

[30] Heinrich von Staden, "Spiderwoman and the Chaste Tree: The Semantics of Matter," *Configurations* 1 (192): 23–56.

[31] Galen, *De sanitate tuenda* 1. 36 (Kühn ed. 6:446); *De locis affectis* 6. 6 (Kühn ed.: 8:439).

Dioscorides said that the chaste tree "destroys generation."[32] Several modern science sources show that the chaste tree not only has abortifacient qualities when fed to female mice but, when given to male dogs, the sperm production is disrupted.[33]

Jewish sources do not specify what the substance was that men may have been taking for sterility, but classical sources validate that the Jewish tradition was followed in other ancient societies. Medieval sources do not continue a tradition for male antifertility agents, so what began in antiquity ended there, as best we can learn. The crucial point is that the Jewish culture believed that both male and female reproduction could be controlled by chemical agents. Whether Jewish men were successfully taking male contraceptives is an open question.

The identity of the root drugs mentioned in the Hebrew sources is not known, but some clues are provided. Rabbi Joḥanan/Yochanan explained that the cup of roots or cup of barrenness [or unfruitful, *ikarin*] consists of a ground mixture of one *zuz* [a measurement] each of Alexandrian gum, alum, and garden crocus served in grape wine or beer.[34] The Hebrew word here for gum is *komos* (Aramaic: *kuma*), possibly a loan word from the Greek, *kommi*.[35] The Greeks used *kommi* in particular to designate the gum from *Acacia arabica* Willd. (= *Acacia nilotica* Delile).[36] Acacia with dates was employed perhaps in the earliest abortifacient prescription that we have, the Ebers Papyrus (No. 783).[37] Dates will be discussed later. In a modern scientific experiment, the leaf of *Acacia koa* was fed to rats twice a day for five days;

---

[32] Dioscorides, *De materia medica*, 1. 103; Hippocrates, *De mulierum affectibus*, 1.79 (Littré ed., 8:184, 2–5).

[33] C. D. Casey, "Alleged Anti-fertility Plants of India," *Indian Journal of Medical Sciences*, 14 (1960): 594 [590–600]; S. K. Bhargave, "Estrogenic and Pregnancy Interceptory Effects of the Flavoids [VI–VII] of *Vitex negundo* L. Seeds in Mice," *Plantes médicinales et phytothérapie*, 18 (1984): 78 [74–79]; S. K. Bhargave, "Antiandrogenic Effects of a Flavonoid-rich Fraction of *Vitex negundo* Seeds: A Histological and Biochemical Study in Dogs," *Journal of Ethnopharmacology*, 27 (1989): 327–339; S. Christie and A. F. Walker, "*Vitex agnus-castus* L.: (1) A review of its Traditional and Modern Therapeutic Use; (2) Current Use from a Survey of Practitioners," *The European Journal of Herbal Medicine* 3 (3, 1997–8): 29–45.

[34] Sabbath 110a (Epstein trans.).

[35] Jastrow, *Dictionary*, p. 1332; Löw, *Aramäische Pflanzennamen*, p. 197.

[36] Henry G. Liddell and Robert Scott, *A Greek-English Lexicon*, Rev. ed. (Oxford: Oxford University Press, 1968), s.v.; see also Immanuel Löw, *Aramäische Pflanzennamen* (Hildesheim and New York, 1973 repr. of 1881 ed.) n. 148, pp. 148–9.

[37] Ebers 783.

their litters were reduced by 88 to 100 percent, while the seed reduced pregnancy by 100 percent.[38]

Crocus was a component in two recipes for an abortifacient found in the Syriac "Book of Medicines," whose recipes came partly from Galen, while some recipes are similar to those found in the Ebers Papyrus.[39] As late as the sixteenth century European apothecaries sold a compound with crocus for an abortion that was called "Powder of Opopanax from Mesue," presumably a reference to Masawaih (tenth century).

Soranus specified alum as an ingredient in a contraceptive pessary, as did the author(s) of the Hippocratic *Diseases of Women.*[40] The historical continuity of the Talmudic passage is found in the work, *Breviarum practice*, attributed to pseudo-Arnald of Villanova (c. 1240–1311), that gave a birth-control recipe consisting of frankincense, gum arabic (acacia), myrrh, and alum.[41] Acacia gum and myrrh were often mixed.[42] According to Greek mythology, myrrh is the tears of Myrrha who escaped an incestuous relationship with her father, Theias, or Cinyras, who was a legendary king of Assyria, by appealing to the gods, who transformed her into the tree now bearing her name. Her tears were shed for those women who were in her terrible situation.[43] Myrrh would continue as an important ingredient in many "over-the-counter" drugs for birth control through the nineteenth century of our era.

Based on identifications of the plants and other drugs above, one can reasonably postulate that the "root medicines" as translated in the Rabbinic passage consisted of acacia, alum, crocus and even, though less certain, myrrh and dates. A second conclusion is that the drug was reasonably effective as a birth-control agent.

---

[38] Andelina de S. Matsui et al., "A Survey of Natural Products from Hawaii and Other Areas of the Pacific for an Antifertility Effect in Mice," *Internationale Zeitschrift für flinische Pharmakologie, Therapie, und Toxikologie,*" 5 (1971): 67–68 [65–9]; Norman Farnsworth et al., "Potential Value of Plants as a Source of Useful Antifertility Agents," *Journal of Pharmaceutical Sciences* 64 (1975): 550, 565 [535–98, 717–754].

[39] *Book of Medicines* (E. A. Wallis Budge, ed. and trans. [London, 1913] 2. 297–8, 485.

[40] Hippocrates, *De mulierum affectibus*, 1.78 (Littré ed.).

[41] *Breviarum practice* in *Articella* (Venice, 1483) 3. 6 [no numbered foliation].

[42] Dioscorides, *De materia medica*, 1.64, says that myrrh and acacia gum are similar, and explains the manufacture of counterfeit myrrh; see also Löw, *Aramaische Pflanzennamen*, p. 197.

[43] Ovid, *Metamorphoses*, 10. 310–533.

Book of Jasher

The possession of antifertility drugs is confirmed by a passage in the Book of Jasher (*Sefer ha Yashar*, "The Book of Righteousness"), a Jewish account of the creation composed in the thirteenth century. In recounting the generations who came from Canaan (based on Midrash Genesis Rabba 23:3 explaining Genesis 4:19–22) there is this passage:

> And they gave some of their wives to drink a potion of barrenness, in order that they might retain their figures and *whereby* their beautiful appearance might not fade.[44]

This is startling. Here it is confirmed that the oral drugs were for birth control, and also that some purposes were cosmetic, not merely for family planning. Such actions were disapproved in the Jasher passage and implicitly in Talmudic commentaries but there was no absolute prohibition of birth control. The reasons and motivations were all-important. No one can read the Hebrew accounts and believe that contraception and abortion were encouraged, but neither were they banned altogether. There were circumstances in which each was appropriate.

Later sources (Christian, Roman, medieval and early modern) may provide some clues. In Galatians 5:20, Paul provides us with a list of sins of the flesh, among them the sin of *pharmakeia*, often translated into English as "sorcery" or "magic". This is the same word that Socrates through Plato had used in reference to birth control: "drugs (*pharmakia*) and incantations."[45] Revelations 9:21, 21:8, and 22.15 denounce those who employ *pharmakon*, translated "magic," "sorcery," or "drug."

There is likely to be a direct connection between the *pharmakia* of the New Testament and the "root poisons" of Hebrew literature. The *Didache* (or *Teaching of the Twelve Apostles*) 5:1 uses *pharmakia* as a sin labeled "Way of Death," one of several loathsome things that make those who did these things "murderers of children" (Didache

---

[44] Jasher. 20 (Goldschmidt, ed., *Sepher Hajaschar* [Berlin, 1923]). I am grateful to C. Dailey for calling my attention to this passage and to Samuel Kottek for the Hebrew translation into English.

[45] Plato. *Charmides*. 157b.

5:2).[46] The *Epistle of Barnabas* 20:1 speaks of the Way of the Black One who uses "things that destroy their soul (*psychē*): . . . *pharmakeia*" and against those who are "murderers of children" (20:2). The same work placed the abortion issue within the context of loving one's neighbours: "Love your neighbour more than yourself. Do not kill a foetus by abortion, or commit infanticide." (*Epistle of Barnabas* 19:5). The *Apocalypse of Peter* (26) spoke unfavourably about those women who "produced children outside marriage and who procured abortions." As stated before, the *Gospel of the Egyptians* replies to a woman about childbearing: "Eat of every plant, but do not eat a plant whose content is bitter."[47] Many of the birth-control plants are bitter; among them artemisia is intensely bitter, and so is willow bark, which I have shown elsewhere to be 1) effective as both contraceptives and early term abortifacients, and 2) widely used throughout the ancient Mediterranean worlds. The obvious inference is that God prohibited birth-control drugs in this unaccepted Gospel. These passages indicate that among some Christians there had developed a notion of the protection of the foetus and that abortion, at any point, was wrong from the religious standpoint.[48]

"Wretched Surely": Modern Hints about Ancient Lore

References in early modern sources reveal some collaborative evidence about the ancient Jews' use of birth control. Early modern medicine was much closer to ancient medicine than is ours, because, excepting drugs of the New World, classical and early modern medicine employed much the same therapeutic agents.

John Freind began his eighteenth-century midwifery and gynaecology work with the prefatory phrase: "Misera profecto videtur et iniqua foeminarum conditio," translated into a contemporary English edition as "Wretched surely and unequal seems the condition of the Female Sex."[49] The use of drugs to promote menstruation was

---

[46] Noonan, *Contraception*, p. 91; see also *Didache* 2:2.

[47] *Gospel of the Egyptians* through Clement of Alexandria, *Stromata*. 3.66 (John Ferguson trans., 85:297).

[48] Ricks, "Abortion," pp. 31–34; Gorman, *Abortion and Early Church*, pp. 47–62.

[49] John Freind, *Emmenologia: in qua fluxus muliebris menstrui phaenomena, periodi, vitia, cum mendendi methodo ad rationes mechanicas exiguntur.* (London, n.d.), fol. A2; [ditto]

beneficial medically in certain conditions. Also taken correctly they did no harm even in weak women, especially if a paregoric (opium) draught was given at the conclusion. They were found in the kitchen (*culina*) as frequently as they were in apothecary shops (*ex officia*).[50]

Freind distinguished between astringents and emmenagogues (menstrual stimulators). Emmenagogues altered the *crasis*, that is to say the "mixture", because their "attenuating/*attenuatrice*" quality produced "sensible effects/*effectus sensibles*." Many of these drugs could be recognized through their taste, characteristically acrid and bitter.[51]

Elsewhere I have shown that during the early months of pregnancy women from the Egyptians of the Old Kingdom and through the nineteenth century took menstrual regulators that restored the menstrual cycle even if pregnancy were the reason for the interruption.[52] The Bible and Talmudic sources designate that it is after the third month of pregnancy that one can recognize the pregnancy without a declaration from the woman. For a primagravida, the period is often longer.[53] For this reason a period of at least three months was required between the death of a husband and the widow's remarriage in order to distinguish between the fathers.[54]

In 1771, Henry Manning wrote that there were medicines to treat menstrual retention and used a word new to pharmacy, emmenagogues because "those [are the] medicines which strengthen digestion, such as the bark, bitters, and steel."[55] The purpose of administration was to strengthen digestion, but some physicians of his time were quite well aware that, if amenorrhea was being treated and its cause was pregnancy, a miscarriage would occur, thereby restoring menstruation, commonly called in the English of the time, "the monthlies." Listed under medicines from barks were willow and cinnamon, but in the eighteenth and early nineteenth centuries most of the other birth-control medicines were listed under bitter medicines.

Emmenologia. Written, In Latin, By the Late Learned Dr. John Freind, Thomas Dale, trans. (London, 1729), p. (A5).

[50] *Ibid.*, pp. 180–181.

[51] *Ibid.*, pp. 201–205.

[52] John M. Riddle, *Eve's Herbs. A History of Contraception and Abortion in the West* (Cambridge, Mass.: Harvard University Press, 1997).

[53] Genesis 38:24; Niddah 8b; cf. Luke 1:24; Genesis Rabbah 71:9; discussion by Preuss, *Bibl. Talm. Med.*, p. 383.

[54] Yebamoth 42a.

[55] Henry Manning, *A Treatise on Female Diseases* (London, 1771), p. 75.

This causes us to remember the classification in the Gospel of the Egyptians that said "eat not of that which has bitterness in it."

In 1932 the U.S. Department of Agriculture issued a legal restraint against a women's medicine called Blair's Female Tablets which consisted of "plant drugs, incl. a bitter drug."[56] This action came as part of a policy removing from the market place the last vestiges of special female drugs, Lydia Pinkham's Vegetable Compound being the most famous, that restored female regularity. Most women had lost the knowledge of the plants. For example, the rabbi who was the head of the Talmudic Academy in Poland in the seventeenth century saw other rabbis permit the "cup of roots" (contraceptive) to be given to a woman with childbearing problems.[57] The knowledge was present three hundred years ago in Poland. But in the late nineteenth century Rabbi Mordecai Horovitz of Frankfurt-am-Main inquired among physicians about what this drug was, the cup of roots. He was told that it was known and "must have been forgotten in the course of time."[58] The American proprietary medicine Blair's Female Tablets may or may not be directly connected with the Biblical bitter water drunk by the suspected adulteress, and the cup of roots (or barrenness). Directly or indirectly, however, I believe that the preponderance of the evidence shows that ancient Jewish women were much more aware of herbs that controlled their reproduction than their American counterparts who purchased Blair's Female Tablets.

Date Palm

The date palm has contraceptive qualities. Interestingly the date palm was one of the first plants that caused modern science to realize that plants produce compounds that stimulate or replicate sex hormones in mammals. In 1933 Adolf Butenandt and H. Jacobi first reported plant œstrogens. The plant they reported as possessing "female

[56] Arthur Cramp, *Nostrums and Quackery and Pseudo-Medicine*, 3 vols. (Chicago, 1936) 3:62–66.
[57] Feldman, *Birth Control in Jewish Law*, p. 237.
[58] Feldman, *Birth Control in Jewish Law*, p. 237.

hormones" was the date palm, a scientific fact since verified.[59] In 1939 Adolf Butenandt received the Nobel Prize for chemistry, but not for the small article he wrote in 1933 on the date palm. The date palm, he and Jacobi reported, had a compound that they called α-follicle hormone, similar in action to human female hormones. What they were describing was an œstrogenic compound. Œstrogen, of course, is a hormone which promotes or interferes with fertility, depending upon timing and quantity.

The Ebers Papyrus (ca. 1550–1500 B.C.E.) has a prescription using date palm that is for "loosening a child in the belly of a woman", which should be understood more likely as an abortifacient than as a contraceptive (although both are possible interpretations).[60] The Babylonian Talmudic tractate *Sabbath* has a probable mention of date palm as an antifertility plant. The discussion concerns drugs that are forbidden on the Sabbath. A "man," however, may eat any kind of food "as a remedy" or drug except water of palm trees and a cup of roots "because they are [a remedy] for jaundice." The cup of roots is clearly abortifacient, as is mentioned a number of times.[61] The rabbis explained that "water" of palm trees is so called because it is spring water that issues from between two palm trees, with one rabbi saying from two different kinds of palms. If this interpretation is correct, then the water comes from a specific, although unspecified, geographical location in Palestine. But there is no tradition for this otherwise and, instead, a more reasonable explanation is likely.

The Hebrew "water of palms" (*may d'karim*) could be what we would call an extract or solution from the palm tree. The rabbis revealed that palm water is drunk because it allows the gall to function, but it must be taken for forty days.[62] The forty-day treatment would explain why it was allowed to be drunk on the Sabbath. If the water of palms is a water extract from the palm tree, the Mishnah was speaking of a contraceptive plant. It is reasonable to think that

---

[59] Adolf Butenandt and H. Jacobi, "Über die Darstellung eines krystallisierten pflanzliche Tokokinins (Thelykinins) und seine Identifizierung mit dem α-Follikelhormon," *Zeitschrift für physiologische Chemie*, 218 (1933): 104–112.

[60] Ebers 799 in: *Grundriss der Medizin der alten Ägypter*, 7 vols. (Berlin: Akademie Verlag, 1954–62), 4, pt. 1, pp. 279–80; pt. 2, pp. 211–2.

[61] See references in Riddle, *Contraception*, pp. 19–20.

[62] *Sabbath*. 110a (Epstein ed., 1, pp. 533–7); I am grateful to Dr. Samuel Levine and several helpful rabbis for assistance in translating and interpreting this passage.

the rabbis were unaware of the pharmaceutical preparation when they defined "water" of palms. The rabbis knowledge of pharmacy and pharmaceutical preparations was likely to have been superficial. Because the ancient Egyptians, Babylonians and Greeks employed dates as an antifertility agent, it seems likely that Jewish women would have known and employed it as a birth-control agent.

Conclusion

Biblical, Talmudic, and other ancient sources indicate that ancient Jewish women, like those in neighbouring cultures, employed pharmaceutical agents both to promote and to inhibit fertility. References to them were matter-of-fact, presented not as miraculous or bizarre, but rather as routine. Owing to the nature of male authorships of most ancient writings, however, the close detail was not given about the ministrations of the agents, probably because even the scrutinizing rabbis were unfamiliar with matters better known to women.

ANCIENT & CONTEMPORARY MANAGEMENT IN A DISEASE OF UNKNOWN AETIOLOGY

Ellis Douek
FRCS, Emeritus Consultant Surgeon, Guy's Hospital, London

A journalist had to interview an extremely rich lady renowned for her philanthropy. She explained that her fortune had originated from having survived two successive husbands, both multi-millionaires. She said that she got up at around eleven o'clock in the morning when the begging telephone calls began, many from medical charities which focused on particular diseases. Although she had felt irritated by these demands she always gave, she said, as she feared she might get the disease herself.

There must be many reasons for giving to medical causes. What this woman admitted, perhaps with the shamelessness of old age, can not be uncommon. It represents the same impulse that in Babylonian times saw disease as possession by a malign influence.

After all, to fear that snubbing a "disease", refusing to propitiate it with suitable gifts of money, may cause it to invade your own body is tantamount to ascribing to it an intelligent existence. The disease ceases to be the result of organ dysfunction in the way that pot-holes occur in a road or wear and tear may damage car tyres. It has to be respected as an entity with a mind of its own which makes it not dissimilar to the demon of Babylonian medicine.

Western culture would not permit many people to express themselves in the terms of the rich old lady and no-one would suggest that someone was actually possessed by a demon, but this paper investigates the possibility that these deeper feelings are still present in our perception of illness.

The study of medicine in antiquity primarily has to identify the terminology that our predecessors used, to work out their method of classification and to relate it to our own way of understanding disease.

What is presented here is the reverse of that approach. We will select a contemporary disease and look at it in a manner acceptable to that of the doctor in antiquity. The purpose is to understand what lies behind modern management, and this may in turn cast some light on the approach of the ancient physician.

In order to do this we have to choose a disease which is as mysterious to us now as those they had to face in antiquity. There is obviously no point in looking at a condition such as diabetes. We know the cause is a dysfunction of certain cells in the pancreas and we can hold it in check with medication. We should examine a disease that baffles us and yet is common enough to observe patterns in the patients' and doctors' way of handling it.

A good example is what is now called "chronic fatigue syndrome". Uncertainty is such that a joint working group of the Royal Colleges of Physicians, Psychiatrists and General Practitioners in Britain recently issued a report to define it.[1] The term itself first appeared in a proposal by the United States Centers for Disease Control in 1988.[2] The disease consists of a collection of prolonged and debilitating symptoms whose association and relationship are ill-defined. No suggested cause has been without controversy and no treatment has been accepted. Our contemporaries are as near to their professional ancestors as they could be in the circumstances, but before looking at our present attitudes we should consider how the ancient physician would approach a disease including debilitating fatigue and little in the way of specific signs.

We can see immediately that the Babylonian physician and the Greek physician of Hippocratic bent would approach it quite differently.

Although there is considerable similarity in the availability of symptom-lists, with the diseases organised from head to foot, the use of incantation seems to be an integral part of Babylonian medicine though not of Greek. The lists which appear in cuneiform tablets dating from the first millennium and which have become known as the "Diagnostic Handbook" were actually used by the incantation-priest (*āšipu*) rather than the physician (*asû*). The line which states: "when the *āšipu* goes to the house of the sick man" suggests that it is the incantation-priest who first visits the sick and makes the

[1] Report of the Joint Working Group of the Royal College of Physicians, Psychiatrists and General Practitioners. *Chronic fatigue syndrome Cr 54.* London: RCP, October 1996.

[2] Holmes, G. P.; J. E. Kaplan, L. B. Schonberger, L. S. Zegans, N. M. Gantz, *et al.* "Definition of the chronic fatigue syndrome." *Ann Intern Med* 1988; 109: 512–516.

diagnosis. The pharmaceutical recipes would be subsequently made up by the *asû*.[3]

The extensive use of incantation and priests in diagnosis indicates the important role demons were believed to have played in the causation of disease. Many exorcistic Sumero-Akkadian incantations include a formulaic instruction by which the demon is banished through an oath by a god, or by a long series of different gods: "By heaven and earth may you (the demon) be abjured so that you will depart". In other words there is overwhelming evidence that the Babylonians saw disease in great part as resulting from the invasion of the body by a demon. We should add that there is rarely a description of the demon, of its face or of its size. No doubt if the modern doctor were to meet an *āšipu* and tell him that we had found out what these demons looked like and that they were exceedingly small, this would perhaps be unexpected but it would hardly be unacceptable to him.

We know also that antiquity offered another approach. Greek medicine grew to the point of dominating the development of modern medicine, and although it took a great deal from Babylon and Egypt it gradually brought about the transition from magic to science. A very ancient form of therapy which was still well-documented in Roman times was associated with the cult of Asclepius. These temples offered what is known as incubation. Patients would lie down to sleep in a dormitory cubicle or *abaton*, possibly after taking a somniferous potion. It was hoped that they would be visited by the god in a dream and the following morning they would discuss the interpretation with a trained priest. Surrounding the sleep treatment and dream-interpretation there were often other therapies available such as diet, water treatments, massage and exercise. There would also be a theatre and other forms of entertainment.

In Hippocratic times opposition to supernatural causes of disease was the dominant philosophy and "natural" causes were considered an imbalance of the four bodily humours: blood, phlegm, choler (yellow bile) and melancholy (black bile). The statement: "Our natures are the physicians of our diseases" was given great importance and at their best these doctors studied the entire patient in his environment.

[3] Geller, M. J. & S. L. Cohen. "Kidney & urinary tract disease in ancient Babylonia, with translations of the cuneiform sources," *Kidney International* 1995; 47: 1811–1815.

Today's doctor facing a patient with unexplained symptoms centred on chronic fatigue will obviously carry out all the investigations available in our time, if only for medico-legal reasons. When everything has proved negative he will find himself in the same position as the physician in antiquity. He will have to give the patient some sort of plausible diagnosis or explanation as to the causation of the disease. The contemporary patient, like his ancestor, wants to know why he is ill. After that the doctor will have to recommend symptomatic if not curative treatment.

In addressing the first requirement our doctors seem to divide into two approaches. Some will give as a diagnosis "post-viral syndrome". This, they will explain, means that the patient's body has been invaded by a virus. Needless to say this can never be proved and the virus is of course invisible. Yet the patient finds this theory of causation as acceptable as his Babylonian predecessor's acceptance of *his* body's infestation by a demon, suggesting that the concept of possession by an external agent is one of the ways we can view our ills. Although exorcism as a way of getting rid of the invading organism is not part of our culture a recent episode shows how near the surface it is. In 1996, The Royal Ballet put on a very successful ballet called "Dances with Death". The choreography was by Matthew Hart to music by Benjamin Britten. It was a beautiful evocation in dance of the effects of invasion by the AIDS virus: normal T-cells represented by performers clothed in white battling and gradually being defeated and replaced by infected cells dressed in demonic red costumes. It would of course be inappropriate to suggest that this ballet was an exorcism ritual, but the emotion it sought to evoke must have been inspired by a deep-seated and ancient source.

Other doctors and patients are not happy with this viral explanation when they cannot have proof of its existence, in the same way that the Hippocratic physician would be suspicious of "non-natural" causes. Instead they turn again to an imbalance or a lack of harmony in the body although we do not recognise the humours as such. Anger and melancholy are treated through psychotherapy and a holistic type of therapy through diet, water therapy, massage and exercise frequently offered by health farms and similar centres.

This paper suggests that the springs of human perception remain the same through the millennia and through the change and transformation of religions and philosophy. Examination of these impulses in antiquity and in modern times may be mutually illuminating.

INDEX

abdomen, 4
abortion, 201, 209, 210
abscess(es), 2, 3, 59
Abzu, 73, 74
Adad, 106, 121
adulteress, adultery, 126, 161, 173, 203, 204, 205
ageusia, 86
Akkadian, 57, 58, 69, 70, 81, 100, 105, 106, 107, 111, 112, 117, 121, 125, 127, 131, 13, 137, 138, 164, 165, 167, 175, 176–179, 182, 183, 184, 185
Allani-Ereshkigal, 117
Alû (demon), 116, 121, 132
Amarna, el-, 181
amulet(s), 132, 145, 161, 165, 166, 169, 182
anal disease, 55
Anatolia(n), 104, 110, 111, 113
anger, 204
anger (of the gods; see also divine), 151, 158
animal(s), 50, 162, 173, 177
Antu, 145
Anu, 121, 145
anus, 18, 20, 25, 33, 36, 37, 183
anxiety, 78, 96, 151, 152
aphasia, 74, 183
apoplexy, 176, 177, 185
apoplectic, apoplexia, 163, 164, 169
apotropaic, 137, 138, 142, 144, 161
appetite, loss of, 96
Arabic, 3, 57, 58, 72, 81, 163, 168, 183
Aramaic, 2, 51, 57, 58, 164, 165, 174, 179, 181, 183 207
arm(s), 22, 65, 70, 77, 78
Aruru, 145
Arzawa, 103, 108
Asalluhi, 73, 74
Asarluhi, 46
Asclepius, 217
ashipu, 85, 88, 128, 135, 155, 158, 216, 217
Ashurbanipal, 68, 71
Asia Minor, 104
Assyria, 208
asthma, 143, 185
astral magic, 45
astrological (allusions), 65
astrological omens, 14
astronomical, 169, 184
asû (AZU), 37, 76, 77, 101, 102, 103, 104, 109, 112, 116, 128, 135, 155, 216, 217
aura, 135, 142

Baba, 121
baby, 7, 9, 10, 11, 12, 123, 141–144
Babylon, 71, 72
Babylonia(n), 174, 179, 184
Babylonia, 101, 105, 110, 173–185, 213, 214
Babylonian Chronicle, 71
bandage(s), 4, 11, 77, 84, 126
bathing, 89
beer, 12, 17, 26, 27, 30, 31, 34
Bel-uri, 63, 64
belly, 4, 5, 9, 13, 17, 18, 20, 23, 25, 26, 27, 28, 35
bewitched, bewitchment (see witchcraft), 108, 110, 111, 147 152, 153, 154
Bible, 160, 166, 203, 211
Biblical times, 186
bile, 33, 176, 177, 179, 183, 217
bilingual texts, 36, 38, 106
birth (aids, rituals), 102, 114, 117, 141
birth control, 205, 206, 208, 209, 210
blindness, 101
black spittle, 9
bladder, 35, 176
"blast of wind" (disease), 36, 37, 185
bleeding, 11
blood, 29, 32, 34, 35, 92, 94, 95, 113, 132, 170, 171, 174, 176, 177, 180, 182, 185, 217
Boghazköy/Boghazkoi, 101, 105, 148
boils, 19, 23, 30
bolides, 46
bone, 12, 25, 27
Book of Jasher, 209
bowls (magic; see incantation bowls), 178

bound (of demons), 162
bowels, 26
bowls, magic, 165, 166, 167, 169
brain(s), 5, 64, 69, 94, 132, 133, 176, 183
bread, 12, 17, 18, 20, 27, 31
breast, 10, 114
breath, 21, 173–185
burn (by fire), 21
burn (inflame), 19, 20, 21
buttocks, 9

Cairo, 161
Cambridge, 161
carbuncle, 38
catchline, 14
cattle, 44
celestial bodies, 185
celestial (sources of disease), 44
celestial influence, 45
celestial object, 46
charm, 102, 111
cheek, 70, 93
chest, 25, 94
child, 183
child(ren), 114, 141, 143, 167
child-bearing, 4
childhood, 62–66
chill(s), 16, 19, 142
chin, 88
Christian(s), Christianity, 160, 209, 210
cleanse (sick person), 46
clysma, 22, 25, 36, 37
cold (in fever), 2, 3, 8, 9, 12, 13, 16, 23, 28, 29, 31, 142
cold shivers, 13, 19, 31
colon, 175
colophon(s), 33, 50, 68, 103, 104
coma, 69, 85, 86, 89
commentary(-ies, ancient), 8, 9, 14, 38, 62, 65, 86, 87, 88, 89, 209
confusion (fever of; post-ictal), 6, 94, 95
conjurer, 135
constellation demons, 165, 169, 170, 171, 179, 183, 184, 185
constipation, 27
contraception, contraceptive, 201, 202, 203, 206, 208, 209, 210, 213
contusion, 67
convulsions, 31, 62–66; 134
convulsive seizures, 134
cooled (during fever), 7
cough(ing), 2, 28, 35, 106, 182, 183
cramps, 27, 28, 176, 182
crisis (in fever), 10
crutch, 97
curses, 110

Daughter(s) of Anu, 44, 46, 145
deaf, deaf-mute, 177
defecate, defecation, 149, 150, 163, 170, 175, 185
demon(s), 9, 46, 65, 84, 85, 87–91, 94, 95, 105, 108, 113, 116, 132, 137–145; 157, 160–172; 173–186, 215, 217, 218
depression, 90, 96
deranged, 184
diabetes, 216
diagnosis, 20, 22, 23, 28, 31, 37, 38, 78, 79, 81, 127, 135, 137, 142, 147, 148, 149, 150, 155, 177, 181, 217, 218
Diagnostic Handbook (*TDP*), 8, 9, 10, 11, 16, 17, 23, 29, 30, 31, 32, 36, 68, 93, 121–128, 132, 177, 178, 180, 181, 216
diagnostic manuals, 135, 136
diagnostic omens, 144
diagnostic text(s), 15, 21, 52, 58, 120, 122, 125, 127, 132, 133
diaphragm, 175, 176
diarrhoea, 28, 32
diet, 204
digestion, 174, 211
digestive (illnesses, problems), 148, 150, 153
Dioscorides, 206, 207
disorientation (mental), 185
dissection, 173, 174
diurnal fever, 33
divine anger/wrath, 127, 145, 158, 159
dizziness, 178, 179
doctor(s), 135, 142, 154, 174, 215, 217, 218
dog-bite, 53
dreamy state, 91
dream(s), 101, 217
drinking (during fever), 7
dropsy, 204
drowsiness, 74
dysarthria, 69, 74, 94
dysphasia, 69, 74

Ea, 111, 123
ear(s), 4, 9, 37, 38, 89, 90, 94, 96, 107, 115

eating (of fire), 2
Ebers Papyrus, 207, 208, 213
eclipse, 45, 63
Egypt, Egyptian(s), 173, 201, 202, 211, 212, 214, 217
ejaculation, 151
Elam, 71, 72
emasculation, 159
enema(s), 83, 149
Enki, 46, 73
entrails, 7, 8, 17, 25
epidemic, 2, 15, 33, 103
epilepsy, epileptic 173–186
epilepsy, 51, 67, 86, 88, 89, 91, 92, 93, 94, 95, 96, 124, 131–136; 160–172, 176, 177, 182
epileptic, 86, 167
equal (of fever), 9
ergot, 54
Ereshkigal, 14, 117, 121, 166
Eridu, 73
Esagil-kin-apli, 50, 120
Esarhaddon, 117
esophagus, 176
Ethiopia, 171
etymology, 10, 24, 60, 72
even (of fever), 9
excrement, 110, 185
exorcism, exorcist, 74, 127, 158, 162
extispicy, 173, 175
eye disease, 54
eye(s), 4, 5, 11, 13, 17, 34, 81, 82, 84, 89, 106, 107, 114, 134, 178, 179, 185

face(s), 4, 17, 57, 59, 81, 88, 92, 141
facial palsy, 67–99
falling sickness, 131
fatigue, 28
fear, 101, 141, 152
feet, 4, 8, 11, 13, 22, 28, 88, 89, 92, 162
fertility, 186–214
fever(s), 1–39; 51, 108, 134, 138, 139, 142, 185
fingers, 13
fire, 162, 168
fire, burn like (skin problems), 19, 109
fire (feverish heat), 1, 3, 138
fire incantations, 1
flatulence, 107, 182
flesh, 12, 34
foetus, 186, 201, 210
foot, 78, 87, 88, 92, 181
foot disease/trouble, 55, 66
forehead, 82, 115
Frankfurt-am-Main, 212
frost, 19
fumigation(s), 11, 83, 84, 109, 132
fungal skin infection/disease, 51, 52

galactosemia, 133
Galen, 133, 173, 174, 183, 206, 208
gall (see bile)
gall-bladder, 140, 143, 175, 183
gall disease(s), 23, 25, 34, 144
gallû-demon, 141
Ge'ez, 171, 185
Genizah, 161, 165, 168, 172
Gemini, 183
genitals, 115
Geniza, 174, 184, 186
germs, 110
ghost(s), 37, 85, 90, 91, 95, 101, 174, 178
ghost diseases, 95
gland, 176
gnawing pain, 20, 25, 26, 38
gossip, 100, 110, 113
Greek, 1, 82, 86, 132, 164, 168, 173, 174, 176, 178, 179, 181–185, 201, 206, 207, 208, 214, 216, 217
guilt, guilty, 159, 204
Gula, 7, 12, 24

haemoptysis, 32
haemorrhage, 69, 91
haemorrhagic (stroke), 84
haemorrhoids, 55
hair, 3, 5, 34, 107
Hammurabi (Code of), 132
hand(s), 11, 13, 78, 87, 88, 89, 90, 115, 162
hand of a ghost, 25, 26, 36, 37, 90, 121–127
hand(s) of the god(s), 7, 12, 32, 33, 120–130; 132, 179, 185
Hand of Gula, 24
Hand of Oath, 33, 36
Hattian (language, rituals), 101, 103, 114, 115
Hattusha, 103, 116
Hattushili I, 111, 112, 113
head, 4, 5, 9, 10, 13, 23, 28, 34, 38, 57, 58, 106, 114, 164, 181
headache(s), 53, 69, 70, 87, 91, 96
healer, 58, 154, 155, 157, 158
hearing, 4

heart, 109, 162, 175, 176, 181
heart attack, 94
heat, 21, 23, 142
heat stroke, 24
heavy (of hearing/ears), 4
Hebrew, 3, 57, 58, 162, 163, 164, 166, 176, 178, 205, 207, 209, 213
hemiparesis, 69, 82
hemiplegy, 176, 177
hemiplegia, hemiplegy, 69, 71, 78, 80, 82, 91, 94, 96, 163, 164, 165, 169
Hesiod, 18
hip(s), 4, 20, 70, 79, 92
Hippocrates, Hippocratic, 17, 131, 173–185; 208, 216, 217, 218
Hittite (language, incantation literature, rituals, witchcraft), 100–119
Hittite Empire, 117
hostile (feelings), 159
hot (feverish conditions), 1, 3, 9, 10, 11, 12, 13, 19, 20, 33, 34, 38
hot (like an inflammation), 21
humours, 177, 178, 179, 181
Hurrian (incantations, language, rituals), 101, 115, 116, 117
hypoglycemia, 133

Ibn Ezra, 169, 184
Igigi, 46
impotence, impotent, 101, 111, 146–159
incantation(s), 1, 6, 9, 13, 14, 38, 40, 44, 46, 47, 49, 50, 53–55, 58, 73, 83, 104, 107, 110, 111, 113–117, 126, 127, 138, 139, 141, 142, 143, 151, 153, 157, 161, 165, 184 216, 217
incantation bowls (see magic bowls), 175, 178, 180, 181, 184
incantation priest, 178
incantation texts, 186
incubation, 217
Incubus, 132
infancy, 152
infarct, 69
infected (person), 60
infection(s), 11, 14, 53, 140, 185
infectious disease, 14
inflamed (by fever, sun-heat), 7, 12, 19–20, 31
inflammation, 51, 180
inflammation of the eyes, 22
inflammation by sun-heat, 21, 25, 31, 32, 34, 36, 37, 38, 39
inflammatory diseases, 46, 47
innards, 7, 12, 25, 26, 27, 36
inner organs, 47
insanity, 168, 183
intercourse (marital), 201
internal disease, 54
intestine(s), 18, 175, 176
ischaemia, 69, 96
ischaemic stroke/event/attack, 77, 91, 94
Ishhara, 121
Ishtar, 115, 116, 117, 121, 122, 124, 125, 135
Islamic medicine, 177

Jasher, Book of, 209
jaundice, 37, 53, 213
jaws, 115
Jesus, 167, 168, 183
Jewish (sources, etc.), 166, 179, 186–214
joints, 79, 96
jug demons (see vessel demons), 165, 179, 184

Kamrushepa, 114, 115
Kanish, 104
kicking, 133
kidneys, kidney disease, 175, 176, 180
knees, 17
Kubu (demon), 121
Kumarbi, 111
Kuyunjik (texts), 139

Lamashtu (demon), 9, 105, 121, 137–145
Latin, 164, 168, 205
lead roll, 182
leg(s), 22, 65, 70, 90
leg tendons, 71
leprosy, 169, 185
lexical lists, 47, 49
lexical texts, 36
lexical tradition, 10, 50
library catalogues, 106
lice, 90
limbs, 16, 18
lips, 27, 88
literary texts, 50
liver, 133, 140, 143, 144, 175, 176
liver omina, 35, 36
loins, 92
Lugal-urra, 63, 132, 183, 184

lunacy, 160, 169, 185
lunaticus, 167, 168, 183
lungs, 11, 35, 115, 147, 174, 175, 176
lurking spirit/demon, 17, 92, 124
Luvian (incantations, rituals), 101, 102, 104, 111, 114, 115

madness, 168, 177, 183
magic, 40–61, 80, 82, 100, 103, 105, 108, 111, 113, 114, 116, 117, 127, 139, 152, 154, 155, 157, 160, 161, 165, 178, 183, 202, 209, 217
magic, astral, 45
magic bowls, 51, 165, 166, 167, 169, 174, 181
magical formulae, 58
magical instructions, 44
magical procedures, 53, 82
magical ritual(s), 12, 104
magical (treatment), 6
magician, 101, 102, 103, 104, 106, 108, 110, 113, 114, 115, 116
Maimonides, 206
malaria, 10, 13, 15–18, 19, 24, 33, 51
malignant malaria, 24
Mandaic, 163, 165, 166, 169, 174–179, 181, 182, 184
mantic, 104
Maqlû (incantation series), 111
Marduk, 121, 153, 169
Mari (incantations, letters, texts), 23, 37, 44, 51, 53, 60, 148, 156
massage, 74, 82, 83, 96
materia magica, 103, 104, 105, 110, 117
mathematical problems, 179
medical corpus, 24
medical incantations, 40
medical literature, 65
medical text(s), 11, 22, 23, 36, 37, 38, 53, 80, 106, 108
medicine(s), 40–61, 177, 186–214
melancholy, melancholia, 132, 176, 177, 217, 218
menstruation, 106, 203, 210, 211
mental (disorders, disorientation, illness, symptoms), 100, 160, 172, 185
Mercury, 182
Midrash, 209
midwife/wives, 114, 201
migraine, 164, 176
mild illness, 33
miscarriages, 101
moon, 63, 90, 132, 168, 169, 182, 183, 185
moon, strike of, 22, 33
mother, 152
mountain, seizure of the, 11, 12–15, 16, 19
mountain fever, 11, 12, 13
mountains, 114
mouth, 18, 20, 32, 33, 55, 69, 70, 72–76, 82–84, 86, 88–90, 93, 115, 147, 171, 177, 178, 185
mouth seizure, 73–76, 89, 171
mouth washing, 113
mucus, 185
mummification, 173
mumps, 38
muscular dysfunction, 79
muscle(s), 8, 30, 33, 36, 37, 65, 69, 70, 82, 83, 95, 96, 131, 133, 135, 184, 185
Mushezib-Marduk, 71
mycetoma, 51
mycotoxicose, 14
myctome, 54
mythological (demon, figure), 138
mythology, 208

Nabû-bel-shumate, 72
namburbi-rituals, 127
name (of disease), 128
Namtar (demon), 184
Naram-Sîn, 112
nausea, 12
neck, 70, 84, 94
Neo-Assyrian letters, 8
Nergal, 14, 121, 164, 166, 180
Nergal and Ereshkigal, 181
nerve(s), 82, 176
Netherworld (see Underworld), 14, 117
neurological disorders, 64
neurophysiology, 79
New Testament, 168, 185
nightmares, 101
Nimrud, 88, 89, 93
Ningirsu, 121
Ningishzida, 15
Niniveh, Ninevite (tradition), 115, 116, 117
Nippur, 2, 8, 9
nocturnal fever, 33
nose, 4, 13, 29, 32, 34, 107, 115, 178

nosology, 85, 181
Nusku, 121

oath (curse), 110
Oath (fever), 8, 25, 33
obstetrics, 186
oil, 13
ointment, 74
omens, 14, 100, 101, 102, 105, 120, 127, 144, 165, 173, 175
omina (liver), 35, 36
Ortaköy, 102

pain(s), 5, 20, 26, 27, 94, 96, 134, 164, 184
Palaic, 104
Palestine, 213
palm tree, 175
palm(tree) demons, 165, 170, 171,179, 185
palsy, 66, 67–99, 163
paludisme, 16
pancreas, 216
panic, 31
paraesthesia(e), 96
paralysed, paralysis, 36, 37, 69–71, 76, 77–79, 82–85, 87, 88, 94–97, 101, 160, 163–165, 169, 182, 184
paralysis, 176–178, 185
paraplegia, 177
paranoid schizophrenia, 85
paraplegia, 71, 164
paresis, 77
pathogenesis, 44
pelvis, 92
penis, 7, 20, 35
Persian, 168, 183
personal god, 127, 158, 159
Peshitta, 167, 168, 183
pessary, 202, 203, 208
pest, 180
pest, pestilence(s), 15, 166
pharmaceutic(al), 109, 205, 214
pharmacological handbook, 21, 32
phlegm, 173–185; 217
phylacteries, 83, 84
physician(s), 76, 85, 173, 178, 211, 212, 216, 217, 204
physiognomic (texts), 15
physiognomy, 107
pills, 25
pimples, 51
plague, 164
plant(s), 11, 20, 21, 25, 26, 32, 37, 39, 82, 84, 109, 110, 144, 148, 149, 156, 157, 165, 205 206, 208, 210, 212
Plato, 209
pneumonia, 185
poison(s), 150, 152, 154, 157, 183, 205, 209
Poland, 212
pomegranate, 202, 203
possession, 89, 95, 179
potency, 35
potion(s), 4, 8, 148, 157, 209
poultice(s, -ing), 11, 39, 77, 78, 83
pox, 49, 51, 54
prayers, 127
pregnancy, 102, 114, 141, 201–204, 211
prescription(s), 31, 66, 73–76, 78, 80, 83, 84, 92, 108, 127, 138, 142, 148, 150, 151, 156, 171
priapism, 206
priest(s), 175, 178, 206
princess, 23
prognosis, 22, 47, 80, 88, 92, 120
prophylactic, prophylaxis, 137, 138, 142, 144
Provider of Evil, 9
psychological (aspect), 96
psychological (deterioration), 146
psychosomatic (disorders), 100, 101, 139, 151
psychotherapy, 218
puerperal fever, 139, 142
pulmonary tuberculosis, 25
pulse(s), 22, 90, 174
pus, 3, 11, 180
pustules, 59

quadriplegia, 85
quotidian fever, 8

rash(es), 142, 143
Rashap, 166
recipe, 202, 208
rectal treatment, 18
rectum, 175, 180
red (skin), 30
remittent fever, 8, 13, 17
Righteous Sufferer, 85
ringworm, 55, 59
ritual(s), 100–107, 109, 100–119, 126, 127, 138, 141, 142, 146, 151, 152, 154, 178, 204

roof, roof-demon(s), 160–172–186
rubbed (with evil oil), 153

saliva, 26, 28, 133, 182
salve(s), salving, 11, 15, 22, 126, 153–155
sandhi writing, 38
Saturn, 185
scars, 143
schools, 103
science, scientific, 160, 173, 174, 176, 179, 204, 207, 217
scorpion-bite, 53
scribes, 104
scurvy, 54
seize(d), seizure (by demon, fever, god), 4, 6, 11–14, 22, 33, 90, 94, 125, 171
seizure(s, of mouth, etc.), 64, 72–76, 89, 90, 171
seizure of the mountain, 11, 12–15, 16, 19
star(s), 184, 185
Star of Marduk, 184
Syriac, 174, 177, 178, 180, 183
Seleucid period, 37
Seleucid (text), 183
Semitic, 180
seven-day fever, 17
Seven Sages, 84
sex, sexual, sexuality, 126, 140, 152, 201, 204, 205, 206, 212
sexual intercourse (illness of), 20, 159
sexual performance and dysfunction, 151, 158
sheep, 44, 174, 175
shivering fever, 13, 19, 39, 51, 52
shiver(s), 31, 95, 144
shoulder(s, -blades), 20, 26, 35, 77, 87
Sinaitic, 183
Sîn (moon god), 90, 117, 121, 124; staff of, 97
Sirius, 16
skin, 19, 20, 24, 25, 90, 95, 96, 109
skin disease(s), 11, 14, 15, 37, 47, 51, 52, 54, 160, 168, 169, 172, 183, 185
skin problems (burning), 19, 21
skull, 3, 4, 5, 19, 34
smoke, 46
snake(s), 45, 50, 107
snout, 115
Socrates, 209
Solomon, 171
Soranus, 203, 208
sorcerer, sorceress, 101, 154, 155
sorcery, 11, 13, 53, 116, 209
soul, 100, 210
spasm, 184
spawn of Shulpaea, 132, 134
speech, 134
spell, 74, 101, 108
sperm, 207
spirit, 127, 162, 165
spitting (at substitute images), 113
spittle, 11, 27, 35
spleen, 175, 177, 181
spots, 12
sputum, 14
staff of Sin, 97
star(s), 46, 76, 121, 126, 148, 169
stadium frigoris, 19
sterility, 206, 209
stiff(ness), 14, 17
stillbirth, 141
sting, 96
stinging pain, 20
sterility, 205, 209
stomach, 4, 7, 25, 37, 147, 148, 175, 181
stop bleeding, 11
strike (by a god), 125
stroke, 66, 67–99, 164, 172, 177
strong fever, 6, 12
stupor, 95
substitute king, 105, 112
Succubus, 132
Sufferer (Righteous), 85, 86
Sumerian, 122, 131, 184, 185
Sumero-Akkadian, 217
sun, 22, 24
sun-heat, 3, 5, 7, 8, 12, 16, 17, 18, 19, 20, 22–39
sunstroke, 24, 28, 39, 53
surgeon, 37
surgery (eye), 54
Susa, 59
sweat(y), 3, 4, 7, 8, 9, 13, 14, 16, 17, 30, 33, 90
swollen(ness), 12, 26, 27, 37, 179
symptom(s), 4, 7, 12, 13, 18, 22, 23, 28, 29, 31, 59, 69, 81, 88, 90, 92, 93, 120, 121, 124, 12, 131, 134, 135, 138, 141–143, 146, 148–151, 160, 168, 181, 184
syndrome(s), 139, 146, 147
Syria, 104
Syriac, 51, 58, 81, 163, 165–168, 208

Shamash, 7, 121
Shimatu, 148
Shulag/Shulak (demon), 88, 92, 121
Shulpaea, spawn of, 132, 134
Shumma Alu, 14
Shuppiluliuma I, 117
Shurpu (incantation series), 110, 111

taboo(s), 173, 174
Takultu, 117
Talmud, Talmudic, 51, 92, 160, 162, 164, 166, 170–172, 174, 178, 180, 185, 186–203, 205, 208, 209, 211–213
tampon, 202
TDP (see Diagnostic Handbook)
teeth, 10, 184, 185
Telipinu, 115
Tell Haddad text, 40
temperature, 3
temple (building), 102, 114, 158
temples (head), 17, 30, 31, 34
tendons (leg), 71
tertian fever, 2, 9
Teshup, 111
Therapeutic Handbook, 31
therapeutic plants, 157
therapeutic series, 67
therapeutic tablet, 70, 72
therapeutic text(s), 6, 10, 15, 34, 36, 40–61, 109, 120, 122, 124, 125, 127, 128, 154, 156, 158
therapeutics, therapy, 125, 132, 136, 144, 146, 148, 158, 210
thirst, 144
throat, 106, 107, 115
thrombosis, 69
Tiamat, 84, 153
tinnitus, 94, 96
toes, 13
toothache, 53
"touch by the divine", 125
touch(ed by fever, sun-heat), 17, 18, 20, 26, 33
touched (in a stroke), 77
tongue, 86, 93, 113
torpidity, 178
trauma, 24
tremble(ing), 11, 14
trunk, 9, 10
typhoid (fever, infections, rashes), 140, 142, 143

Ugarit, 38, 180
Underworld (see Netherworld), 121, 166, 180, 181
Ur, 65
uraemia, 24
Urash, 121, 126
urethra, 175, 176
urinate, urine, 20, 32, 35, 180
urine, 183
Urshu, 112
uterus, 204
Utukku (demon), 116

vagina, 202, 203
veins, 31, 34
vertigo, 17, 28, 178, 179
vessel demons (see jug demons), 169, 184
virus, 218
vomit(ing), 12, 25, 27, 33, 148, 150, 183
vows, 126

water, 17, 20
weather god, 102, 103
wind, 25, 26, 35, 36, 37, 107, 174, 182, 183, 185
windpipe, 28
witch(es), 154, 157, 158, 159
witchcraft (see bewitched), 101, 104–107, 146–159; 183, 184
woman, women, 107, 186–214
worry, 26, 27
wounds, 36

Zimri-lim, 148
ziqqurat, 44
zodiac, 169, 182, 184